GASPARE TAGLIACOZZI AND EARLY MODERN SURGERY

This book uses the work of Bolognese physician and anatomist Gaspare Tagliacozzi to explore the social and cultural history of early modern surgery. It discusses how Italian and European surgeons' attitudes to health and beauty – and how patients' gender – shaped views on the public appearance of the human body.

In 1597, Gaspare Tagliacozzi published a two-volume book on reconstructive surgery of the mutilated parts of the face. Studying Tagliacozzi's surgery in context corrects widespread views about the birth of plastic surgery. Through a combination of cultural history, microhistory, historical epistemology, and gender history, this book describes the practice and practitioners considered to be at the periphery of the "Scientific Revolution." Historical themes covered include the writing of individual cases, hegemonic and subaltern forms of masculinity, concepts of the natural and the artificial, emotional communities and moral economies of pain, and the historical anthropology of the culture of beauty and the face and its disfigurements.

The book is essential reading for upper-level students, postgraduates, and scholars working on the history of medicine and surgery, the history of the body, and gender and cultural history. It will also appeal to those interested in the history of beauty, urban studies, and the Renaissance period more generally.

Paolo Savoia is Assistant Professor of the History of Science at the University of Bologna.

The Body in the City

Series Editors: Peter Howard
Monash University, Australia
John Henderson
University of Cambridge, UK

This series aims to intersect and to energise two strands in historical studies: the pre-modern city as an historical subject (encompassing political institutions, rituals, built environments, religious activities, etc) and histories of the premodern body with their debates about how bodies are shaped by discourse and context. The series will highlight approaches which emphasize the vernacular as revealed by new sources and novel approaches to them. While there are numerous studies of the body in history, this series will explore critically and in innovative ways the relationship between bodies and environments. This will allow scholars involved to analyse how particular spaces, locations and physical *milieux* affect understandings of the body and govern responses to particular problems. The multi-disciplinary approach to the topic places the series at the leading edge of its field.

In this series:

Plague and the City
Edited by Lukas Engelmann, John Henderson and Christos Lynteris

Gaspare Tagliacozzi and Early Modern Surgery
Authored by Paolo Savoia

For more information about this series, please visit: https://www.routledge.com/The-Body-in-the-City/book-series/BOCY

GASPARE TAGLIACOZZI AND EARLY MODERN SURGERY

Faces, Men, and Pain

Paolo Savoia

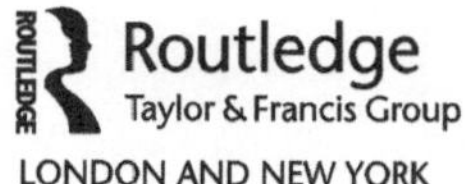

Routledge
Taylor & Francis Group
LONDON AND NEW YORK

First published 2019
by Routledge
2 Park Square, Milton Park, Abingdon, Oxon OX14 4RN

and by Routledge
52 Vanderbilt Avenue, New York, NY 10017

Routledge is an imprint of the Taylor & Francis Group, an informa business

British Library Cataloguing-in-Publication Data
A catalogue record for this book is available from the British Library

Library of Congress Cataloging-in-Publication Data
A catalog record for this book has been requested

ISBN: 978-0-367-20174-6 (hbk)
ISBN: 978-0-367-20173-9 (pbk)
ISBN: 978-0-429-25994-4 (ebk)

Typeset in Bembo
by Apex CoVantage, LLC

This book is dedicated to Linda and Nora.

CONTENTS

ACKNOWLEDGMENTS

As a philosopher-turned-historian, I very much appreciated the collective dimension of historical research.

The first person I wish to thank is Katharine Park, for being a model of scholarship, an extraordinary teacher, and an extremely perceptive mentor and for trying to teach me how to write like a historian.

Exchanges with the following persons over two continents and at different institutions have been crucial in developing my work and in improving as a scholar and, I hope, as a human being. I warmly thank, in no particular order, Cara Kiernan Fallon, Laura Schmidt, Leena Akhtar, Devin Kennedy, Joelle Abi-Rached, Deidre Moore, Allyssa Metzger, Ardeta Gjikola, Shireen Hamza, Marco Viniegra, Jacob Moses, Alexander More, Ann Blair, Ahmed Ragab, Alex Csiszar, Janet Browne, Bruce Moran, Chin Jou, Charles Rosenberg, Allan Brandt, Florin-Stefan Morar, Jean-François Gauvin, David Jones, Anouska Bhattacharyya, Susanne Schmidt, Tal Arbel, Anne Harrington, Alessandro Pastore, Ottavia Niccoli, Giancarlo Angelozzi, Domenico Bertoloni Meli, Nir Shafir, Allen Grieco, Lucio Biasiori, Dario Brancato, Monica Azzolini, Laura Moretti, Francesco Borghesi, Paola Ugolini, Alessandro Polcri, Jonathan Nelson, Paula Findlen, Sheila Barker, John Gagné, Rosario Moscheo, Michael Rocke, Hannah Marcus, Marta Cavazza, Alisha Rankin, Roberto Brigati, Raffaella Campaner, Roberto Poma, Maria Conforti, Elena Canadelli, Leah DeVun, Monsterrat Cabré, Michael McVaugh, Jill Burke, Marco Annoni, Bonnie Gordon, Andrea Carlino, Marica Setaro, Fernanda Alfieri, Giovanni Gondoni, Kathleen Walker-Meikle, Evelyn Welch, Juliet Claxton, and Natasha Awais-Dean.

A very special thanks to Gianna Pomata, Steven Shapin, Noam Andrews, Cynthia Klestinec, Lisa Haushofer, Hannah Murphy, and Marco Beretta. Another special thanks to the series editors, John Henderson and Peter Howard.

Libraries and archives – and all the people who work there and have been so patient and helpful – deserve to be mentioned, as they are the material tools with – and the working environment in – which this book has been researched and written. In Bologna: Biblioteca Comunale dell'Archiginnasio, Archivio di Stato, Biblioteca Universitaria, and Biblioteca Umberto I-Istituto Ortopedico Rizzoli. In Boston and Cambridge, MA: Countway Library of Medicine and Widener Library. In Florence: Berenson Library, Biblioteca del Museo Galileo-Istituto e Museo di storia della scienza, and Biblioteca Nazionale. In London: the Wellcome Library.

This book has been written thanks to the support of Harvard University, the Council on Library and Information Resources (Washington, DC), the Wellcome Trust, and King's College London.

And the biggest thanks to Linda Martini for being with me through the many events that shaped our life together in the past years.

ABBREVIATIONS

ASB	Archivio di Stato di Bologna
BCAB	Biblioteca Comunale dell'Archiginnasio di Bologna
BUB	Biblioteca Universitaria di Bologna

FIGURES

INTRODUCTION

This book is about why the Bolognese anatomist, surgeon, and physician Gaspare Tagliacozzi (1545–1599) desired to be remembered as a "plastic surgeon" and how medical knowledge mediated his desire to realize his patients' wish to have their faces restored to their original beauty and dignity after having suffered disfiguring injuries.[1]

In order to answer these questions, I have followed the traces and clues in Tagliacozzi's book *De curtorum chirurgia per insitionem*, published in Venice in 1597, and I tried to look at what the author left out of it by turning to archival sources, medical books, and cultural history. Tagliacozzi's book is a unique example of a hybrid between the humanistic medical treatise and the technical surgical manual. Tagliacozzi focuses on the surgical procedure of reconstructing mutilated parts of the face – lips, ears, and especially noses. The author describes a procedure of grafting. It consists of cutting and preparing a skin flap on the upper region of the arm, making it adhere to the defective nose by keeping the two parts bound together for about three weeks, severing the flap from the arm, shaping the new parts of the nose, and finally making sure that the outcome would last by using special molds. The procedure has to take place in a well-illuminated room, and at least two strong assistants have to hold the patient. The best season in which to perform it is the spring, but it can be done in the summer too, when the weather and the natural heat of the body help in attaching the flap. The best patients are strong young men ready to undergo such a demanding operation. Finally, Tagliacozzi describes a set of surgical tools and a special vest with a hood and bandages that kept the arm fixated to the face, of which he is very proud (Figures 0.1–0.4).

De curtorum chirurgia per insitionem was published in two volumes in Venice in 1597 and immediately had a pirate edition in Florence. The year after, another unauthorized edition was published in Frankfurt with the title of *Chirurgia nova*

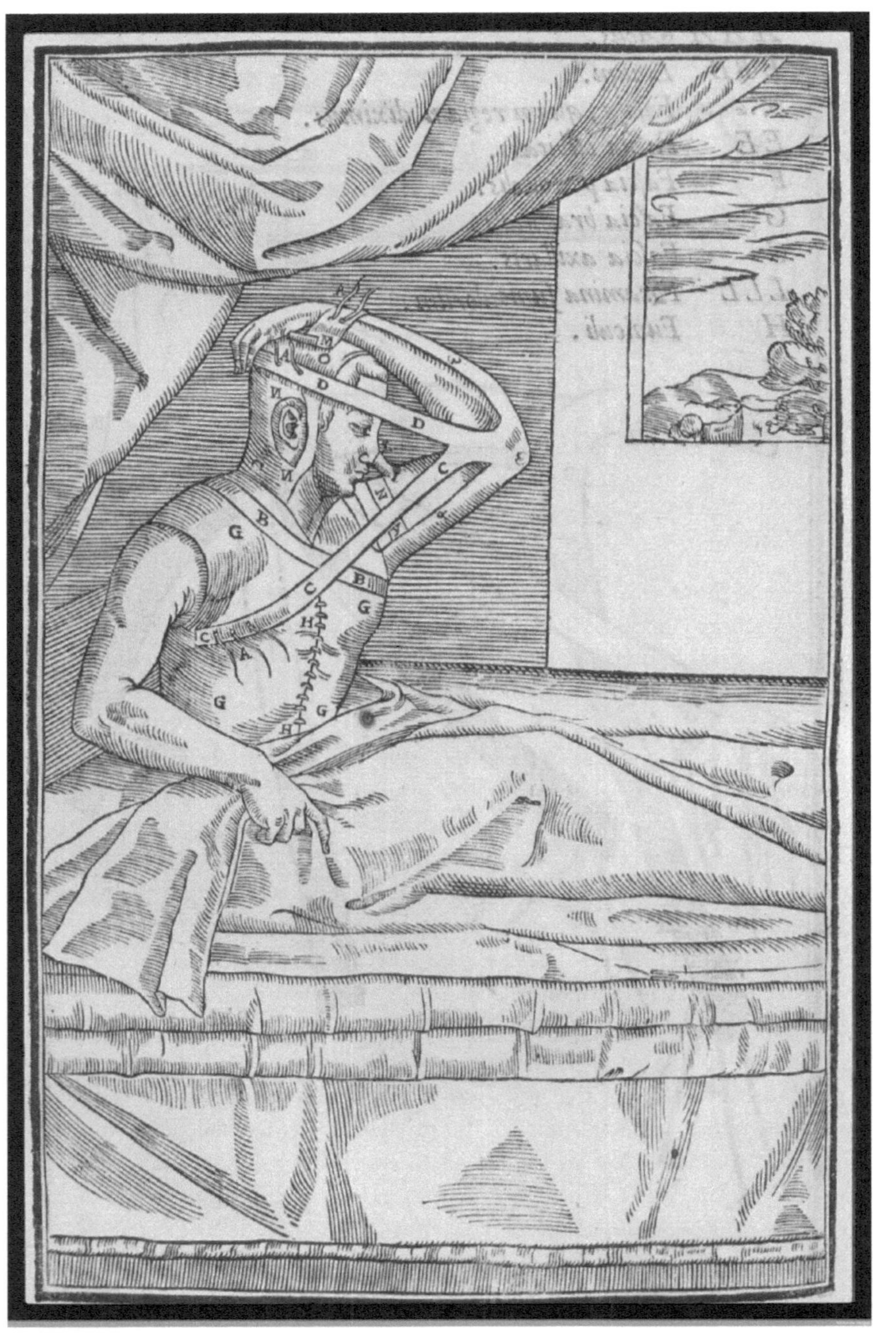

FIGURE 0.1 Gaspare Tagliacozzi, *De curtorum chirurgia per insitionem* (1597): nose reconstruction.

Source: Courtesy of the Wellcome Collection

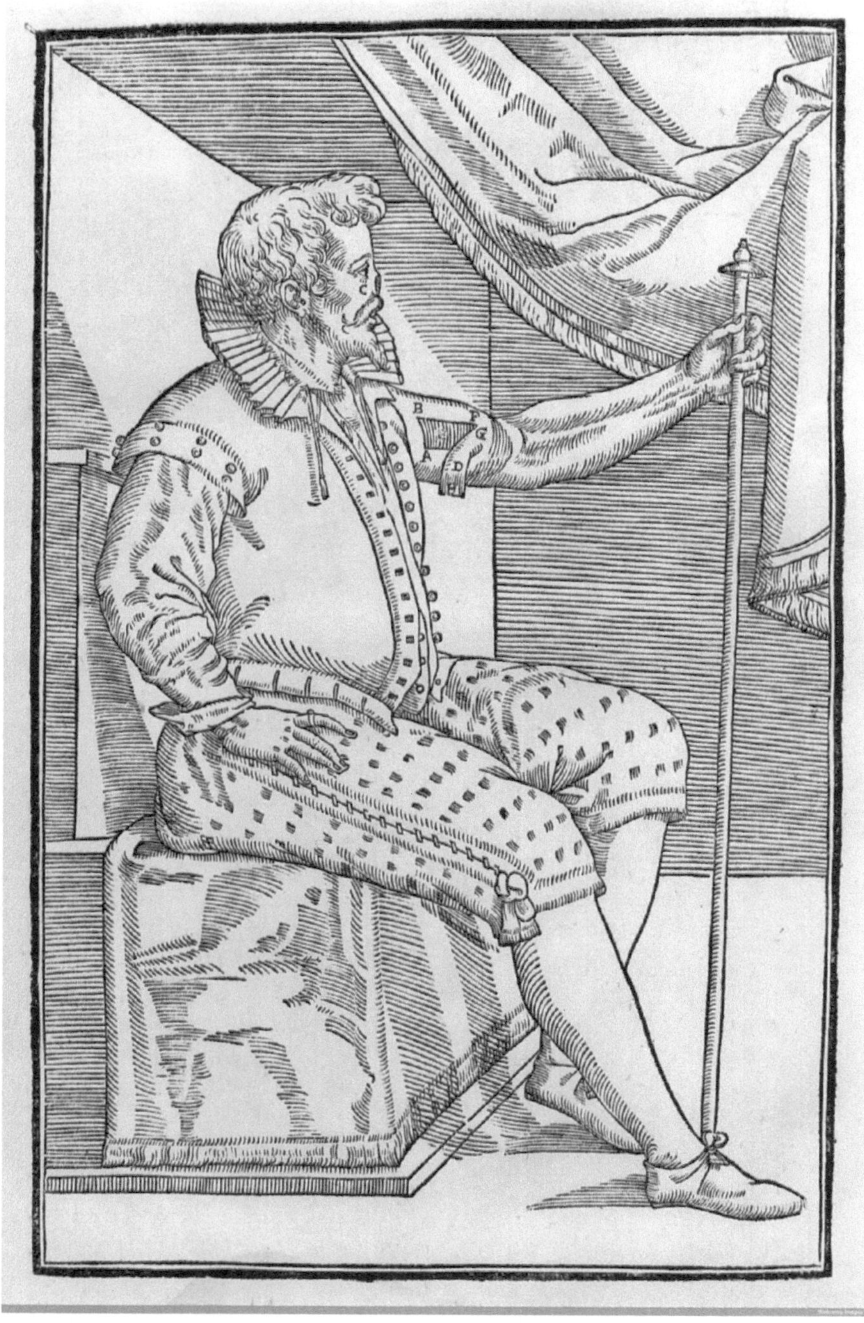

FIGURE 0.2 Gaspare Tagliacozzi, *De curtorum chirurgia per insitionem* (1597): a noseless patient in gentlemanly clothes.

Source: Courtesy of the Wellcome Collection

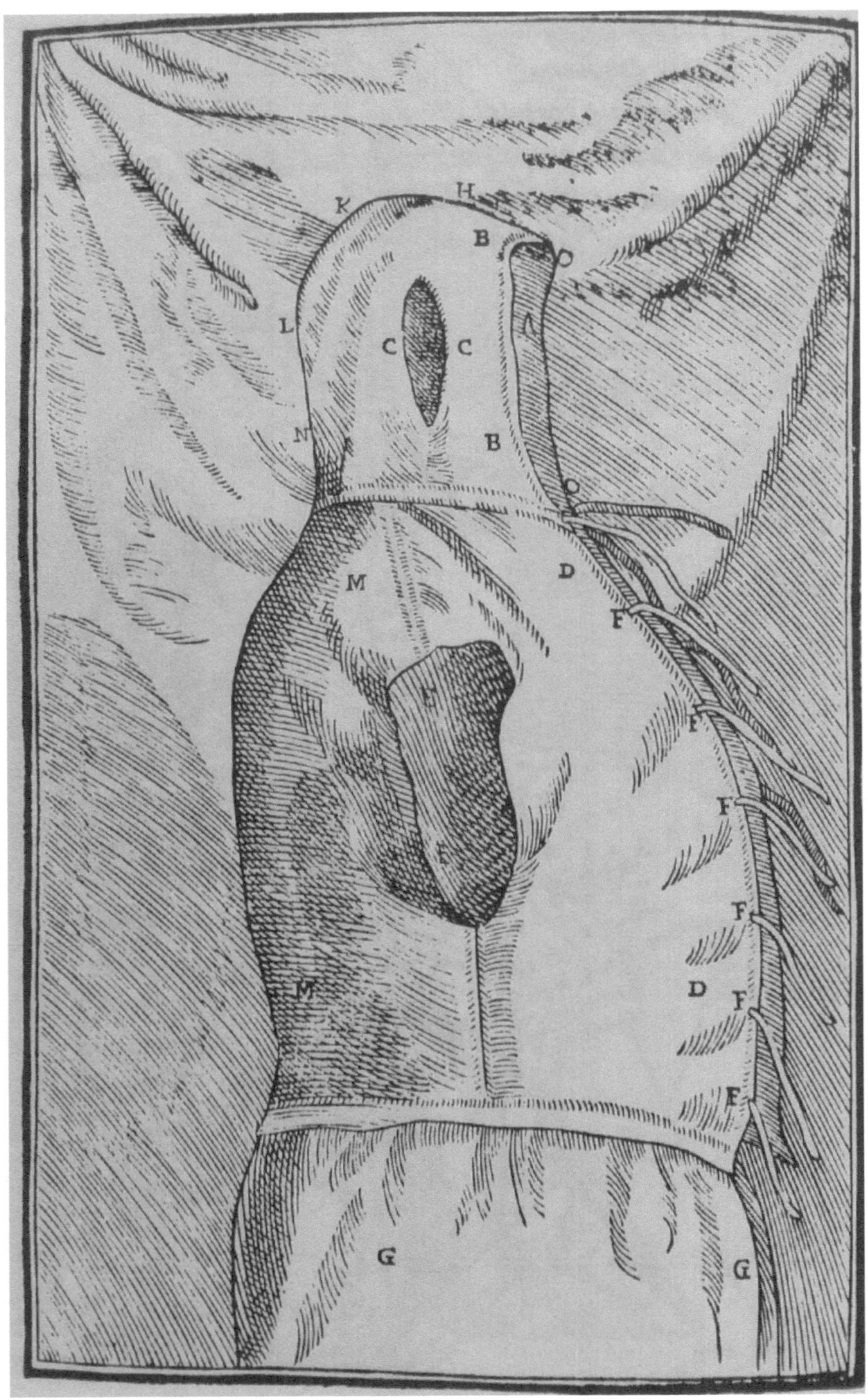

FIGURE 0.3 Gaspare Tagliacozzi, *De curtorum chirurgia per insitionem* (1597): a "machina" or vest designed by Tagliacozzi.

30 CHIRVRG. CVRT.

Icon Decimaquarta.

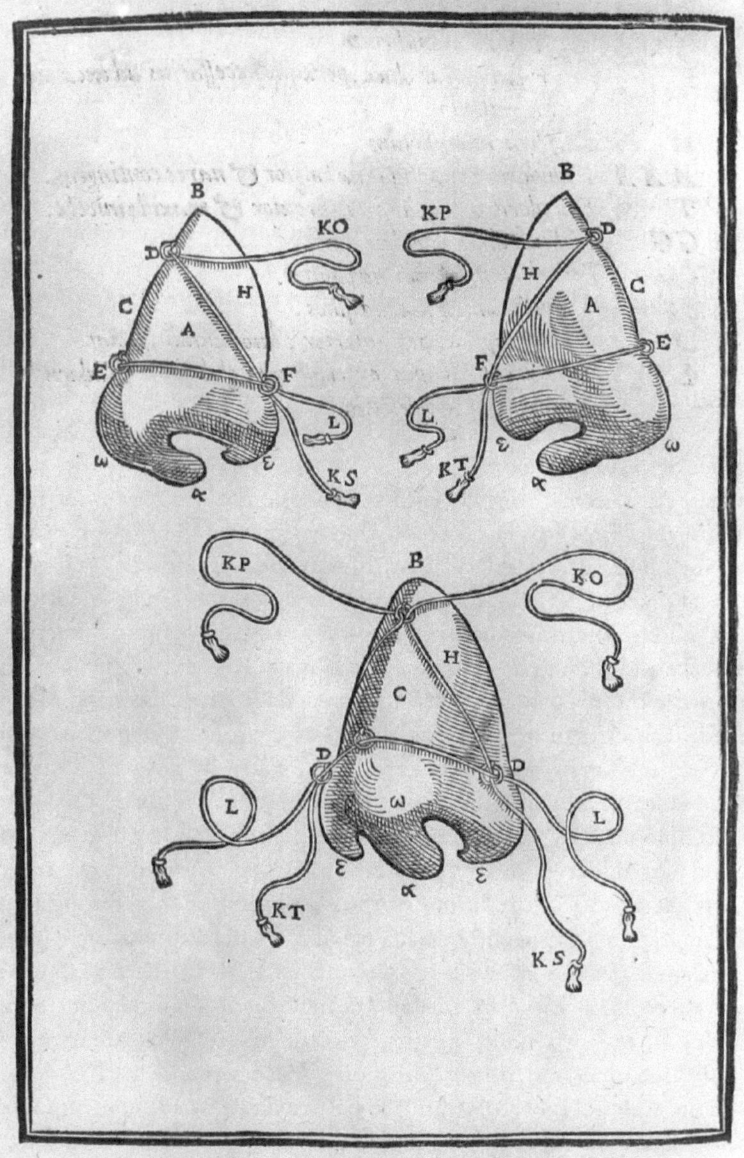

FIGURE 0.4 Gaspare Tagliacozzi, *De curtorum chirurgia per insitionem* (1597): molds for reshaping the nose.

Source: Courtesy of the Wellcome Collection

de narium, aurium, labiorumque defectu.[2] The first volume is the longest. It consists of 23 chapters approaching the human face from a wide variety of points of view, all reflecting the erudition and the humanistic culture of the author. Tagliacozzi discusses the medical and literary tropes concerning the face and each of its parts; physiognomy and the art of reading character through facial features; a natural history of the human face; the history of grafting; a review of the most painful procedures in the history of surgery; the difference between cosmetics and reconstruction; and the relationships between beauty and health. The second volume is the technical one and focuses on a detailed description of the major steps of the operation. It is accompanied by 20 illustrations of the procedure and of the new instruments necessary to perform it.

Tagliacozzi's version of the procedure was a very specific one, because by the late sixteenth century different opinions and descriptions of the procedure circulated throughout Europe. It was well known that the procedure was perfected by two families of "empiric" surgeons from Southern Italy, the Branca in Sicily in the fifteenth century and the Vianeo in Calabria in the sixteenth century. Nonetheless, Tagliacozzi was the first one to put on paper the details of the procedure, and therefore historians of medicine and surgery have celebrated him as the father of "plastic surgery."[3]

In fact, the artisanal and the learned dimensions of surgery are strictly intertwined in the history of facial reconstructive surgery. This book explores this intertwined history by emphasizing that early modern surgeons and other kinds of surgical practitioners had to deal with the appearance and the health of their patients' bodies. But this is not simply a story of a secret empiric practice traveling in space and time to be considered "rational." Rather, the focus of this book is on how, why, and when a textual printed tradition concerning this practice emerged. Rather than treating Tagliacozzi as the solitary genius who invented "plastic surgery," my work tries to explain how and why this practice became the subject of a learned monograph in the last decades of the sixteenth century in a city like Bologna, the second most important city of the Papal state. This is the only, and partial, exceptionality one can find in the history of facial surgery and concerns the historical conditions of the possibility for the coming into being of a monograph on this technique at a particular time and in a particular place.

Tagliacozzi decided to write about such a difficult, daring, and spectacular operation not because he invented a new field of surgery but because he was living in his own times. For several reasons – such as time, cost, length, uncertain outcome, and risk of infection – the procedure itself was not practiced many times. Tagliacozzi came to be perceived by his contemporaries as a specialist of the human face in general, as someone capable of treating several kinds of surgical and medical facial issues. Nonetheless, he chose to write only about this particular procedure. This was a conscious decision: he desired to be remembered for this operation. This is not to say that this surgical procedure was merely a literary *topos* or, worse, that all that matters in the history of medicine are textual representations. It is not by chance that Tagliacozzi and the other learned surgeons and physicians who wrote about the operation mentioned only cases regarding men and duels, because in this period the ideology of noblemen centered precisely around this ritual. Such a decision can be understood only by exploring the ideology of honor and duel proper of the aristocratic classes of the courts around the Po valley and the Papal state in the sixteenth century. It is true that this operation became visible only when integrated into a textual tradition, the subject of a published monograph authored by a learned surgeon and physician in one of the most important medical schools of medieval and early modern Europe. But I anchor this emergence of texts within multifarious social, political, cultural, and medical contexts. The present work explores how a fluid oral tradition transmitting a "secret" solidified into a public textual tradition, which in turn became the point of departure for another history of practices and receptions.

I have envisioned this book as a kind of "total history" pulling together such various threads and methodologies as political history, social history, intellectual history, microhistory, and the history of science in order to track down the many facets of a practice and a discourse. The roots of what the moderns still call "plastic surgery" lie not only in the ingenuity of a surgeon but also in a series of interactions between different historical phenomena. Specific academic settings; the dynamics of early modern state building; shifts in scientific concepts; gendered perceptions of male and female beauty and public roles; practices of manipulating nature; the evolution of genres of medical writing; the art and rhetoric of pain management; the encounters between the ways of living of different social classes; and the anthropological, theological, and aesthetic meanings attributed to the human face are all factors that figure in this total history. At first sight, this might seem like a list of haphazard topics. The task I gave myself is to give these topics order and coherence, to see the early history of reconstructive surgery through a magnifying glass.[4]

Historians of "plastic surgery" – both surgeon-historians in search for professional origins and, more recently, cultural historians – seem to agree in suggesting that after Tagliacozzi the procedure fell into oblivion for two centuries. In the seventeenth and the eighteenth centuries, Tagliacozzi's methods would simply have become the object of ridicule and satires, becoming attached to a story of noses grafted from slave-donors that would fall down when the donor died. Among the causes mentioned for the disappearance of Tagliacozzi's method are the fact that the practice became associated with syphilis and the opposition of the Counter-Reformation Church to aesthetic procedures.[5] Others insisted on the limited circulation of *De curtorum*, on the early death of Tagliacozzi, on theological-religious opposition, and, above all, on a general European decline in the art of surgery by the end of the sixteenth century as reasons for the disappearance of Tagliacozzi's method.[6]

Twentieth- and twenty-first-century historians have taken up this theme of the oblivion and bad reputation of Tagliacozzi's method from the supposed rediscoverers of plastic surgery of the nineteenth century. These early historians of plastic surgery claimed that the oblivion was due to the paucity of cases of such wounds; to the fact that European civilization was all too advanced to allow for the legal practice of punishing people by cutting off their noses; to the lowly origins of the practice among the semi-barbaric peoples of Southern Italy; and finally to the fact that the operation was too arduous and demanding for the patient.[7] It has been argued that the oblivion and bad reputation were ended by an anonymous report from the Indian colonies published in 1794 in the *Gentlemen's Magazine* describing the so-called Indian method (Figure 0.5). This report supposedly spurred a renewal of interest in the "Italian" method as well. In a way, this document lies at the origin of modern historiography of plastic surgery. From this passage, nineteenth-century European surgeons – especially German surgeons – would have slowly but firmly placed Tagliacozzi's technique within the modern rational and scientific method, which was still practiced to treat the damaged faces of World War I soldiers coming back from the trenches. This book challenges many of these historical explanations.

I had to ask again why the stage for Renaissance facial surgery is late sixteenth-century Bologna? And what motivated Tagliacozzi, a man who graduated in medicine, a man coming from the middle class with hopes of climbing the social ladder, to embrace such a shaky, artisanal, oral tradition of surgery?[8]

First of all, Tagliacozzi was involved in a debate around Galenic ideas concerning the relationship between health and beauty that went on in the last decades of the sixteenth century among a group of professors of anatomy, surgery, and medicine in Bologna and Padua. These two cities were also the places where surgery as an academic tradition had taken root earlier. Indeed, between the late thirteenth century and the first decades of the fourteenth century surgery was already taught in academic settings in Bologna, when what Michael McVaugh called "rational surgery" flourished.[9] Contrary to what happened north of the Alps, in Bologna learned graduate physicians could specialize in surgery and still be part of the medical elite that gathered in the College of Medicine. Only in such an academically friendly space could someone like Tagliacozzi write a learned monograph on one single surgical operation. Also, the professional boundaries between surgeons, barbers, and empirics were not as clear-cut as one might think, and a large spectrum of practitioners of the body dealt with both health and appearance.

But one of the core arguments of this book is that the emergence of a textual tradition of facial surgery is to be seen as one of the many fruits of an encounter between the needs, desires, and ideological mind-set of the noblemen and the social ascension of the sons of the lower classes who used reconstructive surgery as a means of attracting fame, cultural capital, wealth, and patronage. Noblemen wanted their public appearance restored; surgeons wanted to be able to offer this service.

Facial disfigurement took a peculiar turn in sixteenth-century Italy, when it became firmly associated not only with traditional imagery of punishments for female adultery and political treason but also with the culture of honor and duel

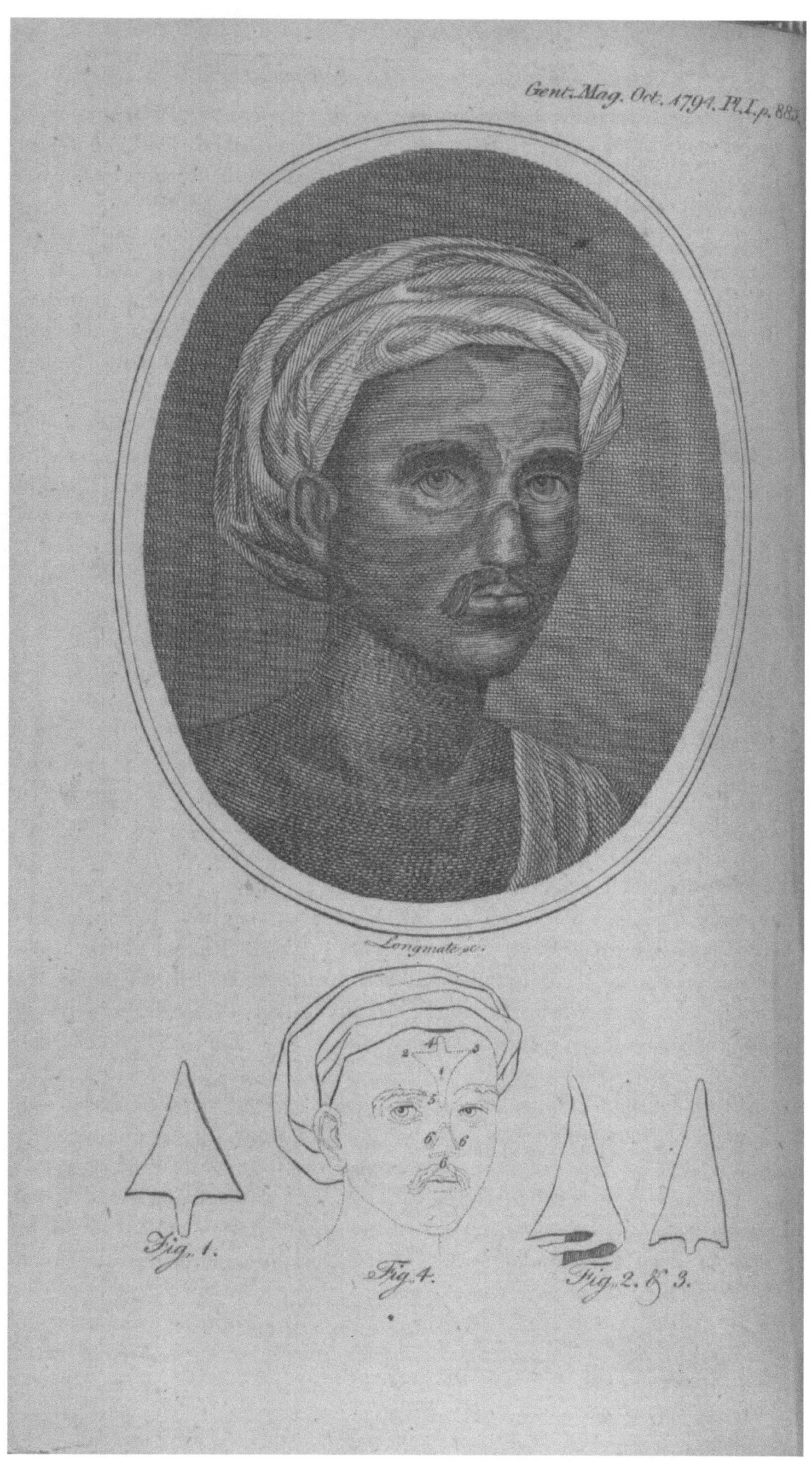

FIGURE 0.5 *Gentlemen's Magazine* (1794): the "Indian method" for restoring noses.

of the aristocratic classes. It is not by chance that the courts of Piacenza, Ferrara, and Mantua keep appearing in this history. Patrons and patients looking for Tagliacozzi's skills came from these places and sought out that wondrous surgical operation that restored noble noses lost in duels. Moreover, the Po valley courts of this period became the centers of the elaboration of a subtle literature on the rules of honor and of duel, considered as the quintessential activities and cornerstones of the lifestyle of the noble class and the masculine identity of its members.

At the same time, in this period the noble classes of the central and northern Italian courts and the Papal state found themselves in a predicament. The late sixteenth-century lords, popes, and government officials were looking for ways of establishing a more certain rule by centralizing authority and creating a new class of civil servants different from the noble class. Male aristocrats responded by elaborating a renewed isolationist culture centered on rules and rituals that had to escape secular justice systems. Authors began to assert forcefully that the way of living of the former ruling classes had to be placed above the state apparatus and the social discipline of the state. How could people coming from the middle classes dare to inflict punishments to noblemen in a court of law? Even if this process of statalization and centralization of the Papal territories were far from complete and successful, phenomena of noble violence can be read as a response to this new political climate.

Bologna was in the middle of this process; it was governed together by the Legates of the pope and by the most powerful local patrician families who gathered in the Senate. Bolognese noblemen of ancient aristocratic legacy were in part co-opted through the Senate and in part, when they exceeded in violence and unruliness, were punished. Tagliacozzi built an entirely male world in his printed works, leaving out the cases in which he operated on women's faces. In this respect, the emergence of reconstructive surgery is part of both political history and gender history. It was the relationship between different kinds of men and their ideas about masculinity that fueled this emergence. In this book, the history of men, gender history, and masculinity are not confined in a separate chapter, but rather they are diffused throughout it. The ideas of life, bodies, and careers of men are placed on an equal footing with ideas about what the ideal masculine identity of a nobleman was. The encounter between different men in the context of Bolognese political life, with its gendered distribution of power and status, also explains why Tagliacozzi tried to appeal to this kind of aristocratic audience in several ways. One of these ways was a strong moralization of bravely bearing pain in surgery as a mark of higher-class masculinity. The complex of social, political, and technical prescriptions about pain management is what I call the "moral economy of pain."

But the surgical procedure, based on skin grafting and taking its model from agricultural practices, also had a scientific relevance of its own. The emphasis on grafting is linked to the crisis of the boundaries between the natural and the artificial in sixteenth-century culture, of which Tagliacozzi's book was both an effect and a contributory factor. Just as trees, human faces and beauty itself could be natural or artificial. This was a heavily gendered distinction because in Renaissance culture "artificial" beauty was associated with women. In the course of his complex and at times convoluted reflections on grafting Tagliacozzi lost track of the epistemological grounding of the distinction and ended up talking about hybrid faces. It is not possible to understand Tagliacozzi's book without understanding the complex culture of the face of the sixteenth century, namely the system of materially inscribed meaning connected to the dignity and the infamy of human faces. This rich culture made of medicine, physiognomy, gender constructions, theology, and the law was not just a background for Tagliacozzi and the reconstructive surgeons but their living and breathing environment, the space in which they could think and act.

In Chapter 1 I start by telling the history of plastic surgery through the case histories of facial surgery that circulated in a period that goes from the fifteenth to the early seventeenth centuries with special attention to patients' social standing. I then analyze two previously unknown cases that I have found in the criminal court of Bologna in which Tagliacozzi served as medical expert. These are cases of female disfigurement.

Given that no great amount of information can be found on patients, in Chapter 2 I try to reconstruct their culture, namely the culture of the male elite. I then briefly sketch a picture of the social and political stratification of late sixteenth-century Italy with special attention to the culture of the duel and honor in the Papal state. The chapter then explores what it was like to be a learned surgeon in sixteenth-century Bologna. I describe the career paths of Tagliacozzi and a group of learned surgeons in the late sixteenth century. I argue that the emergence of a textual representation of reconstructive surgery is partially linked to the specific social and political conditions of Bologna, to the great prestige that surgery and surgeons enjoyed at that university, and to the encounter between middle-class men who became "graduate surgeons" and the noble classes.

Chapter 3 presents a cultural history and historical anthropology of the human face in sixteenth-century Italy. It deals with attitudes toward the dignity, honor, and integrity of the face as it appears in medicine, law, literature, and the Christian theological tradition. I follow Tagliacozzi's text and highlight three components of reconstructive surgery: the Renaissance revival of classical notions of beauty, proportions, and integrity of the human figure; the growing importance and influence of physiognomy; and the great reputation and cultural salience the human face enjoyed in that period. I show how this particular culture of the face was organized along the gendered and moral lines of the distinction between the natural and the artificial and what the relationships between the face and the self in the sixteenth century were.

In Chapter 4, I approach the topic of the relationships between the natural and the artificial from the point of view of medical debates around beauty, cosmetics, and reconstructive surgery. I describe the debate around Galenic notions of health and beauty that developed in the second half of the sixteenth century. Then I discuss the care of appearance in the writings of the so-called professors of secrets – who targeted both women and men – and in the printed works of barber-surgeons – who took care of those external parts of the body that were located in a liminal space between ornament and health. Then I go back to Tagliacozzi's way of dealing with the distinction between "true" and "false" beauty, showing both the gendered nature of this distinction and the contiguity between health and appearance as represented by the concept of *politezza* – which meant, at the same time, physical and moral cleanliness – that ran across professional distinctions between barber-surgeons and learned surgeons.

Chapter 5 focuses on grafting as it was thought about and practiced across a range of different disciplines in the early modern period and argues that grafting must be put in close connection with the conceptual transformations of the "Scientific Revolution." By following the history of a practice – grafting – rather than a discipline – surgery – I approach Tagliacozzi's text from the point of view of ontology and epistemology. First, I briefly describe the classical distinction between art and nature in the Renaissance. I then discuss the many contradictions and oscillations concerning the natural versus artificial opposition that are to be found in Tagliacozzi's book. I argue that these difficulties were linked to the practical example he chose as the main guide for the operation itself: grafting. I then move on to discuss classical and contemporary practices and theories of grafting that were in place by the late sixteenth century. Finally, I discuss further and clarify the main epistemological and ontological issues in Tagliacozzi's book.

Chapter 6 explores the methodological stakes of writing a history of pain and sketches a history of the techniques of pain management in early modern surgery. I treat pain not as a subjective feeling but as a social event historically determined by the distribution of power, gender, and medical techniques. I introduce here the concept of "moral economy of pain" to account for the social and political dimensions of the epistemological and "clinical" encounter between surgeons and patients in the old regime.

The last chapter offers a conclusion in the form of a history of the reception of Tagliacozzi's book and, more generally, of the reconstructive technique in the seventeenth and the eighteenth centuries. I argue that Tagliacozzi's book was not at all neglected by his contemporaries and immediate followers but rather that it became the subject of a complex and fragmented reception. First, I underline the deep resonances of reconstructive surgery and Tagliacozzi's method in two important branches of seventeenth-century medical and natural philosophical culture: teratology and the debate around mechanism and empiricism. Then I show that in the seventeenth century this surgical method was present in two distinct kinds of medical writings. The first is that of collections of *observationes*, especially in the German-speaking lands; the second is the alchemical literature on sympathies and magnetism, especially in England. In this way I am able to sketch a map of the geographic spread of the technique of reconstructive surgery between the fifteenth and the seventeenth centuries and to emphasize the overlooked role played by surgery in the process of the establishment of the "new science."

The history of facial surgery is a longue durée history, marked by both deep continuities and sudden discontinuities. Besides the undisputable technical progress surgery enjoyed from the middle of the nineteenth century on – above all in the anesthetic and antiseptic methods – the deepest continuities between modern and early modern worlds have to do with the gendered relationships among personal identity, beauty, and integrity of the face. While I was writing this book, the Italian parliament discussed a law concerning "identity murder" (*omicidio d'identità*). Following a series of well-known and intensely debated cases of gender violence centered around disfigurement (such as those involving Lucia Annibali and Carla Caiazzo), the proposed law aims at changing the penal code by increasing the sentence of those explicitly aiming at disfiguring their victims. These are still cases of men disfiguring women for the sake of "honor," in order to make them unrecognizable to themselves and horrible to other men. This book is precisely about the knot of identity, gender, and violence and about the ways in which medical knowledge tried to untie it in the early modern period. Clearly, medical culture never succeeded.

Notes

1 While the etymology of "plastic surgery" points to molding and malleability of body parts, in this book I prefer to use "reconstructive surgery" or "facial surgery." These options are preferable for two reasons: they are more faithful to what the actors themselves were thinking in the early modern period, and they avoid easy anachronism and slippage into modern conceptions of cosmetic surgery, thus helping the appreciation of historical differences.

2 Gaspare Tagliacozzi, *De curtorum chirurgia per insistionem libri duo* (Venice: apud G. Bindonum iuniorem, 1597). Throughout this work I will refer to the English translation: *De curtorum chirurgia per insitionem*, tr. Joan H. Thomas (New York: The Classics of Medicine Library Gryphon Editions, 1996). On the editorial history of the book, see P. Tomba, A. Viganò, P. Ruggieri, and A. Gasbarrini, "Gaspare Tagliacozzi, Pioneer of Plastic Surgery and the Spread of His Technique throughout Europe in *De Curtorum Chirurgia per Insitionem*," *European Review for Medical and Pharmacological Sciences* 18, 4 (2014): 445–450, pp. 446–447.

3 The history of "plastic surgery" has been narrated several times; the best works are M.E. Alfonso Corradi, "Dell'antica autoplastica Italiana," *Memorie del Regio Istituto Lombardo di Scienze e Lettere, classe di Scienze matematiche e naturali* 13 (1877): 225–273; Martha Teach-Gnudi and Jerome Pierce Webster, *The Life and Times of Gaspare Tagliacozzi, Surgeon of Bologna 1545–1599* (New York: Herbert Reichner, 1950), pp. 105–128; Paolo Santoni-Rugiu and Philip J. Sykes, *History of Plastic Surgery* (Berlin/New York: Springer, 2007), pp. 168–198; Luigi Monga, "Odeporica e medicina: I viaggiatori del Cinquecento e la rinoplastica," *Italica* 69, 3 (1992): 378–393; Mariacarla Gadebusch Bondio, *Medizinische Ästhetik: Kosmetik und plastische Chirurgie zwischen Antike und früher Neuzeit* (München: WFink, 2005), pp. 129–182. In addition to these kind of works, there is an abundance of literature on the history of plastic surgery written by surgeons and surgeon-historians, who generally describe Tagliacozzi as the father or a pioneer of modern rhinoplasty and trace a direct vertical line connecting the sixteenth century to the present; examples include Hildebrando Landazuri, "Plastic Surgery Pioneers," *British Journal of Plastic Surgery* 15 (1962): 117–122; Giovanni Micali, "The Italian Contribution to Plastic Surgery," *Annals of Plastic Surgery* 31, 6 (1993): 566–571; Claus Walter, "The Evolution of Rhinoplasty," *The Journal of Laryngology and Otology* 102 (1988): 1079–1085; Iain S. Whitaker

et al., "The Birth of Plastic Surgery: The Story of Nasal Reconstruction from the *Edwyn Smith Papyrus* to the Twenty-First Century," *Plastic and Reconstructive Surgery* 120 (2007): 327–336; Silvia Marinozzi, "The Vianeo and Gaspare Tagliacozzi," *Medicina nei secoli* 11 (1999): 603–610.

4 For the metaphor of the magnifying glass, see Carlo Ginzburg, "Microhistory: Two of Three Things That I Know about It," *Critical Inquiry* 20, 1 (1993): 10–35.

5 See, for example, Sander L. Gilman, *Making the Body Beautiful: A Cultural History of Aesthetic Surgery* (Princeton: Princeton University Press, 1999); Emily Cock, "Lead[ing] 'Em by the Nose into Publick Shame and Derision': Gaspare Tagliacozzi, Alexander Read and the Lost History of Plastic Surgery, 1600–1800," *Social History of Medicine* 28, 1 (2015): 1–21.

6 Santoni-Rugiu and Skyles, *History of Plastic Surgery*, p. 89.

7 Among the most famous, I will mention Joseph Constantine Carpue, *An Account of Two Successful Operations for Restoring a Lost Nose* (London: Longman, Hurst, Reese, Horme, and Brown, 1816); and Kurt Sprengel, *Geschichte der Chirurgie* (Halle: Kümmel, 1819). For a review of this historiography, see François Delaporte, *Figures of Medicine: Blood, Face Transplants, Parasites*, tr. Nils F. Schott (New York: Fordham University Press, 2013), pp. 25–59.

8 Tagliacozzi's biography has been narrated in detail by Teach Gnudi and Webster in their monumental study of 1950, which is surely outdated from a medical history viewpoint but still valid for biographical purposes.

9 Michael McVaugh, *The Rational Surgery of the Middle Ages* (Florence: Sismel/Edizioni del Galluzzo, 2006).

1

PATIENTS AND CASES

Gaspare Tagliacozzi is elegantly dressed with a long robe and sports all the symbols of the College of Medicine of Bologna. He holds a book in his hand, while another one stands on a pile of volumes. The two open books show the key phases of an operation he is known for, the reconstruction of mutilated parts of the nose. The book has been written by the sitter, who is so proud of it that he chose to have it in the portrait (Figure 1.1).

This portrait has not been dated with precision, and its author has not been identified with certainty. The Federico Zeri Foundation attributes it to Bartolomeo Passerotti (1529–1592) and/or his school, while other scholars attribute it to Tiburzio Passerotti (1575–1612), the eldest son of Bartolomeo.[1] Bartolomeo and Tagliacozzi knew each other well. They were part of a circle of physicians, anatomists, artists, and naturalists that gathered at the museum of Ulisse Aldrovandi (1522–1605), one of the most famous naturalists and collectors of *naturalia* of his times.[2] Bartolomeo must have observed dissections practiced by Tagliacozzi several times.

Now, by the second half of the sixteenth century portraits of scholars were not uncommon, and the subjects were most often represented with books or instruments.[3] However, this portrait of Tagliacozzi strikes the viewer because the physician is the author of the book shown in the painting. This was not so common. For example, Bartolomeo Paserotti's portrait of mathematician Ignazio Danti (1536–1586) shows the sitter as appropriately reading Ptolemy's *Almagest* (Figure 1.2). Lavinia Fontana (1552–1614) portrayed in Bologna the eminent physician Girolamo Mercuriale (1530–1606), professor of theoretical medicine there from 1587 to 1592, reading *De humani corporis fabrica* by Andreas Vesalius (1514–1564) (Figure 1.3). Mercuriale also has a pile of books by classical authorities such as Hippocrates, Galen, and Avicenna, as someone equally fluent in the new and the classic medical literature. But Tagliacozzi wanted to be identified so closely with his book on facial reconstructive surgery that he pushed the author of his portrait to break these stylistic rules.

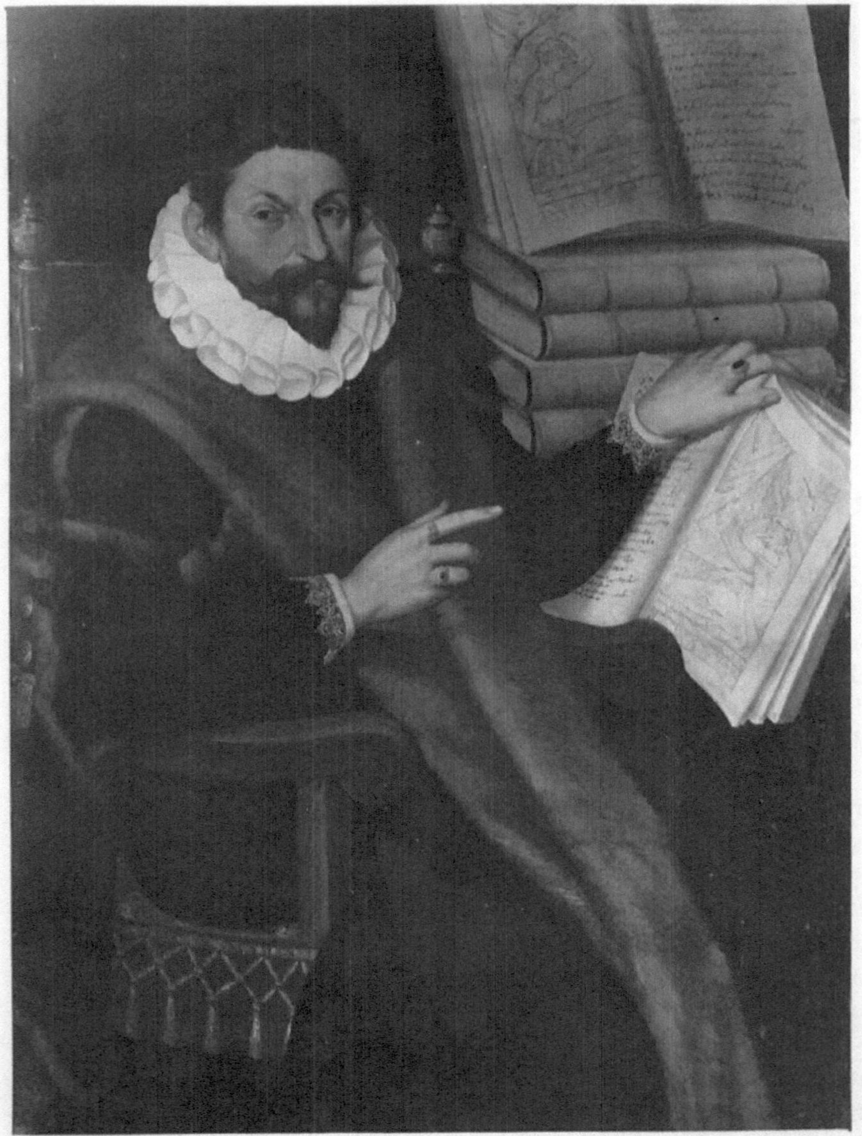

FIGURE 1.1 Tiburzio (?) Passerotti, *Portrait of Gaspare Tagliacozzi* (date uncertain). Bologna, Putti's Donation, Rizzoli Orthopaedic Institute (public domain).

The book on reconstructive surgery came out in 1597. One of the best candidates as the author of the painting, Bartolomeo, died in 1592. This circumstance could of course mean that Tiburzio, who died in 1614, is in fact the author of the painting. But one detail can make us doubt about it. Besides the fact that the two illustrations reproduce quite faithfully those we can find in print, Tagliacozzi's

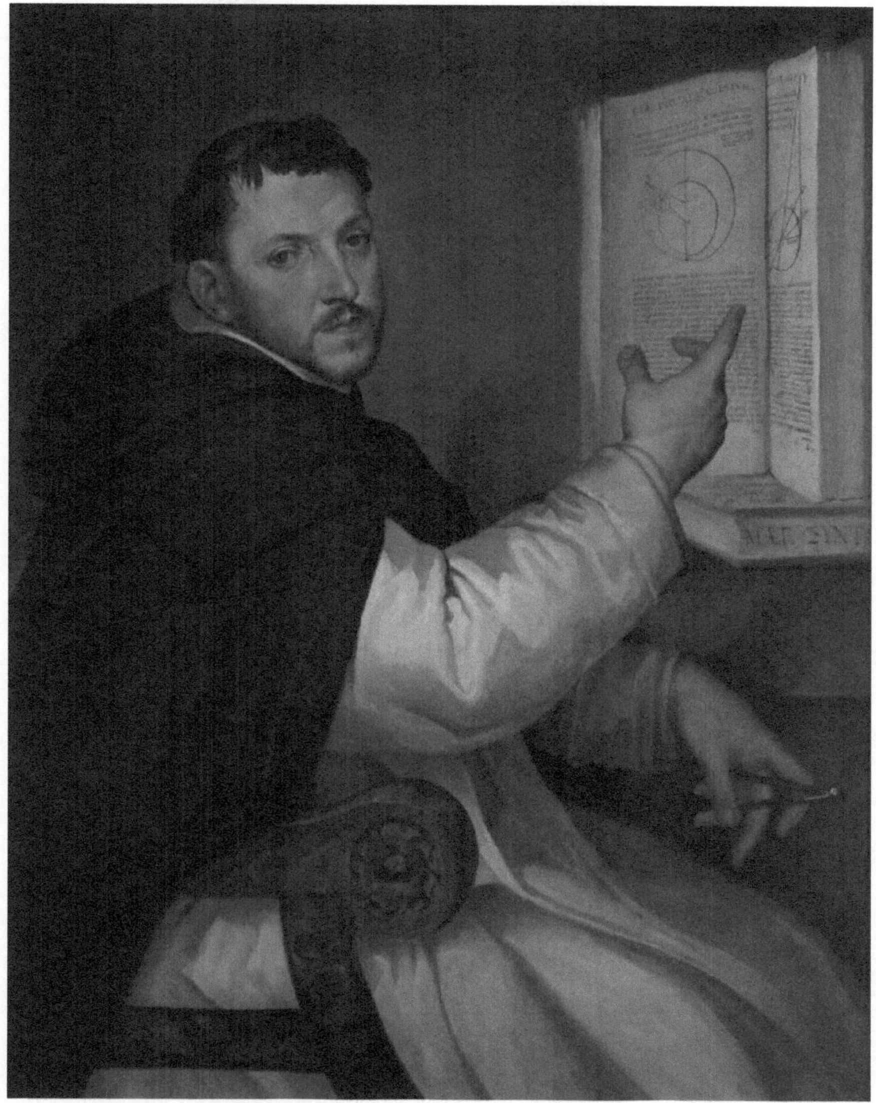

FIGURE 1.2 Bartolomeo Passerotti, *Portrait of Ignazio Danti* (between 1576 and 1586). Brest, Musée des beaux-arts (public domain).

books are here clearly in a manuscript form.[4] We know that a letter sent by Tagliacozzi to Mercuriale, in which the former described in detail the surgical procedure, was printed in the latter's *De decoratione* in 1587.[5] So by that date at least Tagliacozzi was known as an expert on reconstructive surgery. We could speculate that a manuscript of the book – or of some parts of it – circulated well before 1597, even before 1592, accompanied by illustrations. The hypothesis that Bartolomeo is the author is not absurd. If this is the case, the image of a learned physician, anatomist,

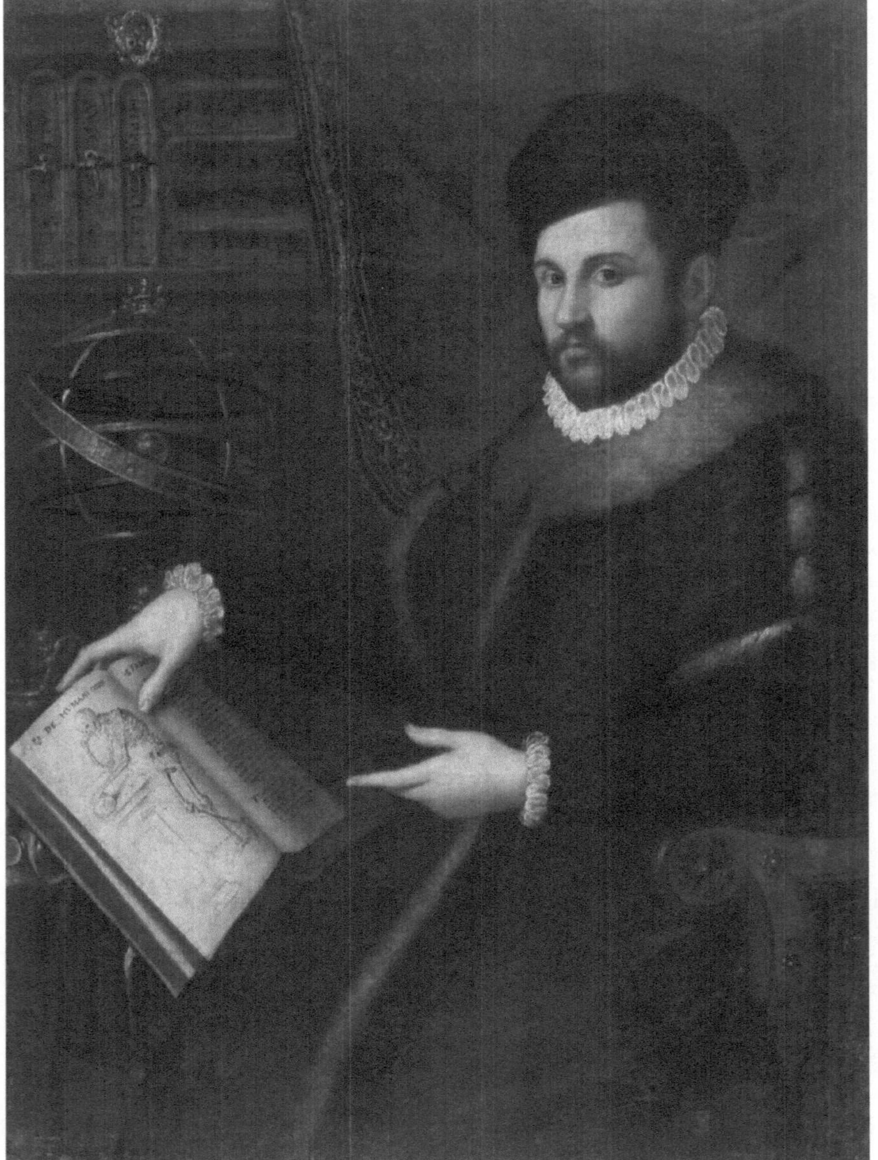

FIGURE 1.3 Lavinia Fontana, *Portrait of Girolamo Mercuriale* (1590). Baltimore, The Walters Art Museum (creative commons).

and surgeon wanting to be immortalized as the author of a book on facial surgery that was not even in print yet appears all the more clear. Also, with this portrait, Tagliacozzi stressed the fact that he was the first one to write the procedure down.

What is missing from the portrait are the surgeon's patients; conversely, the illustrations in the book only represent patients and never the surgeon at work.

Tagliacozzi described very few case histories of patients whose faces he reconstructed. In this chapter I try to understand why.

I describe the patents' identities and culture as they appear from the few cases circulating in early modern Europe from the fifteenth to the seventeenth centuries. Patient stories and culture – which I reconstruct mostly indirectly, because almost no direct, first-person patient account of the procedure survives – provide a first point of entry into Tagliacozzi's book and its context. First, I describe the history of facial reconstructive surgery through these case histories. I then put into question a widespread historical narrative associating the success of plastic surgery with the ravages of the French disease and prove that the known cases concern male patients wounded in duels or war. Finally, I analyze two previously unknown cases that I have found in the criminal court of Bologna in which Tagliacozzi served as medical expert on disfigured women. It appears that the world of reconstructive surgery was a men's world, from which women were deliberately removed. The popularity of facial reconstructive surgery in early modern Bologna is specifically linked to an encounter between learned surgeons and upper-class men.

Cases

In the literature on facial reconstructing surgery, either in the pre- or the post-Tagliacozzi versions, I have been able to find no more than 13 case histories. However, I use here the term "case history" in a rather liberal way. In fact, these cases include episodes in which the physician advised patients not to undertake the procedure and episodes in which we do not even know whether the procedure was performed or not. Moreover, in many instances, we even lack the names of the patients, for reasons that will be discussed later in the chapter.[6] Almost all of these *historiae* are either short anecdotal narratives embedded in longer texts or fragments of a bigger whole. I say "anecdotal" and not anecdotes because however fragmentary, brief, and isolated from their context these narratives might be, in most cases they still retain the function of connecting one single instance to a set of rules or norms.[7] Moreover, all these cases were *historiae* in the early modern sense of the word, in all their broad range of meanings, which went from compilation from learned sources to direct observation, or a combination of the two, from the valorization of firsthand experience to a new sense of the specificity of time and place.[8]

Early witnesses

Procedures of surgical reconstruction of mutilated parts of the face – noses in the first place – are the subject of a long and global history.[9] The earliest mentions of a procedure of surgical reconstruction of facial disfigurements belong to the classic ancient Indian text of the *Sushruta Samhita*, written around the fifth century BCE. This text described a method for covering up nasal mutilations through skin flaps taken from the forefront.[10] A very similar method was described by Celsus (c. 25 BCE–50 CE) in the first century CE in his *De medicina*, which circulated in fragments in the Middle Ages and was published in its entirety only in 1478. While Lanfranc of Milan (c. 1250–1306), Henri de Mondeville (c. 1260–1320), and Guy de Chauliac (1300–1368), three of the "rational surgeons" of the Middle Ages, all addressed issues of nose loss and repair, none of them described a technical procedure for reconstructing missing portions of the nostrils and the soft parts of the nose.[11] Treating facial wounds was also part of the empiric and vernacular tradition of surgery. For example, in a fifteenth-century anonymous Italian manual there appeared a long chapter on the "wounds of the nose caused by swords and arrows" that detailed a complex typology of wounds and the relative ways of treating them with unguents and manual manipulation of skin, flesh, cartilage, and bones.[12]

The first mention of a technique similar to that described by Tagliacozzi comes from the first half of the fourteenth century, when members of the Branca family were practicing surgery in the city Catania, Sicily. They were licensed "empiric" surgeons, without university training, as the family-related nature of their trade attests. In particular Antonio, the son of Gustavo, who had received a license from the King of Aragon in 1412, is credited of having invented the technique of taking the skin flap not from the forefront but from a more discreet, virtually invisible site: the upper interior part of the arm.[13] Many hypotheses have been made regarding where the Brancas might have learned the technique, whether from Arabic sources or from Persian ones via the *Sushruta*, but no plausible explanation has been advanced.[14] As the court historian of the Aragonese king, Bartolomeo Fazio (1410–1457) wrote in the mid-fifteenth century:

> [W]hereas his father had taken the flesh for the repair from the mutilated man's face, Antonius took it from the muscles of the man's arm, so that no distortion of the face should be caused. On the arm that was cut open and into the wound itself, he bound the [site of the] mutilated nose so tightly that the patient might not move his head at all. After fifteen days or sometimes twenty, little by little with a sharp knife he cut away the flap which had become attached to the nose; finally he severed it entirely from the arm and shaped it into a nose with so much ingenuity that it was scarcely possible with the eye to detect the flap that had been added, since the deformity of the face had been entirely removed.[15]

The detail concerning the "muscles" that had to be excised from the arm would be repeated several times in the sixteenth century and would then be corrected by Gaspare Tagliacozzi, who greatly emphasized this difference with respect to the empiric surgeons' technique. By this time the Brancas were famous enough to be remembered in a dialogue of the humanist, diplomat, and courtier of the Aragonese, Giovanni Pontano (1492–1503). In his *Antonius* (1487) one of the characters, Compater, says that "the Catalans" have brought many vices to Naples and among them the "daggers," namely the habit of fighting:

> [N]nor is anything sold more cheaply than a man's life, and if your Branca, a second Asclepius, had not arrived to heal them, you would see the majority of the citizens with their ears and lips cut off, or with their nose mutilated.[16]

Antonio Branca's technique was known by a German nobleman and surgeon with the Prussian Army in the 1460s, Heinrich von Pfolsprundt (c. 1415–1465), who described it in a manuscript published only in the nineteenth century. In this work, the German surgeon made reference to an Italian family of surgeons from whom he had learned the technique.[17]

Traces leading to the actual practice of such an operation on one specific individual come from the fifteenth century. In the 1950s, Ladislao Münster found in the State Archives of Milan a letter sent by Federico I Gonzaga (1441–1484), marquis of Mantua, to the duke of Milan's commissioner for Piacenza, dated January 31, 1470. With this letter, Fererico Gonzaga intended to defend one of his soldiers, Antonio Terzo, who had been arrested for a brawl with a Milanese soldier. Federico Gonzaga mentioned that Antonio was passing through Piacenza en route "to have his nose re-made (*per farsi rifare lo naso*)." In another letter, this time sent directly to the Sforza duke of Milan to ask for the release of Antonio, Federico Gonzaga said that his protégé was in Piacenza with the Bolognese surgeon Gaspare Speranza Manzoli (c. 1410–1475), who "was re-making his nose anew, which had been cut off in a brawl (*gli stave facendo lo naso da novo, che per questione gli fu tagliato*)." Unfortunately, the letters do not go into any further detail about the procedure. Besides appearing once as a medico-legal expert in a 1471 trial, nothing has been found about the surgeon Manzoli, but nonetheless this scant information reminds us that the art of making noses was practiced in Bologna in the late fifteenth century and that the Gonzaga and the Sforza families were well aware of that.[18]

In the same year (1470) a young woman, Catilina García, was disfigured for unknown reasons by a nobleman's gang in Cuidad Rodrigo, in the Kingdom of Castile. Years after the assault, Catilina went to Portugal, where an anonymous surgeon performed a Branca-style rhinoplasty on her using the skin from her arm. The story as it can be understood from the trial document – as in the previous example, I am hesitant to call it a case, because these two stories had no medical circulation – is full of mysteries. Nonetheless, we have here the rare case of a woman. By the second half of the fifteenth century this procedure was known in Portugal, Castile, and Germany.[19]

Humanist physician Alessandro Benedetti (1450–1512), professor of medicine at Padua, discussed the method, crediting Antonio Branca, in his 1502 anatomy book. Even if he never practiced it, Benedetti is the first author who made the technique enter the stage of learned medicine. Benedetti gave a very interesting and detailed description of the procedure and claimed he witnessed the operation:

> [S]ome ingenious minds (*ingenia*) taught how to correct (to make gracious again) the deformities of the nose (*narium deformitatem cohonestari docuere*):

> several times we have seen (*saepe visum est*) that after having cut a little piece of flesh (*carunculam*) from the arm, they fashioned it in the shape of the nostrils and attached it to the mutilated nose (*trunco naso*). Indeed, they separate the skin of the arm with a little razor (*novacula*); after they have made that wound (*facto vulnere*), they scrap the nostrils again, or they cut them anew, they tie the head to the arm in order to make the two wounds to adhere (*ut vulnus vulneri cohereat*). Once the wounds adhere to each other, they cut with a little knife only the part which is necessary from the arm: the little veins of the nose nourish the little piece of flesh take from the arm. Finally, they cover (*superinducitur*) the nose with the new skin: sometimes, given the arm's nature, a few hair grow on the nose. Through this method they fashion new nostrils with admirable zeal, dominating nature with the power of their daring minds (*audaci ingenio naturae imperantes*). The added part (*additamentum*) can barely can withstand cold weather, and patients must be very careful because if they touch their nose at the beginning of the procedure, it is likely to fall down.[20]

This account is interesting for two reasons. Benedetti used the language of nature versus art (a challenge apparently won by art), and he described the same shortcomings of the procedure Tagliacozzi would mention almost a century later.

In the meanwhile, the empirical tradition of reconstructive facial surgery continued in Southern Italy, specifically in Tropea, Calabria, where the Vianeo brothers Pietro and Paolo famously practiced it through the second half of the sixteenth century. Several authors left accounts of their practice, including Ambroise Paré (1510–1590) and Leonardo Fioravanti (1517–1588). Fioravanti described two cases. In his self-portrait as a medical secret-hunter, *Il Tesoro della vita humana* (1570), he recalled that in 1549, while on his way to Naples from Messina, he stopped at Tropea, where the Vianeo brothers were performing that marvelous procedure. In order to induce the Vianeos to tell him all about their secret, Fioravanti invented a story. He told the brothers that he was a "Bolognese gentleman" and that he wanted to talk to them because "I had a relative who had his nose cut off while fighting the enemies at the battle of Serravalle, in Lombardy, and he wanted to know whether he had to come by or not." The lie proved successful because there was indeed a Cornelio Albergati in Bologna who had been de-nosed at the battle of Serravalle "by a Stradioto [a Balkan mercenary] & they [the Vianeos] had heard about him from a letter already." Fioravanti wrote that while he was pretending to wait for Albergati he regularly went to the Vianeos' workshop; finally one day, when they had five rhinoplasty procedures scheduled, he got the chance to see them performing. He then described the very same procedure Tagliacozzi would make famous later in the century.[21] This case of Albergati has been overlooked by historiography, but it looks quite important to me, because it could provide another piece of evidence of a direct contact between the noble classes of Bologna and the Southern empiric surgeons performing the procedure.[22]

Fioravanti connected his ability to master the reconstructive method to other cases, even if he mentioned only one, which was actually the account of a rather different procedure. In May 1551, Fioravanti left Naples with Charles V's army as the physician of Don Garcia, son of the viceroy of Naples Pedro de Toledo.[23] In Egypt he once treated "a Spanish gentleman" called "Andres Gutiero," aged 29, who one day while walking through the camp "started a fight with a soldier, and they took out their blades, and that soldier cut off Mr Andres' nose with a back-hander, and the nose fell in the sand." Fioravanti peed on the nose to clean it from the desert sand and then attached it to the gentleman, healing it in just eight days.[24]

Another case comes from private correspondence. When in Tropea in 1561, the Neapolitan nobleman, jurist, lawyer, and historian Camillo Porzio (1526–1580) wrote a letter to his friend Cardinal Girolamo Seripando (1493–1563), one of the five Papal Legates representing Pius IV at the Council of Trent, describing how the Vianeos had restored his nose. He said that he suffered greatly but that it was absolutely worth it and complained about the fact that no one had published a description of the procedure yet, which deserved to be publicly available for the benefit of the whole mankind. The cause of this missing nose is unknown.[25]

Patients

The most famous surgeon of the Renaissance, Ambroise Paré, is the author of another, more detailed, case. The French surgeon discussed "the making of an artificial nose" in his book on prosthetics (finished in 1575, but some of the material dates back to 1561), correlated with the case of a man he calls the "Cadet de Saint-Thaon." This was a young knight who had his nose cut off in battle and came to him to show his remade nose, claiming that it was a procedure he had underwent in Italy, performed by some unnamed Italian surgeon, probably one of the Vianeo brothers. Paré's description of the method is the one that circulated most frequently before Tagliacozzi and the one that the Bolognese surgeon most harshly attacked. In this version, the procedure lasted 40 days, and it included the use of the muscles and the flesh of the arm, not just the skin. Paré expressed several kinds of doubts on it. He argued that those who had lost their noses needed to have someone make an artificial one for them, be it "silver, or made with paper and glued pieces of cloth, of the same figure and color as the natural nose"[26] (Figure 1.4). Paré believed that

> this operation is not impossible; however, it seems to me very difficult and too demanding for the patient, as much as for the trouble (*peine*) of keeping his arm tied to the head, as for the pain caused by cutting the healthy parts [of the arm] and by removing them for shaping the new nose.

Moreover, the temperature and appearance of the flesh of the arm were nothing like those of the nose, and the result could not be aesthetically satisfying.[27] This

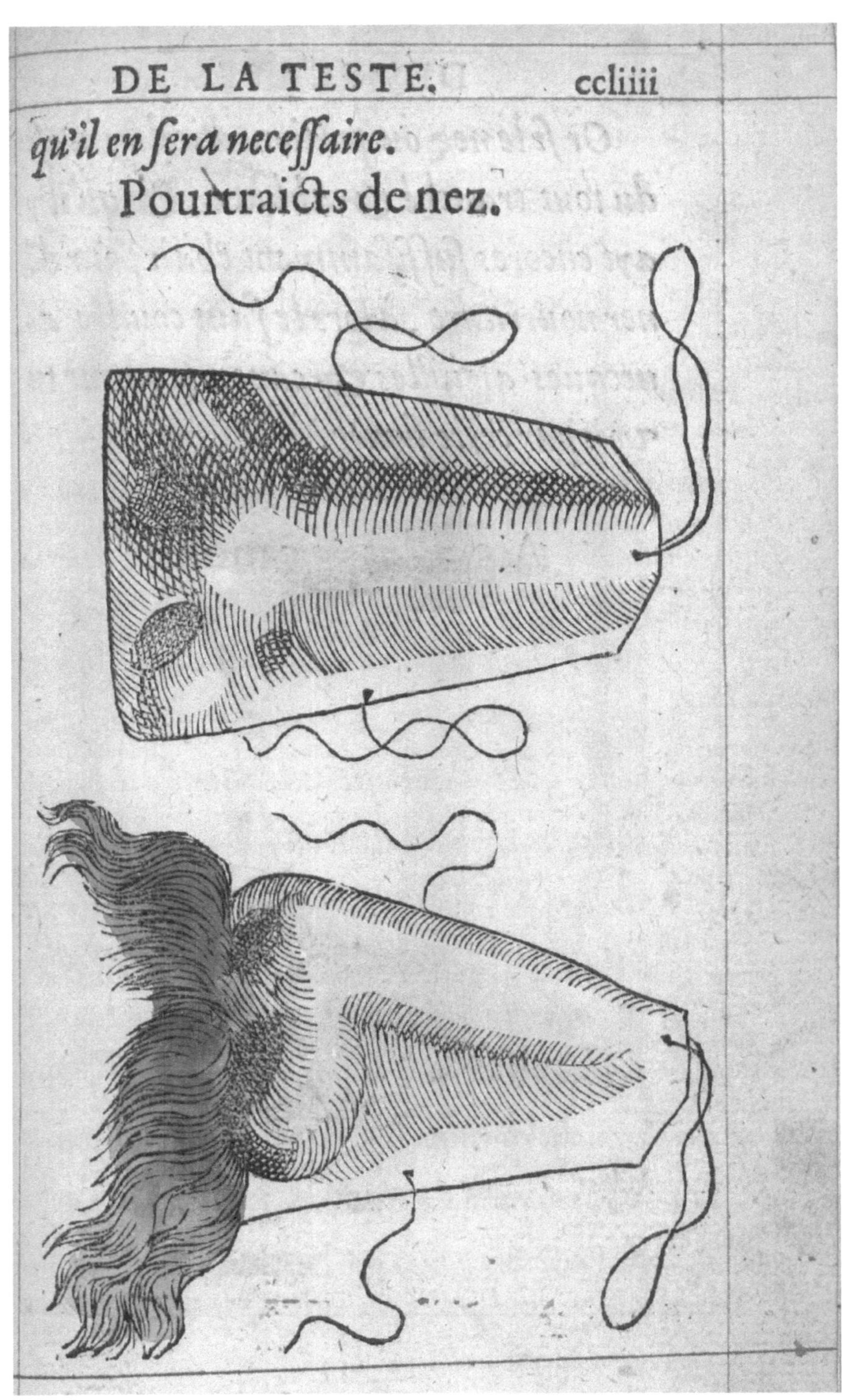

FIGURE 1.4 Ambroise Paré, *La methode curative des playes, et fractures de la teste humaine* (1561): nose prosthetics.

is a very interesting passage, in which Paré seems to imply that it was both ethically disturbing and epistemologically ambiguous to wound the patient in his healthy parts, thus inflicting patients a great pain, given that the outcome would be ugly anyway. One thing was to cut near the wound to directly treat it or to cut for extracting a bladder stone that clearly impaired the normal course of life. Another one was to wound a healthy arm once the wound to treat was already distant in the past and for the sake of a dubious outcome.

In the second half of the sixteenth century several authors claimed, implicitly or explicitly, to have seen, heard, or read about the procedure. The French physician and learned surgeon Etienne Gourmelain (d. 1594) cited in his 1580 *Chirurgicae artis* a letter written by the Roman poet Elisio Calenzio to his friend Orpianus, first printed in Rome in 1503, and therefore referring to the Brancas. In this letter, Calenzio praised the art of remaking noses and mentioned the fact that a slave could serve as a donor of the skin flap.[28] Likewise, Girolamo Mercuriale; Gabriele Falloppio (1523–1562); Pseudo-Vesalius or Prospero Borgarucci (a work on surgery attributed to Vesalius but written by Prospero Borgarucci [1540-1578]); Johannes Schenck von Grafenberg (1530–1598); the Spanish physician Dioniso Daza Chacon (1510–1596); German surgeon and anatomist (who had studied in Padua) Johann von Jessen (1566–1621); and Fabrici d'Acquapendente (1533–1619) all mentioned the procedure, usually with marked skepticism and insisting on its difficulty and painfulness.[29]

It appears that Giulio Cesare Aranzi (1530–1589), eminent surgeon and anatomist in Bologna and Tagliacozzi's teacher, had bettered the method of nasal reconstruction by correcting the view according to which the muscle of the arm had to be incised and had claimed that only the skin of the arm should serve as the flap to be attached to the nose. The only evidence of this is provided by a Polish physician who had studied medicine in Bologna in the 1560s, Wojciech Oczko (1537–1599).[30]

Tagliacozzi himself cited no more than six cases. In the letter to Girolamo Mercuriale, dated February 22, 1586, the Bolognese surgeon replied to Mercuriale's description of the reconstructive method included in the first edition of 1585. Tagliacozzi named four patients whose noses he restored.

> For there have been several gentlemen – among whom Messer Segismundus Barianus, a noble, Messer Alexander Visintinus, also a noble, both of Piacenza, whose noses were cut off while they were dueling, Octavius Facinus, also of Piacenza, and a Fleming, Messer Henricus von Banesghem of Antwerp.[31]

Tagliacozzi claimed that in all four cases he restored the noses so perfectly that they really resembled natural ones. I have not been able to find any information about these patients. Teach-Gnudi and Webster found an *affidavit* for Barianus written by Tagliacozzi in the State Archives of Milan, dated February 26, 1586, stating that there had been some problem in the cohesion of the parts of the nose caused by "a discharge of bad humors," and so Barianus

> will be obliged to come to Bologna from about the end of the month of March next at least throughout the month of May, during which time he will have to remain in Bologna constantly, if he does not wish to lose what he has regained with so much suffering and loss of sleep (*laboribus et vigilii*).[32]

Two things are remarkable: Tagliacozzi called back his patient in the spring, the period deemed ideal for grafting, because maybe he wanted to remake the whole procedure, and he mentioned the discomfort and painfulness of the procedure, to be repaid by having a whole face back.

Despite the fact that in one passage of *De curtorum* Tagliacozzi mentioned the "multitude of patients"[33] he treated, he presented no specific cases in his main opus. In fact, there were only two of them, brief and scarcely significant. The first one was mentioned within a passage in which Tagliacozzi listed all the kinds of nose injuries one could suffer and how they could be treated with his method. The most serious and difficult one was when

> the hollowing out of the middle of the nose is excavated and [there is] the cutting of the top of the dorsum. This happens sometimes when a sword plunges into the flesh of the nose and, like a forceps, tears some of it away. . . . This type of injury is fairly rare, I myself have only encountered it twice. . . . In fact, during the time when I was concentrating my thoughts on this defect, a certain knight of Malta came to me, having sustained this very injury, coincidentally, in a duel (*monomachia*).[34]

The second one sounded like a moral or cautionary tale, named no names, and aimed at teaching his readership and potential clients that they had to be open to the novelty of such a procedure. It was the story, allegedly reported by an unnamed but "very important" physician, of

> a young nobleman whose nose [the physician] was in the process of restoring. They happened to have some business to deal with a Cardinal, who noticed that the young man's nose was covered. The Cardinal asked if the nose was indeed new and made from flesh. The young man replied in the affirmative, and the Cardinal added that he would be most interested in seeing the nose uncovered, as he had never seen anything like it before. When the young man excused himself to uncover his nose and clear the secretions from it, the Cardinal shouted at him, 'Make sure your nose doesn't come off!'[35]

The skepticism of the Cardinal was recalled here to highlight the wide diffusion of wrong ideas about this practice. Moreover, skepticism also showed a general diffidence and suspiciousness toward novelty and, once again, how incredible was that even the smartest men, like Paré and Vesalius, could be so easily blinded by prejudice.

A different case is very important. Fabry von Hilden (Hildanus, 1560–1634) in his best seller *Observationes et curationes chirurgicae*, more specifically in the second edition dated 1614, mentioned the only woman patient I have been able to track down in this printed literature.[36] The episode took place in 1590, during a war waged by the Duke of Savoy against Geneva. A nun called Susanna N. fell prisoner of the Piedmontese soldiers, who had all intentions to rape her but could not because of her fierce resistance. Completely mad by rage, the soldiers cut off her nose. Two years later – and this detail is important – she went to Lausanne, where the surgeon Jean Griffon was living: Griffon undertook the treatment and remade her nose so beautifully that he earned the praise of the whole town. Hildanus, who had studied with Griffon in Geneva, where his teacher served as surgeon at the general hospital, commented that he himself saw this nun several times at the house of a noblewoman. The nose looked good, except that in the winter it turned a little blue. This girl lived in Lausanne until 1613, and her nose remained in good shape throughout her whole life. Hildanus said that Griffon received a first preliminary instruction by some Italian passing through Lausanne who had his nose remade by Tagliacozzi in Bologna, but then he perfected the method by himself. Griffon was Italian himself: a native of San Miniato in Tuscany, he had moved to Geneva in 1582 after he converted to Protestantism.[37] Griffon thus performed the operation in 1592.[38] Another mention of the case can be found in a letter from Bruxelles dated March 20, 1603, in which Hildanus wrote Griffon that he had seen the girl and urged him to send drawings of the instruments he had used in the procedure.[39]

In his 1602 book on the physiology of the human beard, Paduan physician Marco Antonio Olmi (?)[40] mentioned a case – the twelfth in my sample of cases – he himself had treated in Montechiari, in the countryside of Brescia. He said that he was helped by his sister's husband Giacomo Zenaro, most likely an empiric surgeon. However, no names and no further details about circumstances were mentioned.

> Incidentally, we have performed the nasal surgery quite successfully in Brescia, and so in the town called Montechiari. This is well known to physicians of Brescia and other learned men, and many nobles. We were among the early cultivators of this art, and on the eleventh day we separated the skin flap from the arm, since it had completely united with the mutilated nose, and once in the middle of winter, for it was Saint Lucia's day [December 13], and we informed Gaspare Tagliacozzi of this case. But in performing this operation I always used the help of Giacomo Zenaro, to whom my parents gave my sister Francesca to wife, for he was an excellent surgeon.[41]

The crowd of physicians, learned men, and noblemen gathered to witness the procedure points out to a situation in which the treatment was showcased as a public demonstration of a wonderful and new procedure. Olmi also showed his competence by modifying the length of the operation. Once again, Tagliacozzi was at the center of this network of surgeons.

Tomaso Minadoi (1549–1615), professor of "practical medicine" in Padua, pupil of Mercuriale, and member of the Paduan-Bolognese connection that lies at the heart of the renewal of the medical interest on beauty in the late sixteenth century, wrote a very interesting and really singular case. Minadoi's story changed the geographical setting, because it took place in Syria.[42] Even though he confessed that he had observed the reconstructive operation firsthand very few times,[43] Minadoi was full of praise and admiration for Tagliacozzi and his method. Like Tagliacozzi, he justified the painfulness of the procedure by highlighting the importance of the outcome for personal, civil, and political life. Brave men in need of a restored face needed to be able to endure this effort.[44] But then he surprisingly told the story of a patient whom he advised not to undergo the procedure, even if he was asking for it.

One day Minadoi decided to purchase some silk and started to browse the markets of Damascus. In one of these markets he met "Mustachius," whose upper lips had been disfigured by an unspecified wound. Mustachius was wearing a prosthetic mask attached under the nose, with fake mustaches hiding the disfigurement. Once Mustachius understood that Minadoi was a famous physician from Europe, he invited him to his house with the excuse that his daughter was sick. As soon as they arrived there, he explained that there was no sick daughter and that he wanted the physician to perform the reconstructive operation he had heard about. Mustachius confessed that in private he put off his mask to eat and talk with his family, but in public he was forced to show a different kind of ugliness to his fellow citizens: that of lying by wearing an artificial face. Minadoi described in detail the mask and praised it as bringing a delicate and gracious beauty to the merchant's face. At this point, Minadoi recalled that he persuaded Mustachius not to undergo the operation, explaining that it was very dangerous and painful, and not to despise his prosthesis, which was an honest and decent remedy to his disfigurement, as showed by Paré and Vesalius.[45]

One can speculate about the possible reasons Minadoi refused to perform or to recommend the procedure, besides the fact that this prosthetic mask seemed to him particularly well crafted. Perhaps as a Syrian, Mustachius was imagined as someone who was not able to suffer through the torments of the procedure like a Western nobleman, supposedly a braver and morally stronger kind of man.[46]

The last case was briefly narrated by Giovanni Battista Cortesi (1552–1643), a graduate from Bologna, in the first pages of his *Miscellaneorum medicinalia*. In Sicily, during the second part of his long career, he performed the procedure on several patients but he mentioned only one of them, the most illustrious.

> With God's help I became an expert in this discipline, and I have helped many patients, both in this most flourishing Kingdom of Sicily and elsewhere, among other the most Illustrious Don Federico Ventimiglia from

> Palermo, whose cut-off nostrils I have beautifully restored, so that even after many years in the same city he still sports a more than decent nose on his face.[47]

There are no further details, but clearly Ventimiglia lost his nose in an accident involving sharp and cutting blades, as the use of the word "sectas" attests: once again, a case of duel or battle.

These cases have three things in common. With two exceptions, and despite the fact that de-nosing women had a long history as both a formal and an informal punishment, patients are all men. Despite the lack of details we know that – except Catilina, Susanna N., and Mustachius – they were all noblemen or at least upper-class men. Virtually all of them were injured in the context of fights, duels, or war, and there is no mention of disease as the cause of disfigurement.

What about the French disease?

Several historians of plastic surgery, most prominently Sander Gilman, have argued that Tagliacozzi's procedure became immediately popular but short-lived and even despised in the seventeenth and early eighteenth centuries because it was associated with the "French disease" or "great pox" (also known as syphilis). Gilman argued that this procedure served as a corrective technology for one of the main symptoms of the French disease: the corrosion of the cartilage and bones of the face, causing the nose to be "eaten away" as the illness advanced.[48] But evidence simply shows that this was not the case.

Besides the fact that the procedure of facial reconstruction predated the first outbreaks of the French disease, no case history circulating in early modern Europe referred to that disease. More generally, textual references to the "great pox" were very scarce in the literature on plastic surgery, while references to duels and other forms of more or less ritualized violence among noblemen abounded. There are only two partial exceptions. The first is the Polish physician Wojciech Oczko, cited in the aforementioned discussion. Oczko connected the procedure with correcting the most hideous symptom of the French disease but presented no cases. The second concerns Vincenzo Gonzaga (1562–1612). Historians still debate whether Vincenzo, Tagliacozzi's patron, had contracted the French disease or not, but it is certain that Tagliacozzi never performed any surgical reconstruction on his face.[49]

Tagliacozzi mentioned the French disease only when he discussed the preliminary conditions of patients who were about to undergo the procedure, insisting on the fact that they needed their bodies to be purged and cleansed. Among the most difficult conditions to clear out he listed "the French disease" and the "cacochymic state." The cacochymic state was a bad bodily disposition, characterized by an abundance of bad humors. This disposition had deep roots in the body, and it was very hard to eradicate quickly. It was often associated with "the venereal plague, or French disease," and it had to be treated with special remedies.[50] The reference to syphilis was incidental. Tagliacozzi was merely contemplating the possibility of having to perform the procedure on someone who currently had or had had the French disease. About the syphilitic patient properly, Tagliacozzi first declared that the surgeon had to carefully evaluate whether the outcome could be successful, given the seriousness of the disease; then, if the disease was in an advanced state and

> the poison has crept deeply into the bones causing obvious erosion of other parts, there is only one course to take. The physician must try to mitigate the savagery of the disease so that the power of the poison cannot be restored, causing it to infect the graft or to provoke the formation of malignant ulcers.[51]

In such cases, a four-month-long treatment was due, involving medicaments, diet, sweating, and phlebotomy combined with guaiacum wood and sarsaparilla. Here, Tagliacozzi referred to the possibility that the syphilitic poison infected the grafts, but it was not clear whether he was talking about treating the damage caused by the illness or not. Given the context of the chapter, readers were more inclined to conclude that he was talking about purging the syphilitic body of a patient with a face that had been injured for other reasons before starting the procedure.[52] This would make sense, because such a procedure was so demanding and patients needed to be in their most perfect bodily state in order to endure it.

Tommaso Minadoi wrote that there could be two distinct groups of causes of mutilations: the actions of a corrupted internal disposition and violent external blows. Among the internal causes, one of the most frequent was the French disease: patients mutilated by the great pox were indeed particularly "hideous" and "very hard, or rather desperate cases to treat."[53] And that was it. The collection of medical *consilia* put together by the German physician Joseph Lautenbach (?) mentioned the case of plastic surgery. Among the required conditions for a successful operation, the author said that, first of all, the surgeon had to be "diligent, patient, prudent and very much dexterous" and, second, the patient had to "have a healthy habit . . . not be affected by the Gallic illness, and be eminently obedient and patient."[54]

It is true that the French disease was perceived as dishonoring and shaming and that Tagliacozzi and others might have wanted to protect their patients' identity. But this does not seem to be a very compelling objection, because the French disease was widely and openly discussed in the medical literature of the time and often physicians named names. A quick look at the two-volume collection of writings on the French disease edited by Luigi Luigini in 1566 would testify to the fact that all the symptoms of the venereal disease were abundantly discussed by European physicians, including facial mutilation and disfigurement, without particular moral problems.[55]

Girolamo Fracastoro (ca. 1476–1553) famously wrote in *De contagione* (1546) that in some cases in patients sick with the French disease "the lips, or nose, or eyes were eaten away, or in others the whole genitals."[56] But reading through Luigini's collection, it is clear that corrosion of noses and mouths was not the most common symptom. Moreover, it was a rather late-stage symptom, indicating a very advanced stage of the disease. Therefore, the suggestion most frequently given by surgeons and physicians was to surgically remove the corrupted parts of bones and cartilage and then treat them like regular wounds.[57] Gabriele Falloppio went beyond this and proposed the use of prosthetic devices of his invention, much like those described by Paré, to correct excessive defects of the bones of the palate, but only in extreme cases in which the faculties of speaking and drinking were impaired.[58] In the same years Tagliacozzi was writing his book, his colleague and friend in Bologna, the famous physician Giulio Cesare Claudini (c. 1553–1618), published a collection of cases (*consultationes*), in which the French disease appears as common. Here, we can see that the canonical three-degree scheme of the great pox was applied to the case of "an egregious young man" who remained anonymous. Claudini discussed three different degrees or stages of the "violence of the disease": the "initial" stage (*incipens*), the "progressed" stage (*progressa*), and the "absolute" stage (*consumata & absoluta*). Symptoms included "spots around the penis and newly incepted gonorrhea" for the initial degree; "long-term gonorrhea, pain in the junctures, hair loss, pustules, warts, fissures on the skin (*ragades*), and ulceration of the mouth" for the second degree; the characteristic "*gummata*, and corruption of the bones" for the third degree.[59] Among the pharmacological remedies, divided between diet, pharmacology, and surgery (the surgical therapy being only bloodletting), Claudini argued that some target the "seeds" of the disease, others its "poisonous quality," still others the symptoms. Among the medicaments targeting the symptoms, Claudini gave a recipe against hair loss that made hair grow again – a circumstance that shows how in many cases the borders between cosmetics and medicine were blurred in this period – an unguent made with "laudanum, distilled urine of a child, honey, oil of spikes, clove, and also guaiacum." For the pustules Claudini prescribed washing them with the decoction of guaiacum and alumina if needed. For the pain in the junctures a warm application (*fomentum*) of hemp soaked in the decoction of guaiacum and althea and anointments with oil of guaiacum were in order.[60] Claudini, a contemporary, friend, admirer, and colleague of Tagliacozzi who wrote about individual cases of the French disease, never mentioned his friend's surgical procedure to restore facial mutilation: another sign suggesting that such procedure could not be used to treat the most serious and disfiguring symptoms of the great pox.[61]

To counter the argument on the need of keeping the patients' identity secret, I believe that references to dueling and the culture of honor would not have been a safe topic either. As we will see, books on duels were officially placed on the Index of the Holy Office of the Inquisition in 1596, and duels were outlawed in many Italian states by the middle of the sixteenth century.

Corrosion of the nose was described as one of the most horrifying symptoms of the French disease, but it does not appear to have been the most common nor the most striking for the contemporaries. Observers of the disease appear to have been more shocked by the so-called syphilitic *gummatae*, and genital sores, especially by the late sixteenth century, when the disease was about one century old.[62] In any case, there was no silence surrounding the French disease at all. Surgeons and physicians, like Falloppio, openly talked about remedies for this heinous condition, and there was no reason for Tagliacozzi to keep it secret had his method been useful to treat such a horrifying symptom. Plus, why would a physician try such a demanding surgical procedure on a patient so weakened?

Missing or severely damaged noses were all over the place in sixteenth-century Italy and carried several negative meanings. Stigmatization of the French disease was certainly one of them, but there is no evidence that this played a particularly significant role in the success of facial surgery in the late Renaissance.

Other cases

My research in the records of the criminal court of Bologna – the so-called Torrone – brought to light two new cases concerning Tagliacozzi acting as medico-legal expert and physician.[63] Attacks damaging the face are often mentioned in the records of the court, and there is ample evidence that disfiguring faces and cutting off noses continued to be a form of punishment in sixteenth-century Bologna, both for condemned criminals (more rarely) and for adulterous women or for women involved in issues of male honor.[64] The following cases involved disfiguring injuries inflicted on women. They show that Tagliacozzi was part of the complex culture of noblemen I will describe in the next chapter and that he deliberately avoided talking about women in his printed works.

The first case involves a modest artisan, Fausto dal Lino, a cloth weaver from Modena, his family, and a community of Modenese citizens doing business in Bologna. Several important characters of Modena, including lawyers and the "chaplain" of the Cathedral, were interrogated, because the crime in question happened in broad daylight in the main square, in front of the Duomo. On September 7, 1584, Fausto had been seen injuring with a knife his mother-in-law Caterina Dossi, a seller of "veils" in the *piazza*. The aggression resulted in two wounds to Caterina's head, deemed by many witnesses as potentially deadly. Fausto suddenly disappeared from Modena. He went to Bologna, where he was arrested along with a young tailor, also from Modena, named Ercole Monti. He was charged of having brought prohibited weapons into the city. Interrogated, Fausto said at first that he had gone to Bologna to see a rich tailor who had a workshop there because he needed to buy certain "cloths" from him. But slowly, as the interrogation became more and more aggressive, he changed his version.[65] In fact, Fausto had fled Modena after having injured Caterina, and he went to Bologna because he was looking for another Modenese tailor called Giovanni Battista. He had brought weapons with him because he needed to be very persuasive with this Giovanni Battista. Fausto's parents-in-law had bought a house from Giovanni Battista two years before. Fausto believed that the money used to buy that house was to be destined to his wife's dowry. It then turned out that buying that house had been a mistake. Giovanni Battista had debts: the creditors took the house back "and I am now with no house and no money, and to tell you the truth I came to Bologna precisely to talk to said Mr Gio. and to ask him to give me at least something, even if not the whole sum of 1000 lire."[66]

Tagliacozzi appeared in the trial as the author of a certificate written on September 18 for Fausto's lawyer in Modena, Domenico Ferraris, attesting that Caterina's life was not at risk. He was confirming the diagnosis made by Matteo Colombo, the Modenese physician who took charge of Caterina after Tagliacozzi had left Modena.

> I, Gaspare Tagliacozzi, testify that in the past days I have been called to Modena to visit a woman injured with two wounds in the head; I have visited said woman and I stayed there until after four days passed and then I left; several times the physician there has updated me on her condition, and more specifically the physician sent me a letter yesterday in which he says that given that 14 days have passed by without having discovered any sign of danger of death, she will get her health back and her life is not at risk in any way either now or in the future, if well treated. I have faithfully written this with my own hand, Gaspare Tagliacozzi, physician.[67]

Why was Tagliacozzi called to another city to see a middle-class patient? One small detail in the young tailor Ercole's deposition helps the modern reader to make sense of the surgeon's role in this case. Ercole, arrested with Fausto, had only known him for two days, but he had immediately noticed that Fausto was a bit of a chit chatterer. In fact, Fausto had told Ercole everything about his assault on Caterina.

> [Fausto] told me here in Bologna that he had injured his mother in law by using a small knife on her face and on her head while his mother in law was in the piazza selling veils, and [Fausto] told me this happened on Saturday 1 September at mid-morning.[68]

Tagliacozzi was called to Modena because in late 1584 he was already known as a specialist of facial injuries – after all, the letter to Mercuriale dates from early 1586 – and this case caused a stir in Modena as it happened right in front of the Duomo, for everyone to see. By that date, Tagliacozzi was famous already for the same group of illnesses having to do with facial appearance, disfigurement, and beauty.[69]

Around the same time Fulvia Ballestra, known as Prieta, a rather wealthy courtesan of Bologna, had been disfigured by an unknown youngster one Sunday while going back home from the Mass. Tagliacozzi treated her wound, about which we have a few details. The case has many characters, and it is impossible to summarize: noblemen openly fornicating with mistresses, strongly independent women forming a community with rivalries and solidarities, issues of male honor connected to fighting for the love of a woman, and the shaming nature of disfigurements.

On December 26, 1583, the notary went to Fulvia's home to check her wound, because he was told that she had been injured "with big disfigurement (*cum magno sfrisio*)." He found her in bed, "with one big wound which I could not see as it was all covered by bandages . . . and she had been recently treated, and her face was all covered by bloody linen cloths."[70]

> A little while ago – Fulvia said – when I was coming back home after the Mass with my mother and the servant . . . a young man whom I do not know hit me with a dagger on my face so suddenly that I did not realize what was happening, and he has wounded my face all across my lips cutting my nose and my face so badly that the physician had to put many stitches in it.[71]

Fulvia's mother, Caterina, was more precise in describing the young assaulter:

> [A] beardless, badly dressed young man passed by, a dark face, wearing a green blouse, a black, old, and short, a pair of very tight pants of I don't know which material, and a woollen black hat French style; his face was thin but he was daring, of middle stature, and as he walked by us and Fulvia he raised his hand from under the cloak and he had a dagger in his fingers, and he hit Fulvia on her face with a diagonal blow, and he cut her lips, so that the physician put 15 stitches in it.[72]

The notary reported that her mouth hurt a lot when she talked and that blood came out of her cheek and mouth. Fulvia was in much pain, and the notary decided to come back the next day. The day after Fulvia was a little better, but she warned the notary that doctor Tagliacozzi had told her not to talk too much. On December 29, during the third interrogation, the notary found Tagliacozzi there medicating Fulvia:

> I have arrived at said house at the same time Magnificent Tagliacozzi, doctor in medicine and surgery, wanted to treat her; while said doctor was changing her bandages, I had the chance to see the open wound on her face, which was like this: a wound starting from the corner of the left eyebrow crossing said eye and the nose, and ending on the right side of the face. . . . Tagliacozzi said he treated this wound with 15 stitches, which I have seen and inspected thoroughly.[73]

Even though this was not a case of a lost nose, a disfiguring wound had been deliberately inflicted on Fulvia's face.

Fulvia gave the notary a list of people she considered her enemies and who could potentially hurt her. "Lucrezia Villana" was her enemy because Fulvia testified against her in a trial in which she was banished as "bad woman (*mala femmina*)." From that moment on Lucrezia, once back in town, always went after Fulvia insulting her. Among other things, Lucrezia uttered nose-related insults: "she used to yell at me from the window, on the street, anywhere: 'bad nose', 'take it through that big nose', and similar other insults, and one day because of her envy, she threw urine or something else at me from the window, which ruined my new pink dress."

Democrite Desiderio was the second suspect: he had been Fulvia's "lover, and during Carnival he insulted me in the piazza and he publicly showed his penis to me along with a rain of insults, and I sued him and he was put in prison both for this reason and because he had insulted me."

Giovanni Mele, another suspect, while the Legate was away from Bologna "more than once sent Giulia Rigoni called la Monarina [another courtesan] to tell me to beware since when the Legate would leave something bad would happen to me."

Francesco Maria Sighizano was another former lover,

> and several times he did beat me up, and even if lately we made peace, last summer he beat me up again and bruised my eyes, and even if I did not sue him I do not want his friendship no more and I don't want him around my house.

Giacomo delli Lieti told la Monarina to tell Fulvia "that I was a whore, a grumbling drunkard and many other injuries (*che io ero una poltrona un bugirona una imbriaconaccia*)."

Finally, another prostitute appears on the list, la Renzina,

> a whore who lives nearby . . . because of the insults she told me the last few days, as Your Lordship knows since I did sue her . . . and also because in the past few days, from her front door she told me so that everyone heard that Mr Giuseppe Orsi, his friend, did not want to go to her house anymore because he had heard other whores closeby saying that she has a mustache like a Ramino.[74]

Here we see the Orsi name, one of the most powerful Senatorial families of Bologna, connected to a matter of rivalry among courtesans.

The case ended abruptly and no one got convicted, but interrogations went on until the end of 1585 and a parade of other characters popped up in the pages of the record. Particularly interesting is the interrogation of one major suspect, Annibale Landini (then released), a young "barber and needle maker (*aguchiarolo*)" in the service of the Orsi family and apparently very close to the two brothers Camillo and Giuseppe Orsi. The Orsi brothers were suspected of having commissioned the disfigurement of Fulvia on behalf of their lover, la Renzina, who had had multiple fights with Fulvia. Annibale told the inquisitors he was poor and that he had lost his job at a master barber's workshop because too many times he had not shown up at work. Since then, he worked for the Orsi and he shaved and cut his patrons' hair as a private barber. Annibale revealed an interesting inter-class male relationship with the Orsi brothers, namely, that Annibale's mother had been Giuseppe's wet nurse:

> 'I sometimes frequent the Orsi household. . . . Of these Orsi I frequent one is called signor Camillo and the other signor Giuseppe, and I frequent their houses more often than others because signor Giuseppe has been raised by my mother and therefore he is my milk sibling.'[75]

Annibale had not any problem in telling the notary that he had been 'many times in the courtesans' houses with these *signori*.'[76]

In another interrogation, Fulvia advanced the hypothesis that she had become the object of a dispute of honor between Democrite Desiderio and a young gentleman from Brescia, Giovanni Giacomo Alberici, who was renting a room at her house and probably had fallen in love with her.

> In the past months [Democrite] fought with signor Giovanni Alberici from Brescia, who is this gentlemen I host here in my house, and who is my friend, and said signor Giovanni gave a lie to this Democrite for the sake of my honor, and since then said Democrite has been out of town, and he says he wants revenge, and signor Giovanni has never left the house again . . . and I think he [Democrite] wants to have me disfigured to get his revenge against him [Giovanni].[77]

Alberici's story soon took a tragic turn, because on January 3, 1584, doctor Flaminio Rota – Tagliacozzi's colleague at the studio – and the notary were called to Fulvia's house because Giovanni Giacomo killed himself by inflicting three wounds to his own throat with a razor blade. Witnesses testified that he took his life because he was short of money; moreover, he was feeling so sad because of Fulvia's disfigurement, probably feeling guilty about it.[78]

A men's world

Disfiguring injuries continued to be a frequent sight in early modern Bologna, for both men and women, criminals and prostitutes, noblemen and adulterous women. Not all of them fell into the rather narrow category of injury described by Tagliacozzi in his learned monograph, and in many cases surgeons could intervene right away, suturing and bandaging, without a significant time span occurring between the injury and the treatment. The Bolognese physician was explicit about that.

> For example – he wrote – I ask the reader to imagine a terrible facial injury, the result of a sword blow that almost severs the jaw and causes it

> to hang down to the level of the shoulders. Anyone can see that the jaw is still attached to the rest of the face, however precariously, and that we can restore its integrity with sutures. But uniting the graft with the mutilated nose is another story. It is a laborious and difficult task owing to the distance between the two parts, not to mention the differences in the substance and nature of their integument.[79]

As noted by François Delaporte, Tagliacozzi's procedure could be performed months and even years after the injury had occurred, and in this sense it lacked that sense of urgency that was so characteristic of many surgical procedures.[80] This generous use of time and this lack of urgency were in itself a measure of luxury that indicated that the procedure targeted the upper class and its rituals. Moreover, wounds to the nose, ears, eyes, and lips were generally classified as "wounds which do not involve any of the principal parts of the body [heart, brain, and liver] or any of the parts that serve the principal parts."[81]

Nonetheless, it is significant that Tagliacozzi, who clearly had to deal with disfiguring injuries given to women's faces of different classes for reasons revolving around male honor, money, or both, chose to mention only men and to build an entirely male world in his book. The other surgeons, with the exception of Hildanus, also built narratives of men and swords. Is it because these women could not pay for the treatment? All the evidence points to the fact that Fulvia had enough money to afford Tagliacozzi's reconstructive treatment. More plausibly, disfiguring wounds on women's faces did not have the same public meaning, as women's role was not a public one, especially among the upper classes. And saving a prostitute's face would not have been a good move for a learned and respectable surgeon. Tagliacozzi decided to write his work as a learned surgery monograph on one specific kind of injury and procedure because he observed that daily life was animated by choreography of masculinity in the form of men debating and fighting in public.

Notes

1 For the Fondazione Zeri, see their online photographic archive http://catalogo.fondazionezeri.unibo.it/scheda.v2.jsp?locale=en&decorator=layout_resp&apply=true&tipo_scheda=F&id=83257&titolo=A.+Villani+e+Figli+-+Bartolomeo+ +%28scuola%29.+Ritratto+di+Gaspare+Tagliacozzi.+Bologna+-+gi%C3%A0+coll.+Prof.+Putti+-+insieme. For the attribution to Tiburzio Passerotti, see Martha Teach-Gnudi and Jerome Pierce Webster, *The Life and Times of Gaspare Tagliacozzi, Surgeon of Bologna 1545–1599* (New York: Herbert Reichner, 1950), pp. 258–260.

2 See Angela Ghirardi, "Bartolomeo Passerotti, il culto di Michelangelo e l'anatomia nell'età di Ulisse Aldrovandi," in Giuseppe Olmi, ed. *Rappresentare il corpo: arte e anatomia da Leonardo all'Illuminismo* (Bologna: Bononia University Press, 2004), pp. 151–164. On the connections between artistic and scientific ideas in Counter-Reformation Bologna, see Giuseppe Olmi and Paolo Prodi, "Science and Nature in Bologna Circa 1600," in *The Age of Correggio and the Carracci: Emilian Painting of the Sixteenth and Seventeenth Centuries* (Bologna/Washington/New York: Pinacoteca Nazionale/National Gallery of Art/The Metropolitan Museum of Art, 1986), pp. 213–235; Giuseppe Olmi, *L'inventario*

del mondo: catalogazione della natura e luoghi del sapere nella prima età moderna (Bologna: Il Mulino, 1992), pp. 91–111.

3 Caroline Murphy, *Lavinia Fontana: A Painter and Her Patrons in Sixteenth-Century Bologna* (New Haven: Yale University Press), pp. 50–51.

4 Jerome P. Webster has noticed that the copies of the book represented in the painting are thicker than the actual ones and hypothesized that they were luxury "presentation copies," of which three exemplars survive. He does not take into account their manuscript form; see Jerome P. Webster, "Some Portrayals of Gaspare Tagliacozzi," *Plastic & Reconstructive Surgery* 41, 5 (1968): 411–426, p. 411.

5 Girolamo Mercuriale, *De decoratione liber* (Frankfurt: apud Ioannem Wechelum, 1587).

6 I have left out of the count the stories concerning "sympathetic noses" and donors, discussed in the Conclusion chapter.

7 This is the definition of the case narrative proposed by literary critic André Jolles and taken up for historians of medicine by Gianna Pomata, "The Medical Case Narrative: Distant Reading of an Epistemic Genre," *Literature and Medicine* 32, 1 (2014): 1–23, pp. 1–7. It must be noticed that such short narratives of remarkable cures, often written for the purposes of self-advertising, had been part of surgical literature since Middle Ages, but in the sixteenth century individual cases and particulars attracted the attention of medical and surgical writers with greater intensity and in new ways. The value of descriptive narratives and the importance of first-person accounts and their trustworthiness greatly increased. See Chiara Crisciani, "L'individuale nella medicina tra Medioevo e Umanesimo: i 'Consilia'," in Roberto Cardini and Mariangela Regoliosi, eds. *Umanesimo e medicina: Il problema dell'individuale* (Rome: Bulzoni, 1996), pp. 1–32; Nancy Siraisi, *The Clock and the Mirror: Girolamo Cardano and Renaissance Medicine* (Princeton: Princeton University Press, 1997), pp. 195–213.

8 See Gianna Pomata and Nancy G. Siraisi, "Introduction," in Gianna Pomata and Nancy Siraisi, eds. *Historia: Empiricism and Erudition in Early Modern Europe* (Cambridge: MIT Press, 2005), pp. 1–38.

9 See Note 6 in the Introduction.

10 See also Sanjay Saraf and Ravi S. Parihar, "Sushruta: The First Plastic Surgeon in 600 B.C.," *The Internet Journal of Plastic Surgery* 4, 2 (2006).

11 See Michael McVaugh, *The Rational Surgery of the Middle Ages* (Florence: SISMEL/Edizioni del Galluzzo, 2006), pp. 120–123. Henri de Mondeville told a story about miraculously attaching a severed nose. The French surgeon reported having seen a patient who had his nose almost completely severed, attached to the face only through a little piece of cartilage. While many lay people and one physician told him to just cut it off and to throw it away, his teacher Jean Pitard cut the head of a chicken and let the blood fall on the ill nose for a long time and with great care. Then the master applied the half-cut heart of the chicken on the wounded part, until it cooled down. Finally, Pitard sutured it. The same operation was repeated with a second chicken. The day after the nose had a better color and after proper treatment it healed. See Henri de Mondeville, *Chirurgie*, ed. Edouard Nicaise (Paris: Félix Alcan, 1893), pp. 345–346.

12 BUB, 811, *Practica chirurgica*, fol. 30r: "De la ferita del naxo per spada opur per sayeta."

13 According to the evidence provided by the Bishop of Lucera, Pietro Ranzano (d. 1492).

14 The two families, and especially the Vianeos, are the object of a literature written mostly by local historians. See Manfredi Greco et al., "The Primacy of the Vianeo Family in the Invention of Nasal Reconstruction Technique," *Annals of Plastic Surgery* 64 (2010): 702–705; Franco Rombolà, *La chirurgia plastica in Calabria nei secoli XV e XVI: I fratelli Vianeo* (Cosenza: Galassia 1997).

15 Santoni-Rugiu and Skyles, *History of Plastic Surgery*, pp. 175–176; Corradi, "Dell'antica autoplastica," p. 265.

16 Giovanni Pontano, *Dialogues*, tr. Julia Haig Gaisser (Cambridge: Harvard University Press, 2012), p. 129.

17 Aina Greig, Andreas Gohritz, Max Geishauser, and Wolfgang Mühlbauer, "Heinrich von Pfalzpaint, Pioneer of Arm Flap Nasal Reconstruction in 1460, More Than a Century Before Tagliacozzi," *Journal of Craniofacial Surgery* 26, 4 (2015): 1165–1168.

18 Ladislao Münster, "Un precursore bolognese quattrocentesco della chirurgia plastica," in *Atti del Convegno medico dell'amicizia italo-svizzera* (Bologna: Zanichelli, 1953), pp. 1–5, 3–5.
19 María Isabel del Val Valdivieso, "Catilina García, la Cantorala. Una actitud decidida tras la agresión," in María Jesús Fuente and Remedios Morán, eds. *Raíces Profundas. La violencia contra las mujeres (Antigüedad y Edad Media)* (Madrid: Polifemo, 2011), pp. 255–276.
20 Alessandro Benedetti, *Historia Corporis Humani sive Anatomice* [1502], ed. and tr. Giovanna Ferrari (Florence: Giunti, 1998), p. 291.
21 Leonardo Fioravanti, *Il Tesoro della vita humana* (Venice: appresso gli heredi di Melchior Sessa, 1570), fol. 47r: "io havea un parente che alla rotta di Serravalle in Lombardia gli era stato tagliato il naso, combattendo co i nemici, e che desiderava sapere se dovea venire sì o no [. . .] d'un Stradioto, & costoro già ne havevano avuto nuova per lettere."
22 Cornelio, from the very powerful Senatorial Albergati family, was born in 1523; he later became Senator and served as one of the ten officials who formed the small council of war of Bologna. The battle of Serravalle was indeed a quite important episode in the Italian wars: the Spanish Imperial army won the battle against the French and the "Italian" army (supporting the French) led by the famous Florentine *condottiero* Pietro Strozzi, and with that victory Charles V extended his power over Lombardy. See Pompeo Scipione Dolfi, *Cronologia della famiglie nobili di Bologna* (Bologna: G.B. Ferroni, 1670), p. 33. Unfortunately, I have not found any traces of this episode of nose loss, neither in the correspondence of the Albergati family nor in some of the city chronicles.
23 Fioravanti, *Il Tesoro*, fol. 60r.
24 Ibid., fol. 64r: "venne a parole con un soldato, & messero mano alle armi, & quel soldato con un man roverso tagliò il naso al Signor Andres, & li cadette nella arena."
25 See Corradi, "Dell'antica autoplastica," p. 40; Teach-Gnudi and Webster, *The Life and Times*, pp. 118–119.
26 Ambroise Paré, *Oeuvres completes*, 3 vols., ed. Jean-François Malgaigne (Paris: Baillière, 1840), vol. 2, p. 605.
27 Ibid., pp. 605–606.
28 See Corradi, "Dell'antica autoplastica," p. 36; Teach-Gnudi and Webster, *The Life and Times*, p. 112.
29 Teach-Gnudi and Webster, *The Life and Times*, pp. 255–280; Johannes von Jessen, *Institutiones chirurgicae* (Wittemberg: Samuel Selsich, 1601), pp. 100v–102v.
30 See Teach Gnudi and Webster, *The Life and Times*, pp. 133–134; Raffi Gurunluoglu and Aslin Gurunluoglu, "Giulio Cesare Arantius (1530–1589): A Surgeon and Anatomist: His Role in Nasal Reconstruction and Influence on Gaspare Tagliacozzi," *Annals of Plastic Surgery* 60, 6 (2008): 717–722. In any case, there could have been many ways in which accounts of the technique had reached Tagliacozzi's attention, and this work is not concerned by origin stories or controversies on primacy but on the social and cultural history of reconstructive surgery.
31 Translation by Teach-Gnudi and Webster, *The Life and Times*, p. 139.
32 Teach-Gnudi and Webster, *The Life and Times*, p. 140 (translation modified).
33 Tagliacozzi, *De curtorum*, p. 171 (2:53).
34 Ibid., p. 108 (1:87).
35 Ibid., p. 179 (2:59): "Fuit enim cum nobili adolescent cuidam nares restauraturus ut is ad unum ex purpuratis Rom. Ecclesiae proceribus negotii causa accederet, qui aspiciens eius nares tectas dixit: nunquid sunt nares restitutae, & ex carne factitatae? Aseverat nobilis adolescens. Tunc rogavit si liceret eas detergere: libentissime fore ut detergeret, & à fordibus nares expurgaret; ei clamavit purpuratus: cave ne sequantur."
36 Fabry von Hilden (Hildanus), *Observationum et curationum cheirurgicarum centuria tertia* (Basel: Typis Hieronymi Galleri, 1614), p. 150 (*Observatio XXXI*).
37 Léon Gautier, *La médecine à Genève jusqu'à la fin du dix-huitième siècle* (Genève: Jullien, 1906), pp. 206–210.
38 Hildanus, *Observationum*, p. 150.
39 Fabry von Hildanus, "Epistolarium," in *Observationum et curationum cheirurgicarum centuria tertia* (Basel: Sumptibus Johannis Theodori de Bry, typis Hieron. Galleri, 1619), p. 389 (*centuria* I, letter 62).

40 Very little is known of this physician. In 1598, he was trying to get the chair of medicine that had been left vacant at the University of Bologna: see ASB, Senato, Lettere, Serie I, 20, fol. 226v.

41 Quoted by Teach-Gnudi and Webster, *The Life and Times*, p. 273 (translation modified). See Marco Antonio Olmi, *Physiologia barbae humanae* (Bologna: apud Iannem Baptistam Bellagambam, 1602), p. 233: "Caeterum nasi chirurgiam felicissimis exemplis in Agro Brixiano, atque in Oppido, quod Montechiaro dicitur, praestititmus. Constat apud Birxienses Medicos, & alios Viros Doctos, Patrioti etiam perplures, Auximus & nos priores hanc Artem, & Die Undecima Traducem cutem à Brachio separavimus, quod Naribus Decurtatis omino coaluisset, atque Hyeme rigente, fuit enim Dies D. Luciae sacra, cuius exempli admonimus Gasparem Taliacotium. In hoc autem opere praestando semper usus sui D. Iacobo Zenaro, cui Parentes dedere Sororem meam Franciscam coniugem, hic enim vir consummatus est Chirurgus."

42 Minadoi had in fact repeatedly been appointed ambassador of the Republic of Venice in Aleppo and in that conjuncture he wrote a history of the war between Syrians and Persians. See Nancy Siraisi, *History, Medicine, and the Traditions of Renaissance Learning* (Ann Arbor: University of Michigan Press, 2007), pp. 246–260; Lucia Samaden, "Giovanni Tommaso Minadoi (1548–1615): da medico della 'nazione' veneziana in Siria a professore universitario a Padova," *Quaderni per la storia dell'Università di Padova* 31 (1998): 91–164, pp. 158–159; Mariacarla Gadebusch-Bondio, "I pericoli della bellezza 'mangonica'. Aspetti del dibattito su protesi, trucchi e chirurgia estetica tra 500 e 600," in *Le corps et sa parure/The body and its adornment* (Firenze: SISMEL/Edizioni del Galluzzo, 2007), pp. 425–449, 425–428.

43 Tomaso Minadoi, *De humani corporis turpitudinibus cognoscendis et curandis* (Padua: apud Franciscum Bolzettam, 1600), fol. 122v: "Nos vero in praesentia eam operationem sic paucis complectimur."

44 Ibid., fol. 122r.

45 Ibid., fol. 121r-v.

46 See Figures 6.2 and 6.4. In this case, the interpretation would be supported by the images decorating the final pages of Giovanni Andrea Dalla Croce's (1515–1575) surgery manual, showing a Christian knight tolerating pain and a Turkish soldier in a rather unseemly posture, unbecoming for the iconographic standard of a Christian soldier. See Chapter 6 for a deeper discussion of these images and the politics of pain management.

47 Giovanni Battista Cortesi, *Miscellaneorum medicinalium decades denae* (Messina: ex typographia Petri Breae, 1625), "Ad lectorem," pages not numbered: "Hac in disciplina, Deo dante, tantum profeci, ut non paucos adiuverim, tum alibi, tum in hoc florentissimo Siciliae Regno, ubi inter alios Perillustri Don Federico Vintimillia Panhormitano sectas infortunio nares ita concinne restitui, ut multis ab hinc annis absque villa labe nasus in decora facie decentissimus appareat."

48 Gilman, *Making the Body*; Cock, "'Lead'em by the Nose'"; Nicholas L. Tilney, *Invasion of the Body: Revolutions in Surgery* (Cambridge: Harvard University Press, 2011), pp. 103–105; Valeria Finucci, *The Prince's Body: Vincenzo Gonzaga and Renaissance Medicine* (Cambridge: Harvard University Press, 2015), mentions syphilis as one "major motivation for the preoccupation with nose reconstruction" but correctly adds that there is no evidence of performing such an operation on syphilitic patients.

49 On this debate and in general on the relationship between Tagliacozzi and Vincenzo Gonzaga, see Finucci, *The Prince's Body*, pp. 62–72; Teach-Gnudi and Webster, *The Life and Times*, pp. 165–182. It has been suggested (Cock, "'Lead'em' by the Nose") that Tagliacozzi's dedication to Vincenzo was a maneuver to cover up the fact that the procedure was mostly intended for treating patients with the French disease, but this suggestion should be rejected in light of a complete lack of evidence.

50 Tagliacozzi, *De curtorum*, p. 121 (2:5).

51 Ibid., pp. 125–126 (2:8–9).

52 In his famous 1816 account of a nasal reconstruction, Carpue describes how he had to make sure that his patient with a missing nose did not have syphilis; see Santoni-Rugiu and Skyles, *A History of Plastic Surgery*, p. 201.

53 Minadoi, *De humani corporis turpitudinibus*, fol. 119v.
54 Joseph Lautenbach, *Consilia medicinalia cum mixtim praestantissimorum Italiae medicorum* (Frankfurt: Officina typographica Wolfgangi Richteri, impressis Iohannis Sartorii, 1605), p. 359.
55 Luigi Luigini, *De morbo Gallico omnia quae extant apud omnes medicos cuiuscumque nationis* (Venice: G. Ziletti, 1566–1567).
56 Fracastoro in Luigini, *De morbo Gallico*, vol. 1, p. 173.
57 See Benivieni in Luigini, *De morbo Gallico*, vol 1, p. 345; Ferri in Luigini, *De morbo Gallico*, vol. 1, p. 382; Tomitano in Luigini, *De morbo Gallico*, vol. 2, p. 136.
58 Falloppio in Luigini, *De morbo Gallico*, vol. 1, pp. 718–719.
59 Giulio Cesare Claudini, *Responsionum et consultationum medicinalium* (Torino: apud HH. Io. Dominici Tarini, 1628), p. 420. The first edition dates 1606.
60 Claudini, *Responsionum et consultationum*, p. 421.
61 Teach Gnudi and Webster, *The Life and Times*, p. 276.
62 Jon Arrizabalaga, John Henderson, and Roger French, *The Great Pox: The French Disease in Renaissance Europe* (New Haven: Yale University Press, 1997), pp. 204–212. See also Claude Quétel, *The History of Syphilis*, tr. Judith Braddock and Brian Pike (Baltimore: Johns Hopkins University Press, 1990), pp. 26–27, 50–72; Cristian Berco, *From Body to Community: Venereal Disease and Society in Baroque Spain* (Toronto: University of Toronto Press, 2016), pp. 21–37.
63 The *Tribunale criminale del Torrone* of Bologna represented the extension of the sovereign power of the Pope and operated from 1531 to 1796. In its archives there are about 10,400 volumes of trial records and documents. Each volume contains traces of about 100 cases and complaints. The trials of the Torrone only rarely ended with an official condemnation or a final sentence. Very often they ended abruptly with no apparent reason, with an acquittal, or with the indication of some kind of peace or composition. As I have noted in the aforementioned discussion, the vast majority of cases concerned the artisanal classes of the city, because noblemen thought they were above the State justice system. In the archives of the Torrone there is no thematic index, so it is extremely hard to make representative surveys. See Giancarlo Angelozzi and Cesarina Casanova, *La giustizia criminale in una città di antico regime: Il tribunale del Torrone di Bologna, secc. XVI–XVII* (Bologna: CLUEB, 2008). Luckily, one notary (notaries wrote down all the details of interrogations) called Girolamo Marino wrote a rather complete list of the cases he dealt with from 1584 to 1589, both in the countryside and in the city, with indications of the volumes in which records have been transcribed: see ASB, Torrone, 1674/46 (thanks to Ottavia Niccoli, who mentioned this precious source to me).
64 For the former, see Giacomo Rinieri, *Cronaca 1535–1549* (Bologna: Studio Costa, Fondazione del Monte di Bologna e Ravenna, 1998); for the latter, Giancarlo Angelozzi and Cesarina Casanova, *Donne criminali: Il genere nella storia della giustizia* (Bologna: Patron, 2015); on gendered violence in early modern Bologna, see Sanne Muurling and Marion Pluskota, "The Gendered Geography of Violence in Bologna, 17–19th Centuries," in Deborah Simonton, ed. *Routledge History Handbook of Gender and the Urban Experience* (Abington: Routledge, 2017), pp. 153–164.
65 Fausto's mother-in-law probably used to sell Bolognese silk "veils," a specialty of the city; all this back and forth between Modena and Bologna is understandable in light of the role of Bologna as a proto-industrial district of silk production: see Carlo Poni, *La seta in Italia. Una grande industria prima della rivoluzione industriale* (Bologna: Il Mulino, 2009), pp. 153–227.
66 ASB, Torrone, 1695, fol. 181r-183v: "di maniera che io mi sono senza casa et senza dinari et per dirvi la verità io sono venuto posta a Bologna per parlar con detto m. Gio. et per pregarlo che volesse esser contento di darmi qualche cosa anco che io non havesse havuto a perdere in tutto et per tutto le mille lire."
67 Ibid., fol. 184v: "Faccio fede io Gaspare Tagliacozzo come alli giorni passati fui chiamato a Modena per visitar una donna ferita de due ferite in testa la qual visitai et stette sin che fu passata la quarta appresso di lei di poi me partì et ne ho più volte del medico presente havuto ragguaglio et in particulare hieri per una sua lettera et una fede che ha fatto dove dice essendo passati la decimaquarta senza che se sia scoperto segno di mortale giudicio

che serà per recuperare la sanità et non habbi da incorrer a periculo alcuno della vita al presente et per l'advenire essendo ben curata, così io in fede di ciò ho scritto et sotto scritto la presente di mia mano, Io Gaspare Tagliacozi medico."

68 Ibid., fol. 180v: "[Fausto] me ha racontato qui in Bologna de haver dato delle ferite a sua Madonna madre di sua moglie dicendomi di havereli dato con un falcinello una ferita nel volto et con un altro su la testa mentre detta sua Madonna stava in piaza a vendere li veli et me ha racontato che questo fu il primo di Settembre che fu il sabato a meza matina."

69 For example, in June 1590, Tagliacozzi, along with the family physician and with another eminent Bolognese academic Felice Castelli, was called by the very powerful Senatorial family, the Gozzadini, to treat one of their offspring. The 18-month-old Fabio Gozzadini suffered from a terrible case of smallpox with *petechie* (a skin eruption), and Tagliacozzi and the others "were much diligent in treating him with good remedies." See BAB, Gozzadini, *Documenti*, 3, 3, fol. 7r: "furno diligenti nel curarlo e farli boni rimedii."

70 ASB, Torrone, 1670, fol. 148r: "unico magno vulnere quam videre non potueri propter medicamenta apposita . . . erat medicata de recenti et habebat faciem tota involutam fasciculis lineis sanguinolentis."

71 Ibid., "Poco fa tornando io dalla messa con mia Madre et la serva . . . un giovenotto che io non so chi se sia mi ha menato un colpo con un pugnale alla volta del viso al improvviso che non me ne so accorta et mi ha ferita a traverso del mostaccio tagliandomi el naso e la faccia con si mal fatto modo, che il medico me ci ha dato parecchi ponti."

72 Ibid., fol. 152r.: "passò un giovene sbarbato malvestito menuto bruono in viso che portava una casacha verdona un ferraiolo negro vechio curto un paro de calzoni stretti stretti che me dettero fantesia di che se fossero ed un cappello di feltro negro basso alla franzese magro in viso ma ardito in su la vita di meza statura, et subito che ci ebbe passato et che arrivò la Fulvia che era davanti a noi alzò la mano sotto il ferraiolo con un pugnale tre dita largo sfoderato et tirò un colpo a traverso il volto a Fulvia mia figlia et gli ha tagliato il mostaccio che il medico ci ha messi 15 ponti."

73 Ibid., fol. 156v: "perveni ad dicta domum in essa hora quae Magnificus D. Tagliacotius In chirurgia et medicina doctor ipsa medicare volebat ita quod deletis per praedictus D. Doctor medicamentis quis reprendebat medicata vidi partitum vulnus existente in facie D. Fulviae hoc modo: un sfrescio piglia dal ciglio de fora del ochio manco et tira a traverso di deto ochio e del naso fino alla parte destra della faccia . . . In quo sfrisio praedictus Magnificus Doctor asseruit dedisse quindecim punctos quae sic bene visa et inspecta per me notarium."

74 Ibid., fol. 148r-152r: "me diceva nasaccio, dalli a traverso di quel nasone, e simil altre iniurie dalla finestra, per strada, et per tutto e tra le altre per farmi dispetto per invidia che mi portava mi tirò dalla finestra non se se fu orina o altro che mi machiò una vesta incarnatina nova che havevo . . . amoroso et anco di Carnevale mi disse villanie in piaza e mi mostrò il membro pubblicamente con dirme un mondo di vilanie basta che ne gli detti la querela et fu messo pregione et per questo et ancho perché haveva un precetto di non dirme villania . . . più volte mi ha mandato a dire per Giulia Rigoni detta la Monarina [another courtesan] che io me guardasse perché quando era andato via il Legato me sarria intervenuto male . . . et più volte mi ha date delle botte et gli ho fatto la pace ultimamente questa state mi dette e mi amacchò l'ochi tanto che io senza farli altra querela non volsi più amicitia sua et non ho voluto che me sia venuto più in casa . . . una puttana che sta qui vicino . . . per respetto delle ingiurie che mi disse alli dì passati come VS sa che gli ne detti querela . . . et ancho perché alli dì passati stando sull'uscio dela casa sua et io su l'uscio qui di casa mia disse così forte che ognuno sentì che il sig. Iosephe del Orsi suo amico non voleva più andare in casa sua de dì perché aveva sentito dir a certe poltrone che stavano qui vicino che lei haveva el mostaccio come un Ramino."

75 Ibid., "io pratico alle volte in casa delli Orsi . . . Questi Orsi in casa dei quali io pratico uno si chiama il signor Camillo et l'altro il signor Giuseppe delli Orsi et in casa de questi io prattico più strettamente che in casa delli altri perché il signor Giuseppe è mio fratello da latte che mia madre l'ha allevato."

76 Ibid., "per assai volte con questi Orsi a casa de Cortigiane."
77 Ibid., fol. 156v-157v: "Alli mesi passati [Democrite] venne alle mane col signor Giovanni Alberici da Brescia che è questo gentilhomo che io tengo qui in casa mia che è mio amico et detto signor Giovanni gli dette una mentita a questo Democrite per respetto mio et dal hora in qua detto Democrite se n'è stato fuor di Bologna et minacciaria di volersene vendicare et el signor Giovanni non è mai uscito di casa . . . penso che sia mosso a farmi sfresciarme per poterse vendicare con lui."
78 ASB, Torrone, 1670, fol. 192r-195r.
79 Tagliacozzi, *De curtorum*, p. 174 (2:53–54).
80 Delaporte, *Figures of Medicine*, pp. 57–58.
81 Jean Tagault, *Institutione di cirugia* (Venezia: appresso Giorgio Angelieri, 1570), p. 128. This book by the French surgeon Jean Tagault (d. c. 1546) had been published in Latin in 1543 and then translated into the Italian vernacular in 1570. It was a very popular and influential compendium: indeed, it went through three other editions (1585, 1596, and 1607) in the space of a few decades.

2

PATIENTS AND PRACTITIONERS

Swords, books, and knives

An aristocratic clientele played a very important role in the career of middle-class graduate surgeon Gaspare Tagliacozzi. Just like other sixteenth-century learned surgeons, Tagliacozzi came from the artisanal class. He was the son of a silk worker of some means, possibly the owner of a small workshop, and climbed the social ladder thanks to his medical education and practice. His career was spectacular: he treated very important and wealthy patients, from the Medici to the Orsini families, until he became the personal physician of Duke Vincenzo Gonzaga of Mantua. He served as Prior of the College of Medicine, which he had entered in 1576, and he also was several times *tribuno della plebe.*[1] He published a first description of his work in a book by his friend Girolamo Mercuriale and then in the form of a long, erudite, and even verbose monograph, a quite exceptional work among sixteenth-century genres of surgical writing. Tagliacozzi's career and wealth were built through his private practice with powerful patrons and facilitated by his choosing a rather unusual and "wondrous" subject through which he wished to be remembered as a writer.

In his chronicle of Bologna in the years 1589–1600, Francesco Galliani wrote the following passage on the death of the eminent surgeon:

> Today 7 November [1599] the excellent doctor of medicine Gaspare Tagliacozzi passed away; in our age, he was more famous than anyone else in the art of surgery, and he used to make noses, lips, and ears that had been cut off by wounds or other things . . . he was the son of a poor carpenter, and with his virtue alone he has earned 30.000 scudi.[2]

Galliani thought that Tagliacozzi was born from a "poor" family, the son of a "carpenter." This information – which possibly plays with the religious reference to Jesus as a "carpenter's son" (Matthew 13:55) – is not correct, but it tells a lot about how Tagliacozzi was associated not only with the faces of the upper classes but also with ideas of social mobility.

Tagliacozzi was remembered in several chronicles, and he too translated and wrote parts of a chronicle, a significant circumstance concerning his desire to become a public civic figure, a living monument to the city's political and intellectual prestige. This document is titled *Chronicle of Bologna by an unknown author from 404 to 1585. Translated from Latin into Italian by Gasparo Tagliacozzi in 1594.* However, this is not just a translation, because Tagliacozzi added his own notes. For example, he shows some familiarity with events related to the hospital of Santa Maria della Morte, the center of training for the Bolognese "learned" surgeons.[3] He has also shown some interest for singular human forms when he added a drawing of a "human monster" to the margin of news from 1321.[4]

As we have seen in the previous chapter, direct information on patients is very scarce. Therefore, in this chapter I briefly sketch a picture of the social and political stratification of late sixteenth-century Bologna, the relationships among different kinds of men, and the culture of duel and the practices of violence in the Papal state. I then move to the encounter between these kinds of patients and the graduate surgeons. I describe what it was like to be a learned surgeon in sixteenth-century Italy. I then focus on practitioners, and I describe the career paths of a group of learned surgeons – teachers, colleagues, and pupils of Tagliacozzi – in late sixteenth-century Bologna. I argue that the emergence of a textual representation of facial surgery is linked to the great prestige that surgery and surgeons enjoyed at that studio. Moreover, the specificity of Tagliacozzi's book and the fact itself that he embarked in the enterprise of writing a long, learned, and specialized monograph on one single surgical operation, at a time in which virtually none existed, was closely linked to the specificity of the Bolognese social, cultural, and urban contexts.

Based on the scant evidence of the actual practice of this procedure, I argue that the reconstruction technique was performed very few times during the long sixteenth century, either by Tagliacozzi or by other surgeons. This means that Tagliacozzi chose to write about and to give textual representation to one of the most spectacular procedures among many a surgeon could perform on men's and women's faces. All kinds of skin problems and injuries could affect people's faces, and Tagliacozzi was known as an expert on facial issues in general. Nonetheless, he decided to write about only a tiny portion of the range of operations one could perform on the human face. In other words, surgical reconstruction was a rare, demanding, and expensive procedure that only few men could undergo, but the Bolognese surgeon chose to give, so to speak, a plastic and solid form to fluid information on the reconstructive technique that previously circulated in the form of cases and sparse notes. However, this rarely practiced procedure was connected with several important trends concerning developments in medicine and surgery and social and political phenomena. Only a self-confident learned surgeon, backed by a century-long tradition of academic surgery and immersed in a culture of aristocratic honor and violence, could have written a learned monograph on one single surgical procedure.

Social stratifications

Reconstructive surgery in the sixteenth century was an elite and a male business. At least, this was the representation the authors wanted to convey to their readership. This tradition predated Tagliacozzi's monograph, but it was both exploited and further carried on by the Bolognese physician. Tagliacozzi consciously targeted noblemen, their culture of the face and honor, and their ethos of aggressive masculinity.

Historians of early modern noble culture generally share the idea that around the middle of the sixteenth century a unified and homogeneous ideology of the noble class took shape. Claudio Donati defined this period as a "time of oligarchical closure and cultural and social aristocratization."[5] Nobility became a "trendy topic" for discussions and writing, and a flood of books, pamphlets, treatises, manuscripts, correspondence materialized on the subject. At the same time, the number of the noblemen increased all over Europe, and the magnitude of the process of class separation and distinction intensified as well. This process of change within the ruling class triggered a widespread social tension. Finally, this was also the period in which noble ideology clashed and negotiated with theories and practices of political "absolutism." The late sixteenth century is recognized as the period in which this process began in Europe and beyond.[6]

If we narrow the focus on Bologna, we have at hand a striking document concerning the definition and role of nobility and social stratification. The author is Camillo Baldi (1551–1637), a very important figure in Bolognese academic and political culture.[7] It does not present by any means an objective view on the social composition of the city, because it was written by a member of the local noble class who enthusiastically supported the central government of the Roman court and for this reason would probably have been considered as a traitor by some of his fellow patricians. Nonetheless, it is a precious source of information if read "between the lines."

In the sixteenth century, after the Church regained effective control of the city, the pope formally ruled Bologna. He exercised his jurisdiction through a Cardinal Legate, who ruled the city with the Senate, or the Reggimento as it was also called, expression of the most powerful, rich, and influential patrician families of Bologna. The Legate had to oversee the justice system and the public order, while the Senate had the power of managing the finances and the general administrative matters. This political balance was called "mixed government (*governo misto*)."[8]

Baldi described the five orders of people of Bologna, associating them with five types of men: knights, gentlemen, merchants, artisans, and the "plebs." The definition Baldi gave of the noble, or chivalric, order was rather standard for the early seventeenth century and followed half a century of debates on the essence of nobility.

> They say that Knights surpass all other citizens by virtue of their nobility and wealth. The Bolognese call noblemen those who are born from an old and honored family, that always had great wealth, and just like without light one cannot see a painting, however beautiful, in the same way they [the Bolognese] do not call one a nobleman if he is not wealthy, and those who were noble and became poor are called fallen noblemen. This is perhaps not without reason, since a nobleman must be generous, liberal, and munificent, and when he has nothing he cannot do any of these things. Therefore, if a nobleman becomes poor, he also becomes ignoble, because he cannot act in a noble way. The other reason is that there are neither nobility nor virtue when there are no wisdom and good judgment in a man: throwing away one's wealth and becoming poor for whatever reason are signs of poor judgment and limited intellect. Therefore, with his wealth a nobleman loses his nobility too; and it is useless to blame bad luck or some other misfortune, since men are the makers of their own fortune.[9]

Noblemen had to meet two requisites if they wanted to be "real" noblemen: they had to be born from an ancient aristocratic family and they had to be wealthy. In other words, they lived without working, and they – at least in theory – cultivated a noble ethos and way of living.[10]

From Baldi's description – certainly biased by the fact that this was the group to which he himself belonged – it emerged that graduates of the studio and members of the Colleges of Law and Medicine occupied a liminal space. "Doctors" were one of the few social ranks that allowed for a certain degree of social ascension, and for this reason they were potentially in conflict with the knights and the gentlemen. Baldi reflected the opinion of the minority of the lecturers and intellectuals who felt discriminated and excluded from real political power. He also voiced the fact that their relationship with the patrician class composing the Senate was not easy at all.[11] Practically speaking, by becoming a doctor a man could jump two or more orders. Baldi had already claimed earlier in his treatise that "as an old habit, doctors have a higher status than knights, and among the lay people they have the higher status after the magistrates."[12] Clearly, a certain tension and competition existed between doctors and knights. Baldi also argued that it was not possible to move from one order to the other but by following two very narrow paths: "on the one hand, the path of the letters and sciences which are useful and necessary, on the other, the path of wealth." The first one was by no means always successful. For example, doctors were entitled to public signs of honor such as that of having precedence on the streets, but in practice

> besides according them precedence when they meet on the street, noblemen do not hold doctors in high esteem, except when they need them; and it has now been a while that people from the first order do not care about the letters, unless they believe them to be the fastest way to access the

> Roman court and the offices that are distributed there; otherwise, noblemen despise the letters, and they laugh about them.[13]

Philosopher and scientist as he was, Baldi complained about the fact that even if wealth did not formally grant access to the first orders, rich people of lower birth were much more respected than learned people.[14]

Noblemen's culture of violence

Baldi's description gives the modern reader a glimpse of the social tensions that could interfere in the doctor-patient relationship, especially for a procedure like facial reconstructive surgery.

By the middle of the sixteenth century, the culture of honor and the elitism of nobility increased as their political privileges became more and more questioned. The discourse on nobility at mid-century established itself around the pairing of honor and the duel. Both honor and the duel were concepts and practices that potentially conflicted with state authorities, especially in the Papal states.[15]

True noblemen had to protect their honor. But what was honor? The famous Portuguese theologian and jurist Luiz Beja de Perestelo (1539–1610) in his *Responsionum casuum conscientiae* (1597) defined honor as "a condition of perfect dignity, proven by the life and customs . . . the fully clear notion that others have of us."[16] Early modern honor was an ephemeral and almost impalpable male value defining the worth of a man in the eyes of others. Honor was a matter not primarily of actual deeds but of perceptions of virtue, social status, and the intrinsic nobility of a person.[17] For a nobleman, a life without honor was worse than death. This was the reason why those whose honor was under threat had to put their life at risk in a duel. When recognition of the other's reputation and virtue failed, a duel should take place in order to restore the broken honor, to which everything else was subordinated. Honor had nothing to do with the law: it was above the law. One of the most famous definitions came from a bestseller of the sixteenth century, *Il duello* (1550) by the writer Girolamo Muzio (1496–1576):

> The knights' opinion is that there is no law, neither of a State nor of a prince, no wealth, no life which should be preferred to honor; and that despite what some constitutions say and whatever the dangers, knights must obey only the law of honor. Such a law says that the one who is called to the challenge of the arms must immediately reply to that call with a brave soul, and that the one who does not, does not deserve to be counted among the honored knights.[18]

In fact, it is hard to grasp what honor consisted in if it is examined apart from duel, its twin.[19] Francois Billacois has defined duel as a "total social phenomenon." The duel was indeed a juridical institution, a vector of social differentiation, a political manifestation, a work of art, and a religious ritual, and it worked according to laws of a "symbolic" economy.[20] Early modern duel was a form of cultural resistance to the rise of the centralizing states or at least the principal expression of a desire of independence from the judicial systems by the noble classes. The sixteenth-century duel for honor was constitutionally linked to the business of men of honor taking care of their affairs as a true "symbol of aristocracy's autonomy and privilege."[21] Duels and chivalric values became the expression of the community of the noble warriors threatened by state developments.[22]

Moreover, duels were socially and culturally linked to war. The periods of the maximum fortune of duels coincided with periods of war, in our case the Italian wars. The specific developments of the art of war also played a part in the phenomenon. The advent of infantry, fire arms, light cavalry, and armies filled with people of lowly origins who could become more "noble" through their service pushed forward the social system of honor with its signs and rituals.[23]

The worst sin for a noble knight was to lie, and especially to lie – or, better, of being accused of lying – about another knight's honor. The most frequent cause of duel was thus an insult *(ingiuria).* In turn, one of the most serious insults was accusing someone of lying *(mentita).* The accusation was even more serious if those insults touched upon honor and the body at the same time, like inflicting punches and stick blows.[24] The culture of duel was a cult of the sword. For example, while the *mentita* was insulting per se, a knight wounded with a sword could not consider himself injured, because the sword was the purest noble-class weapon. On the other hand, the stick and the hand as instruments of offense expressed disdain for the insulted, a sign that he was believed to be of a lower class. But the sword had to be used to cut, not to inflict blows with its flat surface.[25] Therefore, certain kinds of wounds and injuries were typical of the nobleman.

The literature on dueling was not uniform throughout the sixteenth century. Indeed, unlike judiciary duels, which were regulated procedures for establishing the legal truth of a matter in the presence of a representative of the king or the local lord, and tournament duels – training exercises for knights who had to be prepared for war – duels "in point of honor" became clandestine in the second half of the sixteenth century.

The paradox was that at the time of its golden age, the practice of duel was also condemned and outlawed by secular and spiritual authorities. While the courts of the Este at Ferrara and of the Gonzaga at Mantua became the best-known centers for the chivalric sciences of sixteenth-century Italy, in the Papal state, where the spiritual and the secular powers were unified in one single person, the matter became particularly delicate. On December 4, 1563, the twenty-fifth decree of the Council of Trent was issued, titled *Detestabilis duellorum usus.*

> The detestable custom of dueling, introduced by the contrivance of the devil, that by the bloody death of the body, he may accomplish the ruin of the soul, shall be utterly exterminated from the Christian world. Any emperor, kings, dukes, princes, marquises, counts, and temporal lords by

> whatsoever other name entitled, who shall grant a place within their territories for single combat between Christians, shall be thereupon excommunicated. . . . As to the persons who have fought . . . they shall incur the penalty of excommunication, and the confiscation of all their property, and of perpetual infamy, and are to be punished as homicides, according to the sacred canons; and if they have perished in the conflict itself, they shall be for ever deprived of ecclesiastical sepulture. Those also who have given counsel in the ease of a duel, whether for the question of right, or fact, or have in any other way whatever persuaded any one thereunto, as also the spectators thereof, shall be subjected to the bond of excommunication, and of a perpetual malediction; any privilege soever, or evil custom, though immemorial, notwithstanding.[26]

Secular state authorities agreed with the core arguments of this condemnation. Duels were assimilated to *lèse majesté* crimes and banned in most of the Italian states.[27]

The severity of Counter-Reformation ideas did not translate automatically and immediately into practice. For example, sixteenth-century confessors' manuals were soft on duels. One of the most influential of such manuals, the *Enchiridion sive manuale confessariorum et poenitentium* written by the Augustinian monk Martin de Azpilcueta called El Navarro (1492–1586), published in Venice in 1584, clearly stated that violence and homicide for self-defense had always been admitted and that honor was the most precious of all goods. Duels for honor had to be tolerated: "Honor is more worthy than other goods given by fortune."[28] Navarro argued that natural law of self-defense could not be altered by positive law, an opinion which was very similar to that of the most radical members of nobility. The Trent decree did not have any strong immediate effects, even though it expressed both the idea that duels were nothing better than homicides and that the state needed to exercise a "monopoly" on violence.

In any case, literature opposing the chivalric sciences, the culture of honor, and duels existed and multiplied, without ever reaching the editorial peaks of its foe, after 1563. One very interesting case is Fabio Albergati's *Del modo di ridurre alla pace le inimicizie private*, published in Rome in 1583. Albergati (1538–1606) graduated in law in Bologna and had a brilliant career at the Papal court. In his book he argued for a new ethos of the good civil servant that reflected new ideas about the state and citizenship. Albergati explicitly claimed that chivalric virtues were not compatible with a well-ordered state and that honor was indeed a value but "true honor" was given by personal virtue, which in turn was linked to the welfare of the state, the *res publica*. Honor was therefore an attribute not just of "active men" but of all men who had a role in the organization of a good society (politicians, the clergy, soldiers, judges, those who practiced the mechanical arts, philosophers, etc.). Honor was not only restricted to nobility, and it was not especially linked to physical prowess or to the ability in using weapons, because the state and the Prince were the only criteria for conferring honor.[29] Learned physicians and surgeons must have felt included in this new class of honorable citizens and civil servants.

However, the impression of tolerance and compromise toward duel is confirmed not only by the cases of duels reported by chroniclers throughout the peninsula and the continuous flow of books, new or reprinted, on chivalric science and duels but also by the fact that the literature on duels became the object of a serious project of expurgation by the Congregation of the Inquisition only in 1596 and with several attenuating provisions. In the period that roughly went from the 1560s to the 1590s the Church was busy on many fronts, and opening up a new one against the ideology of the upper class would have seemed unwise, at least until the outbreak of noble brigandage in the 1590s.[30] Books on honor and duel continued to circulate. The 1596 prohibition took some inquisitors by surprise and even raised doubts and criticisms. For example, the project of expurgation in Parma and Piacenza was welcomed lukewarmly by the local Inquisition's examiners. Ultimately, even projects of expurgation and correction failed to see the light and remained unpublished in the Inquisition archives.[31]

A similar tension between condemnation and fascination for noble violence by the emerging states can be found in the case of banditry or brigandage. In the Papal state there was a real outbreak of banditry in the period between the middle of the 1570s and the middle of the 1590s, against which the popes did not hesitate to wage real wars. The phenomenon of banditry, in its specificity related to this time and place, originated when powerful and rich noblemen were banished from their cities for various sorts of crimes considered *lése majesté* – the most common one was murder – thus falling victim to the inquisitorial trial enforced by the state. These bandits then retreated to the countryside, sometimes taking advantage of their county villas or castles, organizing private armies, subjugating peasants, and robbing passersby and entire villages. The current view is more inclined to picture banditry as a higher-class phenomenon. Some historians explained the banditry crisis of this period as the resistance of the feudal class and local lords to the absolutist policy of the popes; others think that the phenomenon was an expression of the permanent weakness of the Pontifical states' power. Popes even tried to integrate noble bandits into the state as military professionals, soldiers, and leaders, and while in some cases they succeeded, many knights of the Papal states preferred to leave to fight against the "Turks" in Eastern Europe, at the service of foreign rulers. The overlap between the knight as a military leader and the nobleman as a privileged citizen in the social life of late sixteenth century was no doubt one of those delicate sites of exchange in which early modern political order was decided. Banditry and nobiliary violence were nuanced phenomena: on the one hand, banditry was the expression of the noble ideology of resistance to the new culture of the state; on the other hand, the Papal states were not an "absolute" monarchy at all in the late sixteenth century. Local noblemen and the upper classes always tried to reach agreements and compromises with the central power. This double process, or double bind, can be seen in banditry, in the use of the army, in the many Bolognese diplomats working in Rome, and in the ambivalence toward dueling and the noble ideology of honor showed by secular and spiritual authorities.[32]

Discourse on duel was heavily gendered and appealed to noblemen's specific virility. One anonymous Bolognese manuscript on the duel from the beginning of the seventeenth century stated that state justice was for women, not real men.

> It seems that in those cities where duel rules the citizens must necessarily practice it not to look dishonored and even impious in the face of others; and this is mainly because soldiers, knights and all the honored men do not think that in such cases it is acceptable to step back . . . they also believe that to call the magistrates and the Prince is by all deemed unworthy of a honored man but only suitable for women, who do not have any strength whatsoever in them and therefore protect themselves under the shield of justice, a shield which is shameful for soldiers and men of honor, whose trial is that of the arms alone.[33]

The very gender identity of someone who refused to duel was put into question.

Violence among noblemen and between noblemen and commoners was a constant feature in the urban and country landscapes of Bologna.[34] A decree on public order published in 1575 addressed, by specifically linking the face to the culture of honor, "disfigurements and injuries" (*sfreggi e debilitamenti*):

> we command that all persons of all status who with weapons or whatever tool will permanently disfigure, mark, or scar someone' face or some other visible body part, or will cut off or injury some other part, will be subject to paying two hundred scudi and to other corporal punishments.[35]

Fencing

Noblemen defending their honor by dueling were part of a coherent and specific culture of violence and physical prowess, which Gaspare Tagliacozzi consciously targeted when he wrote his book. Sixteenth-century Bologna, as noted by Montaigne, was famous not only for its studio but for its schools of fencing, too. The emergence of fencing as a sport, just like the contemporary transformations of jousting, riding, and gymnastics, was part of a wider process of transformation of military techniques into new bodily techniques separated from the purpose of war and associated with the new "civil" needs of the noble class in times of political crisis.[36] *Opera Nova*, by the master of fencing Achille Morozzo (1484–1553), is the most famous and well-received fencing book of the times, reprinted throughout the whole sixteenth century after its 1517 first edition (Figure 2.1). Despite being mostly a manual of bodily technique and training, in book V of his treatise the author ventures into a discussion of the rules of an honorable duel. Morozzo discussed the case of a duel in which one of the duelists cut one

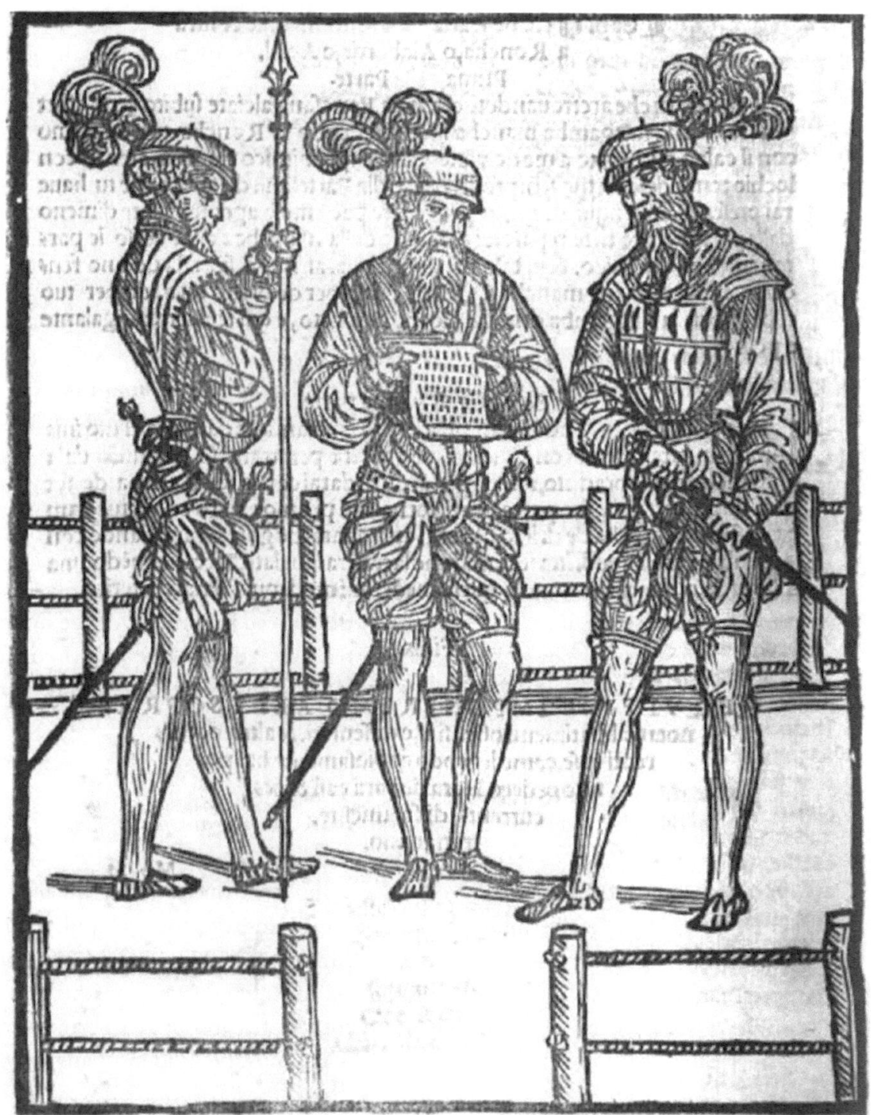

FIGURE 2.1 Achille Morozzo, *Opera nova* (1550): the preparation for a duel.

eye out of the enemy's orbit and the other reacted by cutting off his nose. The question was how to decide who won the duel. The knight who cut out the eye argued that there was no worst thing than to be deprived of sight, because a man was useless if he could not see. He went on by explaining that the eye was the most noble part of the face, placed in a most eminent site, and it was the guide of the whole body as it shed light on its path. Moreover, visual impressions were decisive for human memory and for human pleasure, for example, when one contemplated the vividness of the colors of the world. Eyes could be opened and closed and thus manifested the supreme human feature of willpower. Finally, the eye was most excellent "so much so that if it is hit it causes more pain, and for this reason it enjoys bigger honor." The knight also reviled the nose. It was a "useless and vile part of the head" because it was the vessel of the excrements of the brain and the "stinking vapors of the head" and, finally, because smell was useless for human life. The only merit of the nose concerned its role in the symmetry and beauty of the face.

The nose cutter replied that the nose was unique in the economy of body parts, and therefore its loss was more disastrous, because a face without a nose could not be repaired in any way. If one lost an eye, one did not lose sight, and moreover the sense of sight was made stronger and sharper in the remaining eye. Moreover – the nose cutter went on making reference to the tradition of excluding disfigured people from both civic and canonical offices – the law did not claim that one who lost one eye must be removed from office, thus implying that such a man was not deemed imperfect.

> Losing the nose is a bigger disgrace, because given that the human face is similar to the divine face, it is completely disfigured by the loss of the nose: it loses its beauty, for which there is no remedy, and no one could cover the deformity produced by a missing nose . . . losing the nose is the bigger loss, just like a man who loses his only son suffers more than a man who has two sons and loses one.

The knight recalled that it was a common and shared opinion that

> there is no bigger insult and affront to a living man than cutting his nose, which represents a bigger offence than the simple loss of a foot, a hand, or an eye, because one thing is more apparent [in those men who have lost their nose], namely shame; and for this reason it is considered a very serious punishment when criminals have their nose cut off, because it is a permanent sign of the punishment on their faces, which cannot be hidden in any way.

The conclusion by Morozzo was that cutting off the nose was by far a more serious offence and that the winner would always be the one who cut the nose.[37]

What is a learned surgeon?

Let me now turn to practitioners. Historians of early modern societies have emphasized the fact that the study of surgeons is still in its infancy[38] and, in general, that the history of early modern surgery and surgeons is just about to begin.[39] One of the most puzzling features of early modern surgery is that the title of surgeon seems to describe very different kinds of practitioners: from barbers to bonesetters, from practitioners hired by the city to treat the people for free to university-trained physicians, from specialists on hernia to sellers of unguents and potions. Recent works on early modern practitioners, or "artisans" of the body, have showed that, despite all the differences among Italian cities, at least south of the Alps the conflict between learned surgeons and nongraduate surgeons was not as pervasive and widespread as it has been imagined. In European cities the typical sixteenth-century institutional arrangement could take three forms. The first was a division between a College of Physicians, a College of Surgeons (learned surgeons), and a guild of barber-surgeons (this was the case of Venice and some northern cities); in the second one, learned surgeons were part of the College of Physicians, and non-graduate surgical practitioners were part of the barbers' guild or independently licensed by the College (the case of Bologna and Padua). The third model, more widespread north of the Alps, was a division between a guild of barber-surgeons and a College of Physicians, with surgeons sharing their practice with barbers. However, subterranean and infra-institutional attempts of surgeons to differentiate themselves from barbers were common in the whole continent.[40]

However, there was a cultural and technical contiguity between practitioners of the body in early modern Italy, who all dealt with the care of health and the care of appearance, which will be explored further in Chapter 4. But emphasizing this contiguity does not mean that there were not significant differences, both in the social status of learned surgeons and in their claims to master a more difficult and important set of surgical techniques, informed by theory. While the social and professional gap between surgeons and barbers widened during the course of the seventeenth and the eighteenth centuries, social and cultural categories, as well as the practitioners' social mobility, were more malleable in the sixteenth century. In this period there was a certain mutually acknowledged complementarity between "lower" and "higher" surgery.

Confusion surrounding the early modern meaning of the word "surgeon" did puzzle the early moderns. Scipione Mercurio (c. 1550–1615) was a student of medicine in Padua and Bologna, a Dominican friar, and a medical practitioner. In his *De gli errori poplari d'Italia libri sette*, a 1603 book modeled upon, and partially translating, Laurent Jaubert's French book on popular "medical errors," he acknowledged the confusion of categories between different kinds of surgical practitioners and attempted an explanation. Mercurio asked himself why so many people used to put their trust and lives in the hands of the "ignorants" – barbers, wise women, and empirics of all sorts. In Padua, Mercurio claimed, no one could treat surgical illnesses unless he was licensed, either by the College of Physicians or by the Rectors of the studio. The problem was that

> these men, when they get a license, they think they have a doctorate too, and so believe the people, who begin to call them Doctors, and they [the licensed surgeons] are so charmed by this kind of language that they believe the people . . . and when they have to show where they can be found they say: there is the house of the Doctor Surgeon.

Furthermore, the common people were confused by the fact that they saw "that some Doctors of Medicine practice surgery, and for this reason they are called Surgeons." This is why the empirics become persuaded, and try to persuade the public, that they were surgeons just like the graduate surgeons.[41] A linguistic gray area existed between the semantic reference of the words "surgeon" and "doctor."

With the license came the promise by empiric surgeons not to give any medicament by mouth and not to perform bloodletting without the supervision of a physician. Moreover, "all Doctors of Medicine are doctors of surgery too, and no simple surgeon can be a Doctor too." The fact that graduate physicians used to practice and in some cases chose to specialize in surgery was indeed seen as a peculiar feature of the Italian medical marketplace. English medical student Fynes Morison (1566–1630) recorded with amazement in the travelogue of his trip to Italy in the late sixteenth century that "many famous physicians are . . . in Italy, surgeons as well."[42] Mercurio tried to explain why there were graduate physicians who practiced surgical procedures, an idea that would seem at first glance a little foolish, given the lower status of surgery. The answer was that "this happens . . . because not all of them [the graduate physicians] have the guts to practice surgery: for this reason some licensed manual operators are allowed to treat wounds and aposteme, to clean rotten parts, to bandage, and to apply plasters."[43] Mercurio explained this puzzlement away by referring to the practitioners' guts to find themselves immersed in blood to their elbows, but there was much more at stake for a graduate surgeon: academic prestige, social status, and the possibility of attracting wealthy patrons.

Self-portrait of a graduate surgeon

The second half of the sixteenth century in Bologna was a period of renewal of health-care institutions. The guild of barbers, the College of Medicine, the Hospital for the sick poor of Santa Maria della Morte all renewed their statutes and internal organization. Moreover, a new institution for the care of public health was created in the 1570s, directly dependent on the Senate, a public health board called *Assunteria di Sanità*, dealing specifically with epidemics and hygiene.

The College of Physicians, an institution formed by the elite members of the medical profession, was established in the fourteenth century on the model of the older College of Lawyers and greatly expanded its functions over the course of the sixteenth century. The Protomedicato, a medical magistracy charged with policing the boundaries among health-care providers and medical practitioners which was composed of members of the College, was founded in 1517. By 1563 Protomedicato officials started to be paid with a public salary. By that time, the Protomedicato had acquired full jurisdiction over people who did not comply with its rules in matters of medical practice.[44] Sixteenth-century Italian Protomedicati and Colleges of Physicians all over the peninsula tried to enforce a threefold partition of the medical professions – graduate physicians, apothecaries, and barber-surgeons – with more or less success, depending on time and place.[45]

As explained by Gianna Pomata, the College and the Protomedicato were not professional associations but an aristocracy, a self-affirming ruling medical elite. Their aim was not to ban all illicit practice but to affirm their right to rule and be recognized as the top of the medical hierarchy.[46]

The first statutes of the College date back to 1395; they were reformed in 1507 and then integrated with several punctual additions over the course of the whole early modern period. *Rubrica xviii* of the 1395 statutes stated that no one could practice medicine or surgery without a license. Surgeons in search of a license had to attend the lectures of "public masters" teaching in Bologna or another studio for at least three years. Plus, all those who wanted to practice the medical arts in the city "must be examined, licensed, and approved by the doctors of medicine."[47] Already in the fourteenth century, taking an academic degree in surgery was an option for medical students.[48] It was also made clear that all the physicians of the College and faculty of medicine could teach and practice surgery without any further examination. On the other hand, "those who are matriculated in surgery should not dare or presume to treat the sick as physicians do."[49]

In early modern Italy there were multiple cases in which one single surgical practitioner was empirically trained in a workshop, then attended a few university lectures, and maybe served as assistant to a publicly appointed physician or surgeon.[50] In any case, just as in Padua, surgery in Bologna had a long tradition as an academic discipline.[51] By the fifteenth century, the holders of surgery chairs were also in charge of conducting the annual public dissection, and in 1570 Bologna was the first studio in Europe to create a chair of anatomy, given to Giulio Cesare Aranzi.[52] The oldest statutes of the College thus established three kinds of surgeons: those with an academic degree in surgery; physicians who chose or wanted to practice surgery; people with no academic degree but with a certified path of apprenticeship with a master surgeon. The 1507 statutes repeated these very same points, but by the second half of the sixteenth century the matter became more complex and professional distinctions multiplied.[53]

The most significant innovation in the system of controlling the practitioners of surgical operations came not from a reform of the statutes but from a 1572 public decree issued by the Protomedicato and signed by the Legate, the executive authority. The text of the decree concerning barbers, and directly addressing the barbers' guild, prescribed all barber-surgeons who wanted, or were used, to

> treat all kinds of people, of whatever illness they are affected, and most prominently wounds, aposteme, tumors or other evils . . . not to let blood or authorize someone to let blood, not to allow someone to give a patient something orally, be they men or women, old or young – if they have not been licensed by the signori Priors and Protomedici.[54]

The leaders of the barbers' guild tried to retain control over the examination of barber-surgeons,[55] but a series of subsequent decrees constantly repeated the injunction.[56] Coming from a century-long tradition of including surgery within the academic disciplines, the Collegiates' strategy was to consider barber-surgeons as health-care practitioners in order to place them under their direct control.

In the archives of the College only 15 licenses for the period 1570–1600 survive. Despite the fact that the 1572 decree explicitly contemplated the possibility that surgical practitioners might be women, there are no surviving records of women officially practicing surgery in the Protomedicato files. From an analysis of the licenses, it emerges that in practice the authorities recognized two kinds of surgeons: barber-surgeons or people who practiced other professions but were also skilled in some surgical specialty (often along with a competence in recipes and "secrets" for external medicaments) and those who had some kind of academic training or at least could read some Latin, for whom the professor of anatomy testified they attended the public dissection. This professional distinction was accompanied by a language emphasizing the difference between treating "simple" wounds and "complex" wounds, the latter often involving the human head.[57]

By comparing the two series of documents – the normative and the archival ones – there emerges a complex picture of the practice of surgery in early modern Bologna: (1) graduate physicians who practiced surgery; (2) practitioners with some measure of academic training, who were trained in surgeons' workshops but did not have a doctorate; (3) barber-surgeons, trained in workshops, licensed by the College; (4) empiric surgeons specialized through apprenticeship in some kind of procedure – like the extraction of bladder stones – and licensed by the College; (5) the moving and hard-to-grasp mass of empiric surgeons. Tagliacozzi belonged to group (1) and had to live, and compete, with all the other groups. The question is why a graduate from the studio should decide to practice and write about surgery.

Learned surgeons like Tagliacozzi were not silent at all about their professional identity. After all, the famous anatomical renaissance of the sixteenth century was carried on by graduate surgeons. Nearly all learned and Latin Renaissance surgery books – be they treatises organized according to kinds of illnesses and injuries or booklets built around specific cases or controversies – included a description of the "ideal" surgeon. Usually such descriptions combined elements that remained constant from the times of Celsus and Galen. First of all, they recall the Galenic idea that surgery, which means "manual operation," was one of the three integral components of medicine, along with dietetics and pharmacy. Then, they define the moral, technical, and cognitive qualities of surgeons. In particular, Celsus' definition of the ideal surgeon, together with a passage of the Hippocratic corpus recommending the dexterity of the practitioners' hands,[58] formed the standard picture medieval and Renaissance learned surgeons always repeated. Celsus' surgeon had to be "youthful or at any rate nearer youth than age; with a strong and steady hand which never trembles"; he had to have "sharp and clear sight." As for his moral qualities, which at the same time constituted a scientific equipment, the good surgeon had to have a

> spirit undaunted; filled with pity, so that he wishes to cure his patient, yet is not moved by his cries, to go too fast, or cut less than is necessary; but he does everything just as if the cries of pain cause him no emotion.[59]

The ability to detach from the patients' vocal and gestural expression of suffering was thus inscribed in the very definition of surgery by one of the most important classical authorities. Pain was also something that the surgeon had to be able to understand, to assess, to pay attention to, and to ease.[60]

Medieval, Latin-writing, "rational surgeons" like Bruno da Longobucco (early thirteenth century – 1286) and Guy de Chauliac (1300–1368) put less emphasis on the ability to handle pain and more on the fact that surgeons had to be literate in Latin and erudite. Their effort aimed at establishing surgery as a dignified medical specialty.[61] In the late thirteenth century, Bruno, whose book was part of the curriculum of the arts and medicine in sixteenth-century Italian universities, recalled that surgeons had to learn from other experienced practitioners and that they had to be cautious and ready to adapt to changing individual situations. He stressed that

> those who practice surgery must be erudite men too, or at least they have to learn from those who studied the letters . . . and it has to be deemed hideous and indecent that weak and ignoble women claimed this art for themselves, because they have neither skills nor inventiveness, as Al Mansur says. He also adds that those who practice this art are for the most part idiots, rustic and ignorant men, and that because of this ignorance they cause in their patients permanent damage or even death, since they operate in a superficial manner and with no reason.[62]

In the fourteenth century, Guy de Chauliac claimed that surgeons must be "experienced"; "ingenious" – they must have a good memory, good judgment, good eyesight; skilled, with a sharp intelligence and "a good appearance" (*bonitate forme*), with thin fingers, a steady hand, and clear eyes; and "modest," "pleasant with patients," "a good companion," chaste, sober, pious, and "compassionate" (*misericors*). Finally, they must not be greedy but rather demand a fee commensurate to their patients' occupation and wealth.[63] Guy too, like Bruno, emphasized literacy: surgeons must be literate, not just in surgery but in physic too, both theoretical and practical; they must know all complexions; they must know the causes, because without knowledge of causes healing cannot be achieved; finally, they should have a practical knowledge of diet and pharmacy.[64]

Renaissance surgeons' definitions combined more or less the same elements but, perhaps influenced by the direct reading of Celsus, usually put the emphasis less on Latin literacy and more on technological innovation and abilities in minimizing pain. Giovanni Andrea Dalla Croce described an ideal surgeon who could also be the "inventor of new instruments," while "his way of proceeding must be light, safe, quick, and painless."[65] Another characteristic theme of sixteenth-century descriptions of ideal surgeons is the "learned hand,"[66] a phrase emphasizing the intertwining of theory and practice, manual skill, and medical education. Finally, even learned surgeons did not disdain comparisons with artisanship and the world of crafts: surgeons could learn how to stitch and measure skin from tailors, how to stop the blood flow from executioners, how to design instruments from engineers, and how to bandage damaged limbs from farmers.[67]

The Bolognese surgeon and anatomist Giovanni Battista Cortesi gave the most complete image of the learned surgeon in his surgical manual published in 1633, titled *In Universam Chirurgiam absolutam Institutio*. Cortesi underlined the necessary preliminary education in the *studia humanitatis* and then in philosophy for the graduate surgeon, along with the close study of human anatomy. Surgeons must also study the contemporaries, particularly "Vesalius' anatomical books, Falloppio's observations, Colombo's, Valverde's and Laurenzi's anatomies, and above all Paré, who also most expertly wrote about surgery."[68] But beyond theory, surgeons must pile up a great mass of experiences and observations taken from the patients' bedside and must always be good and gentle with them.[69]

> The surgeon must among other things be young, or close enough to the young age, since this is the age at which the body and the senses are in their prime, and apt for correctly performing all the operations pertaining to the art; so that he is able to carry on the tasks required by the art without being hampered by the weakness of the senses: he should always be ready to use both his hands, and have a strong and effective hand, always steady in making an incision, cauterizing, and cutting off; an acute and clear eyesight; a brave and merciless soul so that he is able to heal screaming, crying, and weak patients, either those who willingly undergo the procedure, or those whom he deems necessary to cauterize and cut. In this way, he will be able to perform his procedures as if he would not hear the screaming, and not be affected by it.[70]

Moreover, a good surgeon had to be a "virile," "pious," and "generous" man,

> confident and brave in uncertain matters and cautious in dangerous ones, not precipitous, a good sport, humane, calm, generous with his assistants and easygoing with his peers, sociable, prudent, most attentive in anticipating future events, neither greedy nor too harsh in collecting his fees.[71]

Almost three centuries of surgical academic education had generated a coherent and widely shared image of the learned surgeon among the experts. This physician who practiced surgery was a product of both humanist education and manual skill, of bookish study and practical training. In cities like Bologna and Padua, the double character of learned surgery could attract middle-class students of medicine wanting to establish their name.

The career of the graduate surgeons

By comparing the lists of the student assistants of the hospital of Santa Maria della Morte in Bologna and that of the professors of surgery and anatomy in the second half of the sixteenth century, a clear pattern emerges. Hospital training was a staple of the careers of learned surgeons like Tagliacozzi. There are significant overlappings in the two lists. The list of student assistants includes Gaspare Tagliacozzi from 1567 to 1570; Giulio Cesare Gessi from 1570 to 1576; Flaminio Rota (d. 1611) from 1576 to 1580; Giovanni Battista Cortesi from 1580 to 1583; and finally Francesco Muratori from 1599 to 1602.[72] There is no way to know whether Angelo Michele Sacchi (d. 1611), lecturer in surgery and anatomy at the studio from 1567 to 1611, had been assistant at the hospital, because the hospital started recording their names only in 1567. But he was nonetheless very much part of the hospital life: by the 1590s he was appointed surgeon of the institution. On the other hand, Giulio Cesare Aranzi had never served as assistant there. But along with Aranzi and Sacchi, all the surgeons in this list, with the exception of Gessi, were lecturers in surgery and anatomy from 1570 to the early years of the seventeenth century. Virtually all the Bolognese surgeons involved in the history of reconstructive surgery had something to do with this hospital. Aranzi, Tagliacozzi, and Cortesi were all involved in the history of reconstructive surgery, while Rota and Sacchi were their colleagues at the studio.

In the period between 1583 and 1599 (the year Tagliacozzi died and Cortesi left Bologna for Messina) these five physicians and surgeons are all listed on the official records of the studio as lecturers in surgery and charged with organizing the annual anatomical demonstration.[73] They were colleagues and rivals, especially for the chair of anatomy, a prestigious position not only for the studio but for the whole city, granted to Aranzi in 1570 and then passed on to his pupils and colleagues. Significantly, Tagliacozzi, when he moved to the much sought-after chair of theoretical medicine in the year 1590–1591, struggled to keep the title of anatomist. These five surgeons had different backgrounds. Aranzi and Tagliacozzi came from the artisanal class, Cortesi was born in a poor family, while Sacchi and Rota were part of medical families of Collegiate physicians. Aranzi, Tagliacozzi, and Cortesi all dealt in various ways with facial reconstruction, and all chose to publish books; Sacchi and Rota never published anything, and it is not clear whether they were involved in the procedure of surgical reconstruction. Two patterns emerge. First, not only many surgery lecturers had received clinical instruction at the hospital of Santa Maria della Morte but those who decided to publish came from the middle and lower classes, while those who did not came from upper-class established families. Second, for those who came from families who had other members in the elite medical profession, university education in surgery passed on among family members.

Aranzi was always listed as "ad anothomiam" until he died in 1589. After that, the other four surgeons were listed all together as anatomy chairs. Salaries varied, reflecting not only social status and seniority but also scientific prestige. In

1587 the Senate listed the following annual expenses: Aranzi, 1100 lire; Tagliacozzi, 600 lire; Sacchi, 590 lire; Rota, 280 lire; and finally Cortesi, 225 lire. Just to make a comparison, the best-paid professor in the arts faculty was Ulisse Aldrovandi with an annual stipend of 1775 lire.[74] Nine years later, in 1596, a document titled *Provisioni che si pagano a' Dottori* recorded by the Assunteria di Studio listed Tagliacozzi, then chair of theoretical medicine and anatomy, 890 lire; Sacchi, 880 lire; Rota, 570 lire; Cortesi, 425 lire.[75] Aranzi had the most important record of academic publications. The second best paid was Tagliacozzi, who was younger than Sacchi and with less seniority, probably on account of his practicing the most spectacular surgical procedure. Sacchi was an eminent person in the city, practicing for a wealthy clientele and for a number of institutions; Rota never published anything but came from a well-reputed family and was very popular among students. The worst paid was always Giovanni Battista Cortesi, the true outsider in terms of social background.

The first thing to understand is what was going on in the hospital of Santa Maria della Morte and how future learned surgeons were trained there.[76] Of the 30 hospitals composing the poor relief and health-care system of Bologna, only two of them – Santa Maria della Morte and Santa Maria della Vita – had a well-structured and hierarchically organized medical staff.[77]

The statutes of the hospital of Santa Maria della Morte were renewed in 1562 as part of the general renovation of health-care institutions of the period. One of the most interesting figures the new statutes introduced is that of the student assistant (*astante*). The *astante* was a complex figure in the social economy of the hospital. He was a medical student of modest means but greatly promising and thus was there to learn. He was at the same time the assistant of the physician and surgeon and ruled over the nurses. He oversaw the preparation of medicaments and the implementation of the dietetic regime, which were typical tasks of the learned physician or surgeon, and at the same time he had to take care of bloodletting, the hallmark of barber-surgeons, an officially subordinated professional figure. He had important diagnostic functions in that his opinion was required in cases of suspect incurable or contagious diseases. He entertained a nuanced relationship with the hospital "guardian": he was hierarchically subordinate to him, because the guardian had to check that *astante* put into practice all the instructions given by physicians and surgeons, but, on the other hand, he had to make sure that the guardian did not let anyone in without his own previous diagnostic assessment.[78]

The Italian sixteenth-century hospital had an educational or proto-clinical function. Jerome Bylebyl has described the innovation in teaching that took place in Padua by the 1540s, including the practice of bedside instruction at the hospital, and emphasized the role of Giovanni Da Monte, whose proto-clinical lectures were recorded and published by his students.[79] The hospital of Santa Maria della Morte – physically contiguous to the Archiginnasio – provided the cadavers for the public anatomical dissection. The cadavers literally passed from the hands of the hospital prior to the anatomist via the written authorization of the official of the criminal court. The anatomist then paid for the funerary rituals of the executed or of the poor who had died in the hospital.[80] A collection of *consilia* by the medicine professor Elideo Padoani (d. 1576) shows that he used to take his students to the hospital to follow him in bedside visits.[81] The Dutch physician and anatomist Volcher Coiter (1534–1576), student and then lecturer on surgery in Bologna in the 1560s, reported in his surgical and anatomical observations that

> in that hospital of Bologna which is called *hospitale della morte* I have dissected the body of a man killed by a long-lasting illness, whose liver was putrid and suppurating, so that I was barely able to extract one fourth of its substance.[82]

We can assume that this was not a singular event and that students and teachers gathered at the hospital to dissect bodies, perhaps in small groups.

It is within this context that Tagliacozzi learned how to open bodies, dress wounds, apply stitches, and perhaps experiment with skin grafting. By looking at his colleagues' career paths we will learn that his own career was not exceptional with respect to patterns of social mobility but only in its intensity.

One of the most important sources in order to sketch a group portrait of learned surgeons are the *civilitatis probationes*, a record of the interrogations of four witnesses conducted in order to admit candidates to the College. In this record, officials verified whether the candidates fulfilled the double citizenship requirement (the candidate plus his father or, better, his father and grandfather had to be Bolognese citizens).

In the case of Aranzi, this document indicates that his father was a simple baker (*fornario*) and that he learned all his Latin and his first medical notions from his maternal uncle, the learned surgeon Bartolomeo Maggi (1477–1552).[83] Aranzi indeed liked to add Maggi to his family name, in honor of his uncle, one of the first innovators in matters of gunshot wounds and professor of surgery at Bologna in the 1540s. Giulio Cesare Aranzi had the best record of publications and was renowned all over Europe. He published on anatomy, on the female organs of generation, and on surgical conditions, particularly tumors, ulcers, and aposteme.[84] Born around 1530, Aranzi made an extraordinary career, graduating, accessing the College of Medicine in 1562, and becoming the first official anatomist of the studio.

From Aranzi's will we grasp something of his fortunes and the kind of sociability he preferred. He had four daughters, for whom he provided a generous dowry; he was also generous with his wife Isabella, to whom he left 5000 lire, 1000 lire from her maternal dowry, plus several pieces of furniture. Isabella was also named the legal guardian of his two male heirs, Ottavio and Angelo, until they turned 20. Had Isabella died before they reached such an age, their legal guardianship would go to Paolo Bucchi, with whom Aranzi owned a silk workshop in partnership. This Paolo Bucchi seems to have been a rather important figure in Aranzi's life: according to the testamentary dispositions, the anatomist's older son, Ottavio, would inherit the silk workshop along with Bucchi's eldest son.[85]

Aranzi and Bucchi owned one of those artisanal workshop, and it is interesting to notice that the capital Aranzi accumulated in teaching and in private practice was invested in the largest proto-industrial productive enterprise of Bologna: in a way, he never cut his ties with the middle class. And his private practice must have been very profitable: Volcher Coiter, his pupil in the 1560s, recalls that Aranzi used to treat the injured members of the Senatorial class, including people from the powerful Senatorial Malvezzi family.[86] He was important enough to be mentioned in the chronicles of the city compiled by Antonio Francesco Ghiselli in the early eighteenth century. Ghiselli describes an important occasion in 1581, in which Aranzi served as lay expert in a case involving the highest civic and religious authorities.[87] Aranzi was in good terms with Ulisse Aldrovandi as well. Together, they wrote a response to a request of advice from the public health board concerning the 1575–1577 plague threat.[88]

Aranzi is a great example of a middle-class man who started a brilliant medical career through his maternal kinship and focused on publishing books of anatomical descriptions based on careful observations. In a way, Aranzi is a typical figure of post-Vesalian anatomy, caught in between traditional Galenism and the new spirit of observation. His *De humano foetu* was published in 1563, at the beginning of his career, and then reworked several times until the third and final edition of 1587; his *Liber anatomicarum observationum* was published for the first time in 1579, when he was already an important professor and influential member of the College, then republished in the edition containing all his works of 1587, and contained important new information on the physiology of blood and the anatomy of the brain.[89] Later in his life, when he was about to retire, he published on surgery. Moreover, he served as Prior of the College of Medicine several times. His career is an example of social mobility based on the prestige of academic writing, quality teaching, and the politics of the College.

Angelo Michele Sacchi and Flaminio Rota were different cases, and they make for an interesting comparison. They both came from families of upper-class physicians, and both never published a word in print. Angelo Michele Sacchi came from a family of *gentilhuomini*; he was not part of the Senatorial aristocracy but of a leisured class that exercised no "mechanical" trade. He occupied the position of lecturer in surgery at the studio from 1567 to 1611, the year of his death. Son of a Antonio Sacchi, a Collegiate physician and lecturer in surgery, he was admitted to the College of Medicine in 1576.[90]

The legacies he charged his son to pay for after his death show his own and his family's commitment to the hospital of Santa Maria della Morte.[91] Indeed, Sacchi appears as "graduate surgeon" of the hospital with the stipend of 110 lire per year for the period 1591–1611.[92]

Sacchi's private practice must have been flourishing too, considering the social rank of the patients he was caring for. An anonymous chronicler reports that on January 31, 1590, Count Andalò Bentivoglio, jousting with one member of the Ruini family, was hit by a splinter, which penetrated the visor of his helmet and lodged itself into the count's eye. One of the bystanders tried to pull it off, but in the meantime Angelo Michele Sacchi was called. The learned surgeon tried to pull off the splinter with his bare hands but finally used a big forceps and removed it. Unfortunately, Count Bentivoglio did not make it and "died because of the spasm and the harsh pain."[93] In another 1598 case, Sacchi worked together with Tagliacozzi and Giulio Cesare Gessi on treating another violent nobleman:

> It happened that Captain Flaminio Ringhiera from Strada Maggiore . . . after about one hour he ledt the Palace [of the Senate] with one of his servants to go home was assaulted near his house by some say four some say more assailants; the servant fled and he was wounded in two parts, one in the head and the other in the face, and the latter crossed his face and cut off his right ear in two . . . the miserable gentleman went to the above mentioned Confaloniere nearby the place he was attacked, and there was treated by Angleo Michele Sacchi, Giulio Cesare Gessi, and Gaspare Tagliacozzi.[94]

Sacchi used to deal with the same kind of disfiguring injuries that affected the faces and bodies of the upper classes of the city, but he never felt the need to publish something on his multiple and probably very interesting surgical practice. As a learned surgeon very well connected with a network of powerful Bolognese families and institutions, Sacchi could treat and observe several kinds of surgical conditions, affecting people of all social classes and genders. Still, or maybe because of this, he did not try to boost his reputation by making use of the printing press.

Flaminio Rota's social background was similar to Sacchi's, but he seems to have left fewer traces in the city archives. He was lecturer on surgery from 1579 to 1611 and the son of another surgery lecturer, Giovanni Francesco, after he had been student assistant at Santa Maria della Morte. In 1576, he was appointed "graduate surgeon" at the Saint Job Hospital of the Incurable and in 1585 was named "supernumerary surgeon" at the hospital of Santa Maria della Vita; finally, in 1592 he was admitted to the College of Medicine.[95] Like Sacchi, he combined the activities of lecturer and of hospital surgeon and recorded the events concerning his family in the chronicles: for example, he made a very good marriage in 1592, the same year he entered the College, with a Lucia Dolcini, who brought him a dowry of about 7,000 or 8,000 scudi.[96] Rota built his career upon his ability as a teacher, both in private and in public, and by exploiting the social prestige he inherited from his family tradition, But like Sacchi, he never published anything.

Giovanni Battista Cortesi explicitly took up the facial reconstructive technique in both his scholarship and his practice. Cortesi's path is the most singular, and it embodies the whole continuity between different kinds of practitioners of the body, in both cultural and social terms. Like Berengario da Carpi and Niccolò Massa in the first half of the century, Cortesi was the last of the sixteenth-century poor barber-surgeons who became learned physicians and surgeons, even if he was accepted as one of the elite only after considerable tribulations. But it is true that social mobility and cultural contiguity between all the professions and practices that dealt with the external parts of the body were much higher in the sixteenth than in the following century.[97]

Early modern and modern biographers of Cortesi report an interesting story about his early years, of which I have not found any archival trace and of which Cortesi himself never says a word in his printed works.[98] The story, first told by Girolamo Ghilini in his *Theatro d'huomini letterati* (1647), goes like this: Cortesi was a poor boy, an apprentice in the art of barbers and a steam bath attendant (*stufaiolo*); he became a barber at the hospital of Santa Maria della Morte when he was about 16, and there he showed his "amazing" will to learn. He started to study Latin and natural philosophy thanks to the generosity of an anonymous grammar teacher who noticed the exceptional intellect of that poor bath attendant; he then studied and acquired medical experience by following the hospital physicians and surgeons in their daily visits; finally, he got his degree in medicine (although not in philosophy) in 1583, and in that very same year he was named lecturer in surgery. That was only the start – if belated – of a brilliant career.[99]

Sources uniformly repeat the fact that he was 16 when he started working at the hospital, so it must have been 1568 or 1570, during Tagliacozzi's tenure as assistant. In any case, what "saved" him from a life of poverty, ignorance, and immorality was the hospital, where he not only studied for about ten years privately and more or less formally but also became assistant in 1580, for the regular three years, until his graduation. Significantly enough, in December 1585, once he had been appointed lecturer in surgery at the studio already, he was paid 18 lire "for letting blood to the poor in the hospital (*per havere cavato sangue alli poveri mentre egli stava nello Spitalle*)," a sign that his ties with the hospital continued, and that he did not disdain to practice the task of a barber-surgeon even after graduation.[100] In 1583 he was made public lecturer in surgery, "even if he had never lectured in logic,"[101] which was the preliminary mandatory teaching for young lecturers.[102]

In the meantime, his career and fame as a teacher and author started to pick up. He was appointed as anatomy demonstrator and started to publish on surgical matters.[103] In the early 1590s Cortesi served as military surgeon for the Bolognese troops in the war several popes waged against the bandits in the countryside in the last decades of the sixteenth century.[104] Cortesi never highlighted the experience he gained on the battlefield in his printed works; on the contrary, in these books he rather stressed his learned training at the studio under the guidance of Aranzi and Tagliacozzi and his animal dissections with the great Ulisse Aldrovandi in the latter's private museum.[105]

In the years 1592–1593 Cortesi got very close to the peak of his professional success in Bologna. In the spring of 1592, between April and July, his candidacy to enter the College of Medicine was taken into consideration and his *civilitatis probatio* examined in the rooms of the College. Cortesi regularly presented four witnesses, all highly respectable citizens, among them Ercole Bentivogli, son of the Senator Antonio. There was a problem though, in that one of the witnesses, the rich merchant Giovanni Battista Avanzi, could not say that Elia, Cortesi's father, was a citizen and instead declared: "I have met Elia Cortesi, tailor, and I know that he was not born in Bologna, but he has lived here for a long time."[106] Despite the fact that Cortesi's grandfather, Bolognino, was a true Bolognese citizen and that Cortesi himself was born in Bologna, the examining board of the College took this problem very seriously. The fact that only Giovanni Battista's grandfather and not his father were verified Bolognese citizens turned out to be a problem, as it is revealed by the other proofs of citizenship, which all insisted on the citizenship of both the candidate's fathers and grandfathers.[107] So, the College ordered a search in the archives of the Duomo of San Pietro for Elia's baptismal record, but this could not be found.[108] Cortesi was not admitted to the College. The missing proof of Elia's citizenship got thrown in the mix with other troubling factors, such as the poverty and low status of Cortesi's family and his lack of degree in philosophy. The Collegiate must have thought that social mobility should be limited somehow.[109]

Cortesi must have been disappointed. Despite all his services to the city and his experience, he was still the least paid of his cohort of surgery and anatomy professors. And of course he was not a member of the College. On the other hand, students must have loved him. There are two memorials dedicated by the students to Cortesi as lecturer in anatomy: one is from 1591 and the other from 1597.[110] In the end of 1598 Cortesi finally accepted an offer from the recently founded University of Messina, in the kingdom of Naples.[111] When he left for Messina, Cortesi definitely had the hope of coming back to finally get what he wanted in Bologna. But that never happened. Cortesi built a new life in Messina. During his travel to Southern Italy he did not miss the chance to visit Tropea, the city where the first and famous reconstructive surgeons had lived and worked, curious to meet them and to see what kind of procedure they employed. He found no more members of the Vianeo family living and practicing, but someone showed him their old instruments, which he judged very rough and "primitive" compared to those designed by his teacher Tagliacozzi.[112] In his 1625 account of the trip, Cortesi presented himself as the heir to the Bolognese tradition of facial surgery, at the same time acknowledging and paying tribute to the inventors of the method, two sons of the Kingdom of Naples. Cortesi became quite famous and respected at that young and dynamic studio, which had an aggressive hiring policy and offered high salaries to its recruits. In 1604, he was admitted to the local College of Physicians in Messina.[113]

A clear idea of his strategies of self-fashioning is given by his constant tactic of recalling his Bolognese training and of embracing one of the most spectacular surgical procedures of the times – that reconstructive surgery of the nose of which he wrote the second most detailed account after Tagliacozzi's – even if a much more dry and technical one. The best example of Cortesi's self-fashioning is given by his 1629 *Pharmacopeia, seu Antidotarium Messanense*, the official list of ingredients and recipes all apothecary shops of the city must comply to in preparing medicaments. In this work, Cortesi recalled that the famous Bolognese jurist and professor of law Andrea Barbato had proposed to him to go to Messina to teach in 1598.[114] But on the frontispiece the most famous Bolognese doctors, most prominently Aldrovandi, who is placed at the center, are at the top: Cortesi lived his whole professional life at Messina while underscoring his Bolognese origins and education.

Between 1618 and 1620, after almost 15 years, the Bolognese studio tried to call back its lost professor.[115] The negotiation did not go anywhere. In 1625 Cortesi decided, perhaps as part of his strategy of self-fashioning – after all, Bologna wanted him back and he refused – to publish a touching 1619 letter to Camillo Baldi, who had written to him relating the Senate's offer. This letter is a document of a life spent in medicine, the life of someone who would have liked to stay in his hometown but ended up building his reputation elsewhere.[116] After his Bolognese beginnings as an author and editor, Cortesi published all his works much later, between 1625 and 1635. Besides the *Miscellanea*, the most original and autobiographical of his books, he wrote a manual of surgery, a manual of practical medicine, a pharmacopeia, and a learned commentary on Hippocrates.

Patients and practitioners

This group portrait of the Bolognese graduate surgeons shows that a certain degree of social mobility was granted to the sons of the middle class when they applied themselves to both manual and intellectual work. These men must have felt a mix of fascination and repulsion for "natural born" noblemen. After all, noblemen could be learned surgeons' best clients, but noblemen must have never lost their sense of superiority toward these "new men" who ascended from a lower class. Tagliacozzi's book, as well as those of the other surgeons who wrote about reconstructive surgery, was full of references to the culture of honor and of the face and to the upper-class masculinity that valued physical strength and bravery in bearing all kinds of suffering. Tagliacozzi mentioned duels fought by gentlemen from Piacenza in the letter to Mercuriale, and we have seen that Piacenza was one of the places where the Inquisition's dispositions against duel encountered strong resistance. Moreover, the surgeon made several references to the "sword" (*ferro*) in *De curtorum*. For example, he said that lips were close to the nose and often they helped it perform its functions, and they were "particularly vulnerable to injuries occurred in dueling."[117] Moreover, the dedication of *De curtorum* to Vincenzo Gonzaga – once again, the Mantua court became specialized in chivalric science in the sixteenth century – said that

> the house of Gonzaga has always been known for its prowess with swords. Because camp followers and those who deal with arms often incur this

> type of injury, I thought it fitting to dedicate a book dealing with martial injuries to military men.[118]

Below the idealized surface of both chivalric science and Tagliacozzi's learned monograph, the early modern graduate surgeon had to deal with more mundane affairs and types of injury. Reading Bologna's chronicles it appears that Tagliacozzi was known among noble circles and often called upon by them for more or less serious episodes of violence and street fights involving firearms as well as knives and swords. In November 1580, after a fight for a futile reason among one member of the Pepoli and someone from the Castelli families, a chain of crossed vendettas started in Bologna and moved to Florence, where Tagliacozzi had to intervene to treat three men injured by firearms.[119] In February 1592, Tagliacozzi was called from Bologna to the nearby small town of Imola to treat local noblemen who injured themselves in a street fight with both swords and firearms and took the time to teach the local barber-surgeons how to correctly dress a gunshot wound.[120] In 1594, at the moment of his greatest renown, the physician traveled all the way to Vienna to treat Virginio Orsini (1572–1615), a very powerful Roman nobleman wounded in the war against the "Turks."[121]

The relationship between doctors and noblemen was not an easy one, and all the more so in cases in which doctors where men who came from the artisanal class. Class interacted with gender. Recent historiography on masculinity in premodern European history has stressed the importance of studying men-men and men-women relations in their historical contingency, without assuming that a fixed male identity would have remained constant throughout history. Historians have insisted on the fact that patriarchy must be historicized.[122] A historical use of the tool of gender and masculinity is most useful to understand the rise of reconstructive surgery.

In the sixteenth century, noblemen lived in a culture of patrilineal kinship structures, of aggressive competition with their peers, and of contempt for lower-class men, and they were used to considering women as "currency." Besides all this, noblemen's political role was a delicate matter in late sixteenth-century Bologna, because in the Papal state, as elsewhere, new ideals of good male citizenship were emerging. On the other hand, the world of crafts, and to a certain extent of health-care professionals, was more open to cognates and horizontal kinship structures (recall that Aranzi received his first medical education from his maternal uncle, Bartolomeo Maggi) and had to deal with women in a different way than noblemen. At least women could work as midwives and could own apothecary and barber shops. Aranzi, Tagliacozzi, and Cortesi had been able to climb the social ladder and to confront themselves with a different kind of men: those of the ruling class. The patients who were financially and morally able to look for this kind of procedure were all members of the noble and ruling class who injured themselves in fights, jousts, duels, and war. Tagliacozzi was a physician coming from the artisanal class who treated noble patients, thus occupying a delicate and liminal social and gender position. As a man, he was not part of the culture of honor and arms by birth, and he raised above those men practicing mechanical arts only by virtue of his education and skills in medicine and surgery. Doctors of medicine were experiencing in a positive way the emergence of new roles of civic officials, while at the same time dwelling in a liminal space between the artisanal culture and the noble culture, of which they were part only because of the formal privileges accorded by Charles V to Collegiate doctors in 1530. This encounter between different kinds of men was mediated by several cultural and scientific factors that I will take into account in the following chapters.

Notes

1 *Tribuni della plebe* were a traditional communal four-month magistracy that had the purpose of balancing the aristocratic side of the city government. Together with the Magistrati dei Collegi, they had economic functions of regulation of food prices.

2 BUB 3839, *Cronica, o sia Diario di Francesco Galliani (1589–1600)*, fol. 83v: "Adì 7 di Novembre [1599] passò di questa vita lo eccellente dottore in Medicina Gaspare Tagliacozzo famosissimo più che alcun altro fosse di nostra età nell'arte della Cirusia, il quale faceva il naso, labra et orecchie a quelli li erano state tagliate per ferite, o altro [. . .] fu figliolo d'un povero falegname, e con la sua virtù ha guadagnato, e lascia il valore di scudi 30.000."

3 Tagliacozzi noticed the remaking of the façade of the hospital between 1565 and 1566, when he was a student about to become assistant (*astante*) of the official surgeons and physician of the hospital: see BUB 1413, fol. 165v-166r. The title of the chronicle listed in the BUB catalogue, *Cronica di Bologna d'Auttore Ignoto che comincia dal 404 e seguita sino al 1585. Portata dall'Idioma Latino In Italiano da Gasparo Tagliacozzi l'Anno 1594*, is doubly incorrect. The manuscript is actually divided into two parts: the first part, up to folio 161v, ends with the reform of the Senate, the end of the Bentivogli rule, and the victory of pope Julius II in 1506, and it is signed: "Laus Deo. Acta Bononiae die quarto mensis Maii anno 1564. Per Gasparem Tagliacotium, ex latino sermone educta." Then there is a second part, undated, which goes up to 1597 but does not record the events in chronological order, which was written by Tagliacozzi himself. So, the correct end date is 1597, not 1594. Indeed, on folio 165r the author recorded the death of the Duke of Ferrara: "In the year 1597 the news came to Bologna that Alfonso d'Este Duke of Ferrara had died (*Nell'anno 1597 vene la nova a bologna della morte del ducha Alfonso da este ducha di Ferrara*)."

4 Ibid., fol. 24r.

5 Claudio Donati, *L'idea di nobiltà in Italia: Secoli XIV–XVIII* (Rome: Laterza, 1988), p. 56; see also Jonathan Dewald, *The European Nobility, 1400–1800* (Cambridge: Cambridge University Press, 1996); Giancarlo Angelozzi, *La nobiltà disciplinata: violenza nobiliare, procedure di giustizia e scienza cavalleresca a Bologna nel XVII secolo* (Bologna: CLUEB, 2003).

6 See Sanjay Subrhamanyan, "Connected Histories: Notes towards a Reconfiguration of Early Modern Eurasia," *Modern Asian Studies* 31 (1997): 735–762; Randolph Starn, "The Early Modern Muddle," *Journal of Early Modern History* 6, 3 (2002): 296–307; Jan De Vries, "The Limits of Globalization in the Early Modern World," *Economic History Review* 63, 3 (2010): 710–733. For the place of early modern Italy within "global history," see Giuseppe Marcocci, "L'Italia nella prima età globale (ca 1300–1700)," *Storica* 60 (2014): 7–50.

7 The manuscript is titled *Descrizione della città, territorio, qualità, costumi e forma del governo del popolo di Bologna, e necessary avvertimenti a chi desidera di ben governare un tal Stato. Il tutto fatto dal dottor Camillo Baldi professore di filosofia nello Studio della città di Bologna l'anno*

di nostra salute 1605. Baldi was born in 1551 from a noble family, and his father was a professor of medicine and philosophy. He became a member of the College of Physicians and Philosophers, was a colleague of Aranzi, Tagliacozzi, and Cortesi, and taught theoretical medicine, philosophy, and logic at the studio for 59 years. He wrote on topics as diverse as practical philosophy, chivalric sciences, and physiognomy, that which makes him a very representative figure of the cultural context of reconstructive surgery and a direct witness to it. Baldi was also named overseer of the Aldrovandi Museum and died in 1637. The *Descrizione* was probably commissioned by a Cardinal Giustiniani, who would become Cardinal Legate of Bologna the following year. See Mario Fanti, "Le classi sociali e il governo di Bologna all'inizio del secolo XVII in un'opera inedita di Camillo Baldi," *Strenna Storica Bolognese* 11 (1961): 133–179. See also Giancarlo Angelozzi, "Nobili, mercanti, dottori, cavalieri, artigiani: stratificazione sociale e ideologia a Bologna nei secoli XVI e XVIII," in Walter Tega, ed. *Storia Illustrata di Bologna* (Bologna: Nuova Editoriale AIEP, 1989), vol. 2, pp. 41–60.

8 On the political structure of Bologna in the early modern period, see Angela de Benedictis, "Il governo misto," in Adriano Prosperi, ed. *Storia di Bologna, Vol. 3.1: Bologna nell'età moderna, istituzioni, forme del potere, economia e società* (Bologna: Bononia University Press, 2008), pp. 201–270.

9 BCAB, B. 3587: *Descrizione della città, territorio, qualità, costumi e forma del governo del popolo di Bologna, e necessary avvertimenti a chi desidera di ben governare un tal Stato. Il tutto fatto dal dottor Camillo Baldi professore di filosofia nello Studio della città di Bologna l'anno di nostra salute 1605*, fol. 64–65: "Definiscono l'Ordine Cavalleresco esser quello, che per nobiltà, per richezze gl'altri Cittadini precede. Nobile chiamano li Bolognesi, colui, che è nato d'un antica e onorata famiglia, dalla quale sempre siano state possedute molte ricchezze, e sicome senza il lume non si vede colore, o Pittura, sia quanto si voglia bella, così senza ricchezza non mirano ne considerano la Nobiltà, e sogliono li Nobili venuti in povertà dire, che già erano Nobili, ma ora sono caduti ed abbassati; e forse non senza qualche cagione, perché veramente il Nobile deve essere magnanimo, magnifico, e liberale, ma quando non ha robba, non può fare alcuna di queste cose: però fatto povero, è fatto ignobile ancora, perché non può Nobilmente operare. L'altra ragione è perché non può esser Nobile veramente dove non è virtù, ne può essere virtù dove non è senno e giudizio: il gittar il suo, e per qualunque cagione diventar povero, è segno di poco cervello, e di mancamento di giudizio, perciò ne segue, che il Nobile con le ricchezze perda la Nobiltà ancora; ne occorre dar la colpa alla fortuna, o ad altra cagione, percioché ogni uomo è fabro della fortuna sua." The narrow correspondence between class and political role of the Bolognese citizens is confirmed by the contemporary manuscript by Ciro Spontone on the governmental organization of Bologna: see Sandra Verardi Ventura, "'L'ordinamento Bolognese Dei Secoli XVI–XVII.' Introduzione all'edizione Del Ms. B 1114," *L'Archiginnasio* 76 (1981): 349–354.

10 BCAB, B. 3587, fol. 75: "Si dilettano questi Signori di abitar nobilmente, vestir bene, aver compagnia quando vanno fuora, alloggiano Forastieri . . . molti si compiacciono si suoni e di canti, di nuove, di ciancie oziose."

11 During the late sixteenth century and the early seventeenth a harsh fight between the Colleges of doctors and the Senate went on in Bologna, particularly concerning the government of the "Gabella grossa," the fund, coming from taxation, destined to pay for the lecturers' salaries; see Gian Paolo Brizzi, "Lo Studio di Bologna tra *orbis academicus* e mondo cittadino," in Adriano Prosperi, ed. *Storia di Bologna, vol. 3, tomo II: Cultura, istituzioni culturali, Chiesa e vita religiosa* (Bologna: Bononia University Press, 2008); Verardi Ventura, "'L'ordinamento Bolognese'," pp. 352–353.

12 BCAB, B. 3587, fol. 19: "precedono per antico uso li Cavalieri, e dopo li Magistrati fra i Laici vengono in primo luogo."

13 Ibid., fol. 70–71: "l'una è quella delle Lettere, e delle Scienze, che sono utili, e necessarie, l'altra della robba . . . oltra quel darli la strada negli scontri, li Nobili poco caso fanno di loro, se non quando e quanto ne hanno bisogno; e da certi anni in qua, molti di questi del primo ordine non attendono alle Lettere, se non quando le stimano scala

per salire alla Corte di Roma, e agl'uffizii, che in quella si dispensano, altrimenti le sprezzano, e se ne ridono."

14 Ibid., fol. 71–72.

15 This was an editorial phenomenon as well: 27 books were printed between 1550 and 1563 on matters regarding the chivalric science of honor and duels; see Donati, *L'idea di nobiltà*, p. 94. The cultural elaboration of the literature on chivalric sciences has been defined as "one of the few avenues for the political debate in Italy," especially because of the problem of "*precedenze*," namely the problem of social and political primacy. Chivalric science literature reflected the fragmented composition of the upper classes, and at the same time it constituted the common language of all these fragmentary components; see Giancarlo Angelozzi, "Cultura dell'onore, codici di comportamento nobiliare e Stato nella Bologna pontificia: un'ipotesi di lavoro," *Annali dell'Istituto Storico Italo-Germanico in Trento* 8 (1982): 305–324.

16 Luiz Beja de Pestrelo, *Responsionum casuum conscientiae* (Venice: apud Io. Baptistam, Io. Bernardum Sessam, 1597), part II, p. 1; quoted by Ottavia Niccoli, *Storie di ogni giorno in una città del Seicento* (Rome: Laterza, 2000), p. 171.

17 One of the most crucial debates running through this literature concerned who could deal with honor, what kinds of men, what social classes. Experts of the chivalric sciences argued that only noblemen had honor to defend. In practice though, historians have showed that the lower classes, and sometimes women too, could fight for their honor and could put their honor at stake in public, even if dominant discourse made honor the upper-class male value par excellence; see Niccoli, *Storie di ogni giorno*.

18 Girolamo Muzio, *Il duello* (Venice: appresso Gabriel Giolito de Ferrari e fratelli, 1550), fol. 84r: "Et la opinione de' cavalieri è, che legge alcuna né di patria, né di principe, né interesse di havere, né di vita, all'honore non debba essere anteposta; e che non ostante alcuna costituzione, né pericolo di perdita, i cavalieri alla legge dell'honore debbano obbedire: la quale è, che dove altri è chiamato per via ordinaria alla pruova di arme, là se ne debba incontanente con prontezza di animo caminare; e che quale altramente fa, non sia degno di essere annoverato fra cavalieri honorati."

19 The literature on early modern duel has grown in the past three decades. These works have been especially useful for this work: Francesco Erspamer, *La biblioteca di don Ferrante: Duello e onore nella cultura del Cinquecento* (Rome: Bulzoni, 1982); Marco Cavina, *Il sangue dell'onore: storia del duello* (Rome: Laterza, 2005); David Quint, "Duelling and Civility in Sixteenth Century Italy," *I Tatti Studies in the Italian Renaissance* 7 (1997): 231–278; Edward Muir, *Mad Blood Stirring: Vendetta in Renaissance Italy* (Baltimore: Johns Hopkins University Press, 1998); François Billacois, *The Duel: Its Rise and Fall in Early Modern France*, tr. Trista Selous (New Haven: Yale University Press, 1990); Thomas V. Cohen, "The Lay Liturgy of Affront in Sixteenth-Century Italy," *Journal of Social History* 25, 4 (1992): 857–877.

20 Billacois, *The Duel*, pp. 8–14.

21 Cavina, *Il sangue*, p. 41.

22 As Mario Sbriccoli has argued, the centralizing model of penal justice ignited a conflict with older modes of communitarian ways of doing justice. Sbriccoli has described a system of *"hegemonic justice" opposed to one of "negotiated justice"* in the early modern states, a regime in which justice lived through an informal network of mediators, negotiators, and peace-makers, which was different, if not always opposed, to a conception of justice as a formal damage to the State. Early modern people used to believe that "justice" was located in the informal and communitarian network, rather than the formal apparatus. See Mario Sbriccoli, "Fonti giudiziarie e fonti giuridiche. Riflessioni sulla fase attuale degli studi di storia del crimine e della giustizia criminale," *Studi Storici* 29, 2 (1988): 491–501.

23 Cavina, *Il sangue*, pp. 43–44.

24 Ibid., pp. 72–73.

25 Ibid., p. 74. Other causes of duel included to defend, exalt, or avenge the honor of a woman, whether she was a wife, a daughter, or a mistress; belonging to rival camps

(mainly to different confessions); fighting for a public office (dueling was a means to prove that the post was not merited); deciding legal cases (when trials were too long and intricate); precedence, or fighting for prestige and material symbols (such as dresses, seating, rank in ceremonies, etc.); fighting just for "fun"; see Billacois, *The Duel*, pp. 8–14.

26 Quoted by Cavina, *Il sangue*, pp. 109–110. Before Trent, several popes had issued similar statements. Julius II in the *Regis pacifici* bull (1509) issued a solemn condemnation of duels for honor as a case of private violence and the propensity to fight long-lasting feuds on the part of the noble class. Leo X's *Quam Deo* bull (1519) confirmed the severe prohibitions and the picture of the duel as a threat to the order of the State, providing for punishments like excommunication, *damnatio memoriae*, confiscation of all property, including the lands, and fines for the spectators. Julius III in the *Cum sicut accepimus* (1554) reaffirmed the need to repress duels, confirming that the practice was far from gone. Pius IV, in the *Ea quae* bull (1556), extended the prohibition to all Christianity, not just the Pontifical State. See Giancarlo Angelozzi, "La proibizione del duello: Chiesa e ideologia nobiliare," in Paolo Prodi and Wolfgang Reinhard, eds. *Il concilio di Trento e il moderno* (Bologna: Il mulino, 1996), pp. 271–308, especially pp. 278–282.

27 Duels were outlawed in Naples in 1540 (passible capital punishment); in Venice in 1541 (passible of banishment); in Milan in 1541 (punishable by death and confiscation of property); in Mantua in 1543 (punishable by confiscation of paternal property); in the Papal States, including Bologna of course, in 1543; and in the Duchy of Parma in 1546 (in both cases punishable by capital execution and confiscation of goods): see Donati, *L'idea di nobiltà*, p. 102. The text of the decree challenged the noble class' customs and ideology. But the decree itself was the outcome of a compromise between two parties within the Church that were divided on the matter, perfectly reflecting a general cultural ambivalence between tolerance and condemnation of aristocratic rituals. The Council fathers devoted very little time to the topic of the duel, but duel was the object of at least three-century-long discussions in Church decrees, canon law literature, and confessors' manuals. Within this long tradition, duels could fall under the rubric of *inculpata tutela*, which admitted the use of private violence in certain cases as a measure of self-defense. And indeed, the text of the decree of the Council had some ambiguous elements and reflected the different views of its extensors. The debate over the text prohibiting duels was marked by a division among the "rigorists," who also wanted to put books on duels to the index and pushed for harsher punishments, and the "laxists," who claimed that Scriptures never forbade it, that the reference to the Devil's work was excessive, and that more tolerance for duels was in order, when such duels were taking place in private. This whole affair did not end in 1563 either. The Bolognese pope Gregory XIII (ruled 1572–1585) in the 1570s and early 1580s made clear that the condemnation referred to all forms of duel, but he never mentioned honor. Furthermore, Gregory made a distinction between duel and fight or brawl (*rixa*), thus leaving a door open for a much more agile and informal form of duel that in the meanwhile had spread across Italy. Clement VIII (ruled 1592–1605) issued his *Illius vices* bull in 1592, a text produced in a very difficult environment marked by a strong preoccupation for public order in the Pontifical State, mostly due to banditry and famine. Clement explicitly connected his condemnation to the knightly (*more cavalleresco)* duel. See Angelozzi, "La proibizione del duello."

28 Quoted by Angelozzi, "La proibizione," p. 268: "Honor pluris valet, quam alia bona fortunae."

29 Fabio Albergati, *Trattato del modo di ridurre a pace l'inimicitie private* (Rome: per Francesco Zannetti, 1583). This seems to be an Italian version of the much more elaborated French debate concerning the nobility of the robe and the nobility of the sword: see Robert Descimon, "The Birth of the Nobility of the Robe: Dignity versus Privilege in the Parlement of Paris, 1500–1700," in Michael Wolfe, ed. *Changing Identities in Early Modern France* (Durham: Duke University Press, 1996).

30 Claudio Donati, "A Project of Expurgation by the Congregation of the Index: Treatises on Dueling," in Gigliola Fragnito, ed. *Church, Censorship and Culture in Early Modern Italy* (Cambridge: Cambridge University Press, 2001), pp. 134–161.

31 Donati, "A Project of Expurgation," pp. 144–145.

32 See Irene Fosi, *La società violenta: il banditismo nello Stato pontificio nella seconda metà del Cinquecento* (Rome: Edizioni dell'Ateneo, 1985); Gherardo Ortalli, ed., *Bande Armate, Banditi, Banditismo E Repressione Di Giustizia Negli Stati Europei Di Antico Regime: Atti Del Convegno, Venezia, 3–5 Nov* (Rome: Jouvence, 1986); Andrea Gardi, *Lo Stato in Provincia: L'amministrazione Della Legazione Di Bologna Durante Il Regno Di Sisto V (1585–1590)* (Bologna: Istituto per la storia di Bologna, 1994); Giampiero Brunelli, *Soldati del papa: politica militare e nobiltà nello Stato della Chiesa (1560–1644)* (Rome: Carocci, 2003); Irene Polverini Fosi, *Papal Justice: Subjects and Courts in the Papal State, 1500–1750* (Washington, DC: Catholic University of America Press, 2011).

33 BAB, A. 1361, *Trattato del Duello*, fol. 11v-12r: "in quella città dove sia introdotto il Duello, parrebbe, che i cittadini per non rimanere, non solo dishonorati, ma ancora empii, dovessero di necessità essercitarlo, et massimamente poiché a soldati, et a cavalieri et a gli huomini honorati non pare in alcun altra maniera convenevole il risentirsi in cotali casi . . . et che il ricorrere a i magistrati, et al Prencipe sia stimata communemente cosa indegna d'huomo honorato; ma conveniente a femina che non havendo in se fortezza alcuna si riprara con lo scudo della giustitia, scudo vergognoso a soldati, et a huomini d'honore, dovendo esser il lor tribunale quello dell'armi."

34 When passing through Bologna in his Italian journey in the 1580s, Michel de Montaigne paused to notice the famous and celebrated schools of arms and fencing, the studio, and the fact that Bolognese noblemen used to divide up in two parties, the Spanish and the French, and to fight against each other; see Michel de Montaigne, *Journal de voyage en Italie* (Paris: Les Belles Lettres, 1946), pp. 154–157. A public decree dated October 1584 forbids to carry the signs and things that mean belonging to a certain "faction" against others, because "non deve esser altro nome, altra Fattione, ne altra insegna, che della Chiesa." Reference to foreign names and symbols, probably the French versus Spaniard parties mentioned by Montaigne; see ASB, Legato, Bandi.

35 ASB, Assunteria di Sanità, Bandi Bolognesi, b. 1: *Bandi generali del Ill. e Reverendissimo Monsignor Fabio Mirto Arcivescovo di Nazarette Governatore di Bologna. Pubblicato in Bologna alli xvii di Febraro, & reiterato alli xviii & xix detto 1575*: "si ordina che qualunque persona di qual si voglia conditione, che con Arme, o qual si voglia instromento farà sfregio, segno, o cicatrice da restarsi perpetuamente in faccia, o in qual altro luoco della persona apparente, o li mozzarà, o debilitarà alcun membro, incorrerà nella pena di scudi duecento d'applicarsi, & c. & di altre pene ancora corporali."

36 Guy Bonhomme, "Le cheval comme instrument du movement humain à la Renaissance," in Jean Céard, Marie Madeleine Fontaine and Jean-Claude Margolin, eds. *Le corps à la Renaissance* (Paris: Aux amateurs des livres, 1990); Georges Vigarello, "The Upward Training the Body from the Age of Chivalry to Courtly Civility," in Michael Feher, ed. *Fragments for a History of the Human Body*, 3 vols. (New York: Zone Books, 1989), vol. 2, pp. 148–199.

37 Achille Morozzo, *Opera nova* (Venice: ad instanza de Melchior Sessa, 1550), fol. 124r-v: "tanto e più quanto che per la sua percussione causa maggior dolore, & per questo ha maggior honore . . . membro inutile, nel capo, e vile . . . puzolenti vapori della testa . . . Perdere il naso, è maggior vituperio, attento che essendo la faza humana assimigliata al volto divino, totalmente per la perdita del naso resta molto deturbata, perdendo la ornate belleza, alla quale non è alcuno remedio, ne potria per coprimento celare tale deformità del naso tagliato . . . è magior pena e incarico per exemplo uno che perde el naso, come quello el quale gli more lo unico figliolo ha magior dolore di quelli che havendone dui, li more solamente uno . . . non si può fare magiore improperio, e ingiuria al huomo vivente, che privalo del naso, per el quale è magiore offesa che se d'un piede, d'una mano, o d'un ochio lo privasse, perché è più manifesta cosa: cioè vergogna, e per questo per una gran pena se sole uno delinquente alla privatione del naso condannare, acioché porta per eternale pena in su la faza de continuo la sua vergognosa punitione, la quale non può in niuno modo coprire."

38 Filippo De Vivo, *Information and Communication in Venice: Rethinking Early Modern Politics* (Oxford: Oxford University Press, 2007), p. 101.

39 On this point, see Sandra Cavallo, *Artisans of the Body in Early Modern Italy: Identities, Families and Masculinities* (Manchester: Manchester University Press, 2010), pp. 1–7. As the bibliography used in this work will show, this is not exactly true. In the last three decades surgeons have become interesting for historians, although generally in light of a history of professionalization more than that of a cultural history of the body. It is true though that surgeons are very rarely the specific focus of monographs on pre-modern science and medicine. This is probably due to the fact that it is often very hard to track down a category that was so multifaceted. On the other hand, there is substantial "internalist" literature on the history of surgeons written by practicing surgeons, at least since the eighteenth century.

40 On the early institutional and academic teaching of surgery in medieval Italian universities, see Nancy Siraisi, *Medieval and Early Renaissance Medicine* (Chicago: The University of Chicago Press, 1990), pp. 153–186; Tiziana Pesenti, "'Professores chirurgie', 'medici ciroici' e 'barbitonsores' a Padova nell'età di Leonardo Buffi da Bertapaglia († dopo il 1448)," *Quaderni per la Storia dell'Università di Padova* 11 (1978): 1–38; Michael McVaugh, *The Rational Surgery of the Middle Ages* (Florence: SISMEL/Edizioni del Galluzzo, 2006). On early modern surgery, see Richard Palmer, "Physicians and Surgeons in Sixteenth-Century Venice," *Medical History* 23, 4 (1979): 451–460; Cavallo, *Artisans of the Body*; David Gentilcore, *Medical Charlatanism in Early Modern Italy* (Oxford: Oxford University Press, 2006), pp. 182–187; Maria Conforti, "Chirurghi, mammane, ciarlatani. Pratica medica e controllo delle professioni," in Antonio Clericuzio and Germana Ernst, eds. *Il Rinascimento italiano e l'Europa. Volume 5: Le scienze* (Treviso: Angelo Colla Editore, 2008), pp. 323–340, especially pp. 324–327. On the institutional settings of surgery in England, see Margaret Pelling, *The Common Lot: Sickness, Occupations and the Urban Poor in Early Modern England* (London: Longman, 1998), pp. 203–229; Celeste Catherine Chamberland, "Honor, Brotherhood, and the Corporate Ethos of London's Barber-Surgeons' Company, 1570–1640," *Journal of the History of Medicine and Allied Sciences* 64, 3 (2009): 300–332. For Edinburgh, see Helen M. Dingwall, *Physicians, Surgeons and Apothecaries: Medicine in Seventeenth-Century Edinburgh* (East Linton: Tuckwell Press, 1995), pp. 34–98. For Paris, see Toby Gelfand, *Professionalizing Modern Medicine: Paris Surgeons and Medical Science and Institutions in the 18th Century* (Westport: Greenwood Press, 1980), pp. 21–27. For the Netherlands, see Daniel de Moulin, *A History of Surgery: With Emphasis on the Netherlands* (Dordrecht: Maryinus Nijhoff Publishers, 1988), pp. 46–94.

41 Scipione Mercurio, *De gli errori popolari d'Italia libri sette* (Padua: ad'Istanza di Francesco Bolzetta, 1645), pp. 208–209: "hora questi tali subbito, che si veggono licentiati, credono di essere addottorati, e così crede anco il Volgo, il quale subito incomincia a dargli del Signor Dottor per la testa, e loro addormentati da queste continue cantilene facilmente lo credono . . . e quando vogliono insegnar lor case, dicono domandate la casa del Dottor Ciroico . . . che alcuni Dottori di Medicina, medicano di Cirugia, dalla quale per il frequente uso sono chiamat Cirugici."

42 *Itinerary written by Fynem Moryson, gent.* [1617], quoted in Edward P. De G. Chaney, "Giudizi inglesi su ospedali italiani, 1545–1789," in *Timore e carità: i poveri nell'Italia moderna. Atti del Convegno "Pauperismo e assistenza negli antichi stati italiani" (Cremona, 28–30 marzo 1980)* (Cremona: Biblioteca statale e libreria civica di Cremona, 1982), pp. 77–101, 80.

43 Mercurio, *De gli errori*, p. 209: "questo nasce . . . perché ognun non ha stomaco da essercitarla: e perciò vien permesso ad alcuni manuali detti cirugici licentiati, che curino piaghe, posteme, nettino martie, facciano taste & stendino ceroti."

44 Gianna Pomata, *Contracting a Cure: Patients, Healers, and the Law in Early Modern Bologna* (Baltimore: Johns Hopkins University Press, 1998), pp. 1–24; Claudia Pancino, "Malati, medici, mammane e saltimbanchi. malattia e cura nella Bologna moderna," in *Storia di Bologna*, vol. 3.2, pp. 683–769.

45 David Gentilcore, "'All That Pertains to Medicine': Protomedici and Protomedicati in Early Modern Italy," *Medical History* 38, 2 (1994): 121–142.

46 The history of the College and the Protomedicato of Bologna has been written in full detail by Gianna Pomata, so I will not insist much on it, except for the parts that are directly relevant to the regulation of the surgical arts.

47 Carlo Malagola, *Statuti delle Università e dei Collegi dello Studio Bolognese*, 2 vols. (Bologna: Zanichelli, 1888), vol. 1, p. 469.

48 Ibid., p. 470. Candidates for such a degree had to "comment upon *puncta* received from the hands of the prior and the doctors of the medical faculty both on lecture I, part III, fen IV of Avicenna's *Canon,* and on lecture II, part I of Bruno's *Surgery*." The candidate must have been able to read and comment upon the passages and to debate them with the examining board of the Collegiate doctors.

49 Ibid., p. 471. A fragment of a manuscript copy of the College statutes of the fifteenth century *restates the requirements for all those who want to practice surgery, adding one year of study*: "no citizen and no foreigner, of whatever status, condition, should dare or presume to practice surgery in the city of Bologna or its countryside if they have not *studied and listened to lectures for four years* with a salaried master of surgery, or someone teaching surgery in the public schools of Bologna or in another place where there is a studio. Our Prior, or the college of the studio in which the candidate studies, should be fully informed of this; as an alternative, the candidate should be examined and approved by the doctors of the college of the faculty of medicine." See Ibid., p. 490.

50 Donatella Bartolini, "On the Borders: Surgeons and Their Activities in the Venetian State (1540–1640)," *Medical History* 59, 1 (2015): 83–100.

51 The 1405 university statutes state that lecturers in surgery "each year, at the beginning of the study [in surgery], they should start lecturing on Bruno's *Surgery* first lecture; once they are done with that, they should read Galen's surgery. For the second lecture, let them teach Avicenna's *Surgery*, then book seven of Almansoris" (see Malagola, *Statuti*, vol. 2, pp. 247–248). As it appears from the *Rotuli* of the studio, the document on which all the lecturers were recorded year by year, by 1586 the whole surgery teaching focused on three books by Galen: *De tumoribus praeter naturam, De ulceribus,* and *De vulneribus*. By the late sixteenth century the chair of surgery was offering lecture cycles of three years on tumors, ulcers, and wounds, one topic each year; see Malagola, *Statuti*, vol. 1, p. xx.

52 Giovanna Ferrari, "Public Anatomy Lessons and the Carnival: The Anatomy Theatre of Bologna," *Past and Present* 117 (1987): 50–106, pp. 66–71.

53 ASB, Studio, 216, *Statuta Collegiorum Medicorum Bononiae 1507*, fol. 92–93.

54 ASB, Studio, 195, *Liber privilegiorum, mandatorum et memorialium*, fol. 29r: "medicare sorte alcuna di persona, di qualunque morbi si sia, et maximamente ferite, apostemi o tumori, o altri mali . . . nemmeno cavar o far cavar sangue in modo alcuno, ne dare ne far dare o consentire sia data cosa alcuna di qualsivoglia sorte per bocca ad alcuna persona maschio o femmina piccola o granda che sia – se prima non sarono stati licentiati dalli sgnori Priori et Protomedici."

55 ASB, Studio, 223, *Bando et Provisione sopra quelli che senza autorità, & licenza dell'Eccellentissimo Collegio di Medicina danno, ordinano, vendono, & applicano medicamenti in alcun modo. Et moderatione rinovata sopra li Spetiali, & Barbieri*. Appresso Vittorio Benacci Stampator Camerale 1594.

56 ASB, Studio, 233, *Provisione sopra il grave abuso di quelli che senza licenza presumono medicare. Moderatione rinovata sopra li spetiali, e barbieri. Pubblicata di XXIX di Dicembre. MDLXXXI.* The situation of barber-surgeons' practice must have been very hard to regulate, since ten years after the first decree the College and the Protomedicato appointed two inspectors, one for the city and one for the *contado* – the country territory subject to the city of Bologna – to verify whether practicing barber-surgeons were licensed by the College or not. The College was taking seriously the barbers' surgical skills concerning bloodletting, cautery and, in some cases, bone setting, pulling teeth, and treating bladder stones.

57 The licenses granted by the College to surgeons I have consulted are in ASB, Studio, 195, *Liber privilegiorum, mandatorum et memorialium*, fol. 26r-v; 53r-54r; 62v-63r; 67r; 76r; 80r-v; 123r.

58 See Giorgio Cosmacini, *La vita nelle mani. Storia della chirurgia* (Rome-Bari: Laterza, 2003), p. 27; Knut Haeger, *The Illustrated History of Surgery* (New York: Bell, 1988).

59 Celsus, *De medicina*, 3 vols., tr. by W.G. Spencer (Cambridge: Harvard University Press, 1935–1938), vol. 3, p. 297: "animo intrepidus," "misericors sit," "ac si nullus ex vagitibus alterius adfectus oriatur."

60 This double feature of the surgeon's attitude to the patient's pain marks the whole history of pre-anesthesia surgery. On this double attitude between dispassion and compassion and its origins in Celsus, see Lynda Payne, *With Words and Knives: Learning Medical Dispassion in Early Modern England* (Aldershot: Ashgate, 2007), pp. 1–7.

61 McVaugh, *The Rational Surgery*, pp. 13–52.

62 Bruno da Longobucco, "Ars Chirurgica," in Alfredo Focà, ed. *Maestro Bruno da Longobucco, chirurgo* (Reggio Calabria: Laruffa, 2004), p. 98.

63 Guy de Chauliac, *Inventarium, sive Chirurgia magna*, 2 vols., ed. Michael (Leiden: E.J. Brill, 1997), vol. 1, p. 3. The reference to surgeons' *bonitate formae* could be linked to the general distrust of disfigured and mutilated people I will examine in Chapter 3.

64 Ibid.

65 Giovanni Andrea Dalla Croce, *Cirugia universale e perfetta* (Venice: Giordano Ziletti, 1583), fol. 52v-53r.

66 See, for example, Tommaso Garzoni, *La piazza universale di tutte le professioni del mondo*, 2 vols., ed. Paolo Cherchi and Beatrice Collina (Turin: Einaudi, 1996), vol. 1, p. 207 (first published in 1585).

67 See, respectively, Cinzio D'Amato, *Prattica nuova et utilissima* (Venezia: Giovanni Battista Brigna, 1669), p. 8; G. Gentili, *La vita e l'opera di Bartolomeo Maggi* (Bologna: Università di Bologna, 1967); Cynthia Klestinec, "Renaissance Surgeons: Anatomy, Manual Skill, and the Visual Arts," in Peter Distelzweig, P.B. Goldberg, and Evan R. Ragland, eds. *Early Modern Medicine and Natural Philosophy* (Dordrecht: Springer, 2016), pp. 43–58.

68 Giovanni Battista Cortesi, *In Universam Chirurgiam absolutam Institutio* (Messina: apud haeredes Petri Breae, 1633), fol. 3r: "libros anatomicos Andreae Vesalii, observationes Gabrielis Falloppii, Realdum Columbum de re anatomica, Ioannis Valverdi & Andreae Laurentii anatomen, nec non Ambrosii Paraei, qui etiam de rebus chirurgicis sapientissime scripsit."

69 Ibid., fol. 3v-4r.

70 Ibid., fol. 5r: "Debet praeterea Chirurgus esse aetate iuvenis, aut saltem iuventuti propinquus haec enim aetas est, in qua, & sensibus, & corpore viget ad ea recte agenda, quae artis propria sunt; atque ut quod ars iudicat, praestare commode possit sensuum imbecilliatate non impediente: manu insuper strenua, & valida ad opus, quod molitur stabili, sive secandum sit membrum, sive urendum, sive etiam excidendum, non minus una quam altera promptus esse debet: oculorum acie acri, & clara, animo intrepidus, & immisericors, ut sanare velit eum, quem accipit non aut clamore, & eiulatu [?], aut mollitie aegrotantis, vel magis, quam res desiderat, properet, vel minus, quam necesse sit fecet aut urat, aut excidat; sed perinde omnia faciat, ac si clamores eius, qui afficitur, non audiret, nullu sue inde in eius animo oriatur affectis."

71 Ibid. "securus & animo intrepidus, in rebus dubiis, periculosisque cautus, ac minime praeceps, comis, humanus, placidusque, circa laborantes facilis, & mansuetus erga suae factionis homines, sociorum amator, prudens, summeque in praesagiendo circumspectus, pecuniae minime cupidus, nec acerbus exactor."

72 ASB, Ospedale di Santa Maria della Morte, VIII, 1, fol. 97r. In another document, an account book of the hospital, there is one Angelo Michele listed as *astante* in 1570 with no family name, but it would be hard to imagine that it is Sacchi, who was already lecturing in surgery at the time.

73 Orazio Bertalotti was also part of the group until 1589. He left no publications. The fact that many professors were listed in the *rotuli* – the name of the official roll of

lecturers – for the same chair was a constant source of concern for the authorities. In 1583 a Senatorial commission reported on this problem and on the frequent controversies among the listed professors. The reformers proposed to divide up lecturers in *ordinarii* (older and more famous) and *straordinarii* (younger), the latter waiting a number of years before entering the former category. Legate Gaetani decreed in 1586 that there could be no more than three teachers for each class, and that if there were more than three, they should be listed as *straordinarii*. Very often, ordinary lectures were based on the most important books and took place in the morning, while extraordinary ones were based on less important books and happened in the afternoon. See Ibid., pp. iv-xv.

74 ASB, Senato, Partiti, 11, fol. 161v-162v and 164r.

75 ASB, Assunteria di Studio, 92, n. 5. In general, professors of arts and medicine make much less than law teachers; among the latter, the highest salary is of 4800 lire.

76 For further details on the organization of this hospital and the role of the student assistant, see Paolo Savoia, "The *Book of the Sick* of Santa Maria della Morte in Bologna and the Medical Organization of a Hospital in the Sixteenth Century," *Nuncius* 31 (2016): 163–235. See also John Henderson, *The Renaissance Hospital: Healing the Body and Healing the Soul* (New Haven: Yale University Press, 2006), pp. 70–110; Sandra Cavallo, *Charity and Power in Early Modern Italy: Benefactors and Their Motives in Turin, 1541–1789* (Cambridge: Cambridge University Press, 1995), pp. 39–97; Giulinana Albini, "La gestione dell'Ospedale Maggiore di Milano nel Quattrocento: un esempio di concentrazione ospedaliera," in Allen J. Grieco and Lucia Sandri, eds. *Ospedali e città: l'Italia del Centro-Nord, XIII–XVI secolo* (Florence: Le Lettere, 1997), pp. 157–178; Salvatore Marino, *Ospedali e città nel Regno di Napoli. Le Annunziate: istituzioni, archive e fonti (secc. XIV–XIX)* (Florence: Olschki, 2014), pp. 3–74; Alessandro Pastore, "Gli ospedali in Italia fra Cinque e Settecento: evoluzione, caratteri, problem," in Maria Luisa Betri and Edoardo Bressan, eds. *Gli ospedali in area padana fra Settecento e Novecento: atti del III Congresso italiano di storia ospedaliera Montecchio Emilia, 14–16 marzo 1990* (Milano: FrancoAngeli, 1992), pp. 71–87; Nicholas Terpstra, *Lay Confraternities and Civic Religion in Renaissance Bologna* (Cambridge: Cambridge University Press, 1995), p. 180; Arrizabalaga, Henderson, and French, *The Great Pox*, pp. 145–170.

77 BCAB, Gozzadini 243, n. 1, *Ordinationi generali per il buon governo di tutti gli Hospitali della Città & Diocesi di Bologna*, fol. 15–16.

78 BCAB, Ospedali 42, *Statuti dell'Ospedale di Santa Maria della Morte (1562)*, fol. 31–33.

79 Jerome Bylebyl, "The School of Padua: Humanistic Medicine in the Sixteenth Century," in Charles Webster, ed. *Health, Medicine, and Mortality in the Sixteenth Century* (Cambridge: Cambridge University Press, 1979), pp. 335–370; see also Henderson, *The Renaissance Hospital*, pp. xxv–xxxiv; Michael Stolberg, "Bedside Teaching and the Acquisition of Practical Skills in Mid-Sixteenth-Century Padua," *Journal of the History of Medicine and Allied Sciences* 69, 4 (2014): 633–661.

80 BCAB, Ospedali 43, *Memoria di quello che debbe fare li Signori Priori della Arciconfraternità dell'Hospitale di Santa Maria della Morte della città di Bologna* [1595], fol. 3.

81 See Stolberg, "Bedside Teaching," pp. 642, 658–659.

82 Volcher Coiter, *Externarum et internarum principalium humani corporis partium tabulae* (Norimbergae: in officina Theodorici Gerlazeni, 1573), p. 120; on this important physician, see Hannah Murphy, *A New Order of Medicine: The Rise of Physicians in Reformation Nuremberg* (Pittsburgh: University of Pittsburgh Press, 2019), pp. 68–96. On hospital dissections, see Monica Azzolini, "Leonardo da Vinci's Anatomical Studies in Milan: A Re-Examination of Sites and Sources," in Jean A. Givens, Karen M. Reeds, and Alain Towaide, eds. *Visualizing Medieval Medicine and Natural History, 1250–1550* (Aldershot: Ashgate, 2006), pp. 147–176; on private surgical and anatomical teaching, see Andrea Carlino, *Books of the Body: Anatomical Ritual and Renaissance Learning*, tr. John Tedeschi and Ann C. Tedeschi (Chicago: The University of Chicago Press, 1994), pp. 188–194; Cynthia Klestinec, *Theaters of Anatomy: Students, Teachers, and*

Traditions of Dissection in Renaissance Venice (Baltimore: Johns Hopkins University Press, 2011), pp. 142–166.

83 ASB, Studio, 196; Giovanni Fantuzzi, *Notizie degli scrittori bolognesi*, 9 vols. (Bologna: Stamperia di S. Tommaso d'Aquino, 1781–1794), vol. 1, pp. 266–272. On Maggi's work, see Chapter 5.

84 Aranzi's scientific record has been described multiple times; see, for example, Raffi Gurunluoglu, Maziar Shafighi, Aslin Gurunluoglu, and Safiye Cavdar, "Giulio Cesare Aranzio (Arantius) (1530–89) in the Pageant of Anatomy and Surgery," *Journal of Medical Biography* 19, 2 (2011): 63–69.

85 ASB, Notarile, fol. 110v-112v. Carlo Poni has described how Bologna occupied a dominant position in Europe for silk manufacture and export throughout the early modern period. Indeed, toward the end of the sixteenth century a very large part of the population of Bologna (about 24,000 people against a population of 60,000 ca) lived off the art of making and selling silk. Production was disseminated in a multiplicity of households, workshops, and manufactures; on the other hand, there were no more than 50–60 powerful silk merchants, and their guild was powerful and influential. The Bolognese silk industry exhibited a clear tendency toward proto-industrial organization, with mechanized mills used by workers in the phase of silk-throwing. The various aspects of silk production can roughly be described as silk-throwing (in proto-industrial and mechanized factories); silk-weaving (mostly done by women in the household); gathering, in large artisanal workshops; and, finally, the sale on the international market. Many women worked in the complex process of silk-making, alongside with their male relatives and co-workers, especially in the household. The high rates of female employment in the silk industry were highly praised by the authorities as they allegedly kept the social order and prevented unemployed women and young girls from becoming prostitutes. All the production of silk in its various stages, except for the cultivation of the silkworms, was concentrated in the urban space. See Carlo Poni, *La seta*, pp. 153–227.

86 Volcher Coiter, *Externarum et internarum*, pp. 110–111.

87 BUB 770, Ghiselli, *Memorie*, vol. 17 (1580–1585), fol. 335: "the bones of the Beata Imelda lambertina were translated from the Church of San Gioseffo to that of the sisters of the Maddalena in Galliera, with the help of Giulio Cesare Aranzi, surgeon and physician, Count Cornelio Lambertini, Senator, Giulio Cesare Lambertini, Alfonso Paleotti, officer of the Cathedral Church, and those sisters' Father Confessor (*furono trasloccate le ossa della Beata Imelda Lambertina dalla Chiesa di San Gioseffo a quella delle suore della Madalena in Galliera, con l'intervento di Giulio Cesare Aranzi medico chirurgo, Conte Cornelio Lambertini senatore, Giulio Cesare Lambertini, Alfonso Paleotti Canonico della Chiesa Cattedrale, e del Padre Confessore di dette suore*)."

88 BUB, Fondo Aldrovandi. They were also correspondents. For example, while in Parma for a patient afflicted by a kidney illness, Aranzi asked Aldrovandi for information about a plant for a medical recipe he confessed he knew nothing about. See BUB 596, Miscellanea CC. 8, *Lettera di Giulio Cesare Aranzi ad Ulisse Aldrovandi*: "Signor Paterno had given a consultation for someone suffering from heated kidney in Parma, in which he proposes the application of a herb called Narisca . . . I was never able to understand what this Narisca is; I have found something with a similar name (Naryca), which is said to be similar to Theophrastus' air and water, coming from a tree in between a oak and a willow, but I am not sure about it. I pray your Excellence to enlighten me about it, because I cannot believe that this name (Neriscae) could mean that other plant (*Il Signor Paterno haveva dato uno consulto a Parma per uno qual patisse calidità di Rene, nel qual propone l'applicatione di un'herba quella nominata Narisca . . . io non ho mai trovato che pianta sia questa se non un nome quale così (Naryca) qual vogliano che sia il simile che Aria, et Aqua Theophrasti che di nota uno arbor mezzo mezzo fra la quercia et salice ma non lo ho certo. Prego V. Ecc. a farmene sicura cognitione perché non posso credere che con quella parolla (Neriscae) voglia significar questa altra in altro modo*)."

89 Gurunluoglu, Shafighi, Gurunluoglu, and Gurunluoglu, "Giulio Cesare Aranzio"; Eugenio Dall'Osso, "Un contributo al pensiero scientifico di Giulio Cesare Aranzio: La sua opera chirurgica," *Annali di medicina navale e tropicale* 61, 5 (1956): 617–627.

90 Giuseppe G. Forni, *L'insegnamento della chirurgia nello studio di Bologna: dalle origini a tutto il secolo XIX* (Bologna: Cappelli, 1948), pp. 89–90; ASB, Studio 196. Chronicler Ghiselli even wrote a brief family genealogy of the Sacchi. He recalled that the Sacchi family was said to have Tuscan origins and that one Pompilio, who had moved to Parma, became doctor of medicine and knight of Charles V, thus starting the dynasty of physicians; see BUB 770, Ghiselli, *Memorie*, vol. 20 (1595–1600), fol. 556–557. The fact that Sacchi's son was part of the Anziani is important: this was a two-month magistracy composed of members of the Senate with the task of running the activities of the Senate and of the guilds.

91 Sacchi left 150 lire to pay for a mass every year "to the Madonna of San Luca in the Hospital della Morte"; 100 lire for one mass every year; 550 lire for provisions of "bed sheets (*lenzuoli*)" for the hospital; 105 lire for wax candles in honor of the procession of the Madonna of San Luca, also organized by the brotherhood of Santa Maria della Morte BAB, Gozzadini 76, n.10 (pages are not numbered).

92 ASB, Ospedali, Santa Maria della Morte, Serie XII, fol. 11: *libro giornale 1591–1612* (pages are not numbered). The Sacchi family donated an altarpiece to the hospital's church, as recorded in a 1606 inventory; see ASB, Ospedale di Santa Maria della Morte, VIII, 5, fol. 6r.

93 BCAB, Gozzadini 287, *Frammento di una Cronaca bolognese degli anni 1588–1595, d'anonimo autore*, fol. 21.

94 BUB 770, Ghiselli, *Memorie*, vol. 20 (1595–1600), fol. 560–561: "Flaminio Capitano Ringhiera habitante in Strada Maggiore . . . avvenne che partito circa un hora di Palazzo con un solo suo servitore e caminando per la volta di casa fu presso quella, chi disse da quattro, chi da più, assalito, essendo fuggito il servitore, di due ferite ferito, l'una nel capo, e l'altra in la faccia, che li traversò, e li tagliò l'orecchio destro per il mezzo . . . e lo sfortunato Gentilhuomo andò in casa del predetto Confaloniere prossimo dove fu ferito, et ivi medicato da Angelo Michele Sacchi, Giulio Cesare Gessi, e Gaspero Tagliacozzi."

95 ASB, Studio 196; Forni, *L'insegnamento*, pp. 95–96.

96 BUB 770, Ghiselli, *Memorie*, vol. 19 (1591–1595), fol. 277.

97 A survey of both the proofs of citizenship necessary to be admitted to the College and of the increased number of barber-surgeons put on trial by the Protomedicato shows that social backgrounds of the admitted members mattered more and more during the seventeenth century and that the politics of licensing became more strict. The language of the notaries recording these documents changed as well, always emphasizing the fact that the candidate and his male family members never practiced any "mechanical arts" and always lived off family revenue. See, respectively, ASB, Studio 353 and 338; on this trend, see Pomata, *Contracting a Cure*, pp. 13–21. I have explored in more detail this figure in Paolo Savoia, "Skills, Knowledge, and Status: The Career of An Early Modern Italian Surgeon," *Bulletin of the History of Medicine* 93, 1 (2019): 27–54.

98 See Stefania Degli Esposti, "Giovanni Battista Cortesi (1553–1636): da garzone-barbiere a illustre chirurgo e anatomico," *Strenna storica Bolognese* 42 (1992): 173–187; Augusto De Ferrari, "Giovanni Battista Cortesi," *Dizionario Biografico degli Italiani* (Rome: Treccani, 1983), vol. 29 gives "1553 or 1554."

99 Girolamo Ghilini, *Theatro d'huomini letterati* (Venice: per il Guerigli, 1647), pp. 139–140; Andreas Ottomar Goelicke, *Historia chirurgiae* (Magdeburg: in Officina Rengeriana, 1713), pp. 218–219; Jean Manget, *Bibliotheca scriptorum medicorum* (Geneva: sumptibus Perachon et Cramer, 1731), vol. 1, part II, p. 120; Fantuzzi, *Notizie degli scrittori Bolognesi*, vol. 3, pp. 209–214; Salvatore De Renzi, *Storia della medicina in Italia* (Naples: Tip. del Filiatre-Sebezio 1845–1848), vol. 4, p. 94.

100 Cortesi is listed in the account books of the hospital as getting his regular annual stipend of 36 lire, but he was also performing other tasks, because, for example, in 1581

the books list a payment to him of 66 lire. See ASB, Ospedali, Santa Maria della Morte, serie XII, 9, *Libro mastro 1572–91*, fol. cclxvi and cclxxxviii.

101 ASB, Senato, Partiti, 11, fol. 24r.

102 I was not able to find much information on Cortesi's family, except that he got married in 1586 with a certain Agata di Pietro Moscatelli; see BAB Cartari B. 900, Matrimoni, 138. Other sources report that he had a numerous family, and Ghilini even says that some of his relatives used to beg in the streets; moreover, in 1589 the Senate started to periodically award him sums of money of 100, 200, and 600 lire because of "rei familiaris tenuitate," a measure repeated in 1591 and 1592; see ASB, Senato, Partiti, 12, fol. 67v, 117v, and 138v.

103 See ASB, Senato, Partiti, 12, fol. 106r. His publications of the period are Giovanni Battista Cortesi, *Epistola qua in simplici sede teli calvariae, os ipsius non abradendum nec perfornadum esse demonstratur, ad Ill.rem ac Excell.mum Virum D. Ioannem Cechium nostrae tempestatis Medicum celeberrimum* (Bologna: apud Faustum Bonardum, 1590); as an editor, Costanzo Varolio, *Anatomiae sive De resolution corporis humani* (Frankfurt: apud Iannem Wechelum & Petrum Fischerum consortes, 1591).

104 ASB, Senato, Partiti 12, fol. 117v: "in curandis militum adversus bannitos missorum vulneribus multum operae ac laboris, idque non sine magno ipsius incommodo impenderit." A special stipend of 600 lire for his military services figures in the account books of the Senate in 1595: ASB, Senato, Partiti, 12, fol. 187v. In 1598 he was appointed to the more official role of military surgeon of the city, a job that depended directly on the Senatorial commission for military affairs, and thus was paid from a special fund allocated to military affairs. ASB, Senato, Partiti 13, fol. 39r.

105 Cortesi, *Miscellaneorum*, p. 1.

106 ASB, Studio 196 (pages are not numbered): "Io ho conosciuto Helia Cortesi Sarto quale so non esser nato a Bologna, ma ha habitato assaissimo in Bologna."

107 ASB, Statuti del Collegio.

108 ASB, Studio 196.

109 Cortesi's disappointment was perhaps mitigated by the fact that he spent a long period of time in Paris from the fall of 1592 to the end of 1593, when he was called to take care of Cardinal Filippo Sega, the Bolognese Papal nuntius in the French kingdom, for an unspecified illness. This must have been a very important occasion for the former *garzone* and *stufaiolo*, who mentioned the episode in print, greatly exaggerating his period of stay in France, extending it to three years; see Cortesi, *Miscellaneorum*, p. 3. The *rotuli* show that this was not true; the Senate reserved his chair for the period Cardnal Sega deemed necessary: ASB, Senato, Partiti 12, fol. 146r. He was still in Paris in November of 1593 though, because he wrote a letter to Aldrovandi from France discussing his observations of the putrefaction of sea shells from the Atlantic Ocean; see BUB, Fondo Aldrovandi, Ms. 136, tomo XXIV. Transunti di lettere, fol. 13v-14r. Biographer Fantuzzi in the eighteenth century wrote that Cortesi was not admitted to the College because he did not enjoy citizenship. This is not correct, but somehow Fantuzzi got close to the truth; see Fantuzzi, *Notizie degli scrittori bolognesi*, vol. 3, p. 210.

110 Gian Paolo Brizzi, ed., *Imago Universitatis: celebrazioni e autorappresentazioni di maestri e studenti nella decorazione parietale dell'Archiginnasio*, 2 vols. (Bologna: Bononia University Press, 2014), vol. 1, p. 374.

111 ASB, Senato, Partiti 13, fol. 47r; ASB, Senato, Lettere, serie I, fol. 20.

112 Cortesi, *Miscellaneorum*, pp. 1–2.

113 Biblioteca Regionale Universitaria di Messina, ms F.N.14, fol. 31v-32r; published by Daniela Novarese, *I capitoli dello Studio della nobile città di Messina* (Messina: Università degli Studi di Messina, 1990), pp. 58–59. On the studio of Messina, see Rosario Moscheo, "Istruzione superiore e autonomie locali nella Sicilia moderna: Apertura e sviluppi dello 'Sudium urbis Messanae' (1590–1641)," *Archivio storico messinese* 59 (1991): 75–221; Paul Grendler, *The Universities of the Italian Renaissance* (Baltimore: Johns Hopkins University Press, 2002), pp. 121–126.

114 Giovanni Battista Cortesi, *Pharmacopeia, seu Antidotarium Messanense* (Messina: ex typis Petri Breae, 1629).

115 ASB, Assunteria di Studio, 36, n.15 bis; ASB, Assunteria di Studio, 8. A negotiation must have taken place, because in June of 1619 the Senate proposed a higher sum, an annual stipend of 2400 lire: ASB, Senato, Partiti 16, fol. 128v; see also ASB, Ibid., fol. 141r.

116 Cortesi, *Miscellaneorum*, pp. 665–666.

117 Tagliacozzi, *De curtorum*, p. 46 (1:33): "quod non infrequenter digladiantibus, altius adacto ferro laesionem incurrant."

118 The letter to Mercuriale is translated in Teach-Gnudi and Webster, *The Life and Times*, pp. 136–139. See Tagliacozzi, *De curtorum*, pp. vii–viii (in the original edition pages are not numbered).

119 BUB 770, Ghiselli, *Memorie*, vol. 17 (1580–1585), fol. 145–146.

120 BUB 770, Ghiselli, *Memorie*, vol. 19 (1591–1595), fol. 212–213.

121 Ibid., fol. 529. All the three cases have been transcribed by Teach-Gnudi and Webster.

122 See Peter Tosh, "The History of Masculinity: An Outdated Concept?," in Sean Brady and John H. Arnold, eds. *What Is Masculinity? Historical Dynamics from Antiquity to the Contemporary World* (New York: Palgrave Macmillan, 2011), pp. 17–34; Diederik Janssen, "Can the Hegemon Speak? Reading Masculinity through Anthropology," in Brandy and Arnold, eds. *What Is Masculinity?*, pp. 35–56; Alexandra Shepard, "Manhood, Patriarchy, and Gender in Early Modern History," in Amy Leonard and Karen L. Nelson, eds. *Masculinities, Childhood, Violence: Attending to Early Modern Women- and Men: Proceedings of the 2006 Symposium* (Newark: University of Delaware Press, 2011), pp. 77–95; Ruth Mazo Karras, *From Boys to Men: Formation of Masculinity in Late Medieval Europe* (Philadelphia: University of Pennsylvania Press, 2003), pp. 1–19; Elizabeth S. Cohen, "Honor and Gender in the Streets of Early Modern Rome," *Journal of Interdisciplinary History* (1992): 597–625; Stanley Chojnacki, *Women and Men in Renaissance Venice* (Baltimore, Johns Hopkins University Press, 2000), pp. 1–24; Cavallo, *Artisans of the Body*, pp. 181–223; Patricia Simons, *The Sex of Men in Premodern Europe: A Cultural History* (Cambridge: Cambridge University Press, 2011), pp. 25–51; Karen Harvey, "The History of Masculinity, circa 1650–1800," *Journal of British Studies* 44 (2005): 296–311. On gender in Renaissance Italy, see also Judith C. Brown and Robert Charles Davis, eds., *Gender and Society in Renaissance Italy* (London: Longman, 1998).

3

THE CULTURE OF THE FACE

Tagliacozzi summarized in one passage of *De curtorum* the centrality of the face for sixteenth-century selfhood.

> For this reason [that the face is the seat of many physiological functions] we will hardly be amazed that Nature has duly bestowed such outstanding qualities on the face and denied them to the other parts of the body. For the face has obtained the highest position; like a citadel, it occupies a high place, especially the area around the eyes, whose action demands a more elevated site than other parts. . . . The face itself is an indication of gender; it distinguishes one person from another and the measure of the entire body lies hidden in it; on the face we can read the foundations of physiognomy. The face reveals age and beauty and distinguishes between the sexes. It displays a man's dignity; finally, it is a true image of our souls and exposes most fully our hidden emotions. . . . Prudent Nature arranged things this way so that individuals could be distinguished one from another by certain special marks and true signs, lest too much similarity of features cause errors in recognition.[1]

This passage opens the way for a deeper exploration of the culture of the face, made both of a network of symbolic meanings attributed to faces and noses and of several practices of the care and the alteration of the face.

In its broadest anthropological meaning, culture can be defined as a system of shared values, meanings, and beliefs inscribed in material supports and expressions. In this sense, there existed an early modern culture of the human face. Without aiming at an impossible all-inclusiveness, in this chapter I discuss the medico-physiognomic culture of the face in Tagliacozzi's times and I place it in the wider context of attitudes toward the dignity, honor, and integrity of the face in medicine, law, and the Christian theological tradition. I follow Tagliacozzi's text and highlight the wider cultural context for the practice of plastic surgery with reference to three components: the Renaissance revival of classical notions of beauty, proportions, and integrity of the human figure; the growing importance and influence of physiognomy; and the reputation and cultural salience the human face – and the nose – enjoyed in that period. In this culture, the human face could be both a sign of prestige and a sign of inferiority and infamy. Renaissance practices of disfigurement built on a rich tradition that consisted in a converging perception of moral character, physical standing, aesthetic appearance, and metaphysical integrity. In the early modern culture of the face, being disfigured meant at the same time being ugly and being morally faulty. This particular culture of the face was organized along the gendered and moral lines of the distinction between the natural and the artificial. I shall show how the face entertained complex relationships with the self in the sixteenth century.

Classical beauty

At the beginning of his erudite discussion introducing the surgical techniques he is presenting to the public, Tagliacozzi includes a straightforward account of what might be called the classical conception of beauty in the Renaissance. Tagliacozzi recalls the opinion of some of the wisest men of Greece and Rome and of their contemporary followers. These men all believed that our face presented a "harmony and a symmetry that, once we know its size, we can conjecture as to the size and proportions of the entire body, since it appears that the other parts are proportionate to the face."[2] A beautiful human face, characterized by symmetry and proportion, was considered the measure of the length, breadth, and depth of the whole human body. Tagliacozzi specifies the rules to recognize a well-proportioned and symmetrical face. "First of all, I must say that the dimensions of this kind are symmetrical and are consistent with a symmetrical body, not at all with a deformed one."[3] Considered with respect to its length, the face was divided into three parts: the forehead, symbolizing knowledge; the medium part (from the eyebrows to the nostrils), the proper seat of beauty; and the lower part (from the nostrils to the chin), the symbol of "honesty." Tagliacozzi's main reference is the famous humanist architect and sculptor Pomponio Gaurico (c. 1482–1530), who had divided the length of the human body in three parts. Each of these parts was threefold, which gave an image of the body as composed of nine parts. The face was the first, and highest, part.[4]

Tagliacozzi shows a good deal of erudition. Erwin Panofsky studied the history of the theories of proportions and defined them as "a system of establishing the mathematical relations between the various members of a living creature, in particular of human beings, in so far as these beings are thought of as subjects of an artistic representation."[5] These systems can be norms for either representing or measuring the actual human body (or both). One of the most influential theoretical conceptions of the normal human body and of beauty in the Renaissance was a loosely Platonic theory of harmony and proportion.[6] Renaissance humanists progressively discovered a whole tradition on geometrical beauty that was more ancient than Plato's. Polykleitos produced his *Diadumeno*, then renamed *Canon*, in the fourth century BCE. The *Diadumeno* is a statue of the perfect human body inspired by this principle of proportion, which became a model not only for artists but for physicians and anatomists too throughout the sixteenth century.[7]

In the first century BCE, the Roman architect Vitruvius – a true Renaissance star – expressed in his *De architectura* the numerical relationship constituting the parts of the body. Vitruvian ideals of ornament and harmony became for Renaissance thinkers the rules not just for art theory and practice but for all the other arts and even for public behavior and social life.[8] The peak of this idea of mathematical beauty was reached in the literature on perspective.[9] Architecture textbooks animatedly discussed harmony and proportion for music, painting, sculpture, and the human body – all together. In particular, the analogies and network of relations between architecture and the human body proliferated.[10] The two currents of technical, aesthetic theory of proportions and of metaphysical harmony merged together.[11]

As we have seen, Tagliacozzi's favorite model was Pomponio Gaurico. In the second part of his 1504 treatise *De sculptura*, titled "On Symmetry," Gaurico had established that all the parts of the body must be compared to the face, which gave them their measure and proportion.[12] Gaurico also gave the ratio for the analogy or proportion between the parts of the face and between the parts of the face and other parts of the body, which he called common measure (*commensum*). "The length of the space between the eyelids and the top of the nose must be the same between the chin and the throat, and in turn it must be the same as that between the top of the nose and the chin: these are the right proportions."[13] Gaurico specified that those peoples who did not embody these rules, such as the African "Pygmies," should be called "monstrous." He went on detailing a complex musical analogy based on the notion of harmony, adding that "measure, or symmetry" was the most wonderful thing God created in nature and especially in man.[14] By uniting all the arts with cosmology and Christianity, the work of Gaurico exemplified the broad scope of symmetry in Renaissance culture.

By endorsing Gaurico, Tagliacozzi also meant to emphasize that there was a parallel intellectual stake in surgery and sculpture: both arts were the outcome of classical culture and manual dexterity. In the second volume of *De curtorum*, devoted to the technical aspects of surgery, Tagliacozzi showed what the theoretical notion of beauty as geometrical proportion meant in practice. While discussing the relation between the skin flap and the mutilated parts to be restored, and the operation of measuring the skin flap itself, the learned surgeon defined the aim of this practice with plenty of references to the classical theme of art imitating nature and to the symmetry of perfect natural shapes.

> The goal of our art – he wrote – namely, that the mutilated part be restored to its former size, will provide the answers to these questions [of

> the relationships between art and nature]. We must do our best to follow Nature's example and provide pleasant sights for mortal eyes.[15]

One of the most telling examples of this conception of beauty, and of its highly intellectualized and abstract character, is to be found in the *Iconologia* by antiquarian and courtier Cesare Ripa (c. 1555–1622) (Figure 3.1). The illustrated 1603 edition of this work shows the quintessential classical conception of beauty as participation of the divine light.

> Beauty is depicted as having her head in the clouds, because there is nothing more difficult to talk about with a mortal speech and nothing which is so hard to grasp by human intellect as beauty, which among creations is – as the Platonists say – nothing else than a light deriving from the splendor of God's face.

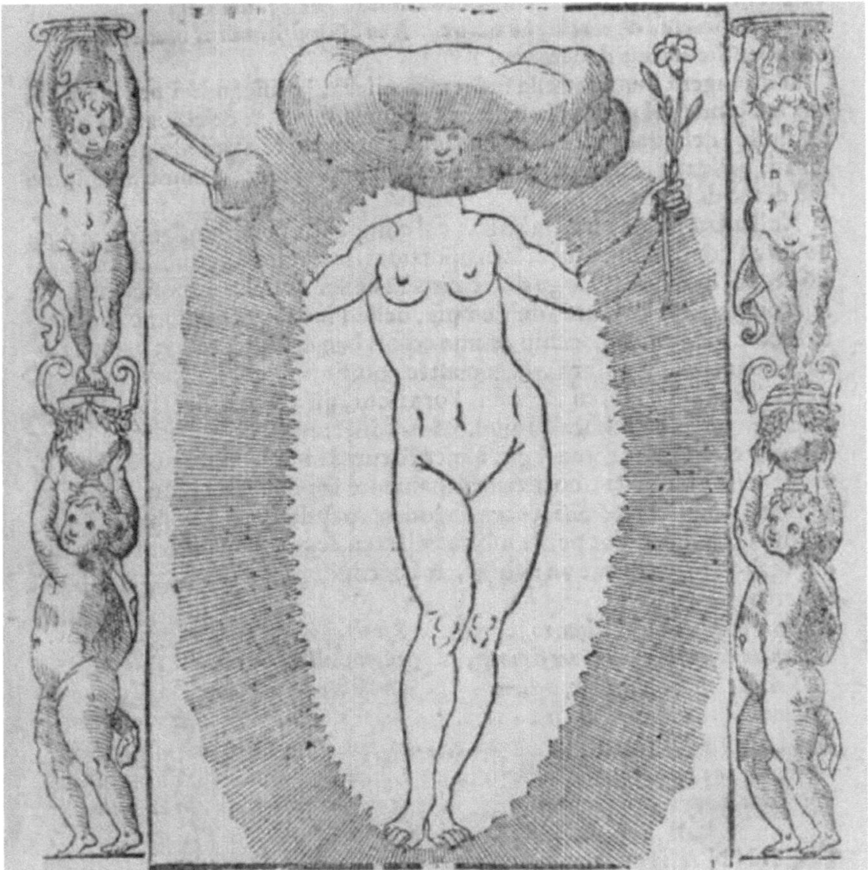

FIGURE 3.1 Cesare Ripa, *Iconologia* (1603): beauty.

Beauty holds a sphere and a compass in her hands

> to show that all beauty consists in measures and proportions, which are harmonized with time and place. Place determines beauty in the dispositions of provinces, cities, temples, piazzas, man, and all things which can be seen by the human eye, such as distinct colors, and with proportioned quantity and measure, and other similar things; time determines harmony, sounds, voices, orations, sadness and other things, which when are performed with good measure are rightly called beautiful.[16]

Ripa's icon of beauty, despite being a woman, is meant to be genderless and universal. However, as we shall see, more realistic and practical conceptions of beauty in the Renaissance were based on gendered conceptions of the human body.

Faces of physiognomy

Physiognomy, understood as the science of interpreting the passions of individual souls through the reading of the external marks on the body, was highly popular in the sixteenth century, both in its philosophico-medical version and in its occult and natural-magical one.[17] Physiognomists were most interested in the human face. Besides the obvious connections between interpreting facial expressions and medical diagnosis, physiognomy played an important role in the literature on facial surgery. All physicians and surgeons who discussed such a technique referred to it. One of the most important tenets of physiognomy was for Tagliacozzi the fact that it showed in the clearest possible way the dignity of the human face. The art of plastic surgery found in physiognomy both an important source of legitimization and a source of operative principles to justify the enterprise of correcting disfigured faces.

In the sixteenth century, physiognomy was one of the factors that contributed to shifting the attention to the face and its traits as key features of social and political life.[18] One of the fundamental axioms of physiognomy – that soul and body can mutually influence each other – became firmly entrenched in the minds of learned writers as well as in institutional practices. Two of the most important and representative texts of the physiognomic tradition are the pseudo-Aristotle's book *Physiognomonika*, central to the medieval institutionalization and scholasticization of the discipline, and the book by Neapolitan natural magician and experimentalist Giovanni Battista della Porta (1535–1615), written in the late sixteenth century. Both are relevant for the discussion of physiognomy made by Tagliacozzi.

By the time of Tagliacozzi, physiognomy had already a century-long tradition, and it was firmly established in the curriculum of arts and medicine faculties. In the 1405 statutes of the University of Bologna, the pseudo-Aristotelian *Physiognomonika* appeared as a mandatory reading in the second year of the arts curriculum, propaedeutic to the medical degree.[19] Similarly to the case of surgery, by the late thirteenth century physiognomy acquired a "rational" structure in the scholastic sense: it became a body of knowledge ruled by a system of knowable causes that could be deciphered through logical thinking. In these new clothes, physiognomy entered the fields of learned natural philosophy, medicine, and astrology. Starting from the late Middle Ages, physiognomy moved from the intuitive and the conjectural to a different kind of knowledge, rooted within a firm theoretical framework and closely associated with medicine.[20]

Pseudo-Aristotle was the most important ally of, and provided the fundamental theoretical ground for, physiognomists throughout the sixteenth century.[21] This book posed the problem of the relationships between the body and the soul in a straightforward manner. Pseudo-Aristotle put the need of a *scientia* of physiognomy in the wider context of human affairs, thus giving this interpretative technique a broad scope from the beginning.

> Dispositions (*dianoiai*) follow bodily characteristics and are not unaffected by bodily impulses. This is obvious in the case of drunkenness and illness; for it is evident that dispositions are changed considerably by bodily affections. Conversely, that the body suffers sympathetically with affections of the soul is evident for love, fear, grief, and pleasure. But it is especially in the creations of nature that one can see how body and soul interact with each other, so that each is mainly responsible for the other's affections. For no animal has ever existed such that it has the form of one animal and the disposition of another, but the body and soul of the same creature are always such that a given disposition must necessarily follow a given form. Again, in all animals, those who are skilled in each species can diagnose their dispositions from their forms. . . . Now if this is true . . . there should be a science of physiognomics.[22]

In the fourth part of the book, the author also discussed the issue of the relationships between body and soul: "It seems to me that soul and body react on each other; when the character of the soul changes, it changes also the form of the body, and conversely, when the form of the body changes, it changes the character of the soul."[23]

Zoological comparison was at the core of Aristotelian physiognomy.[24] Pseudo-Aristotle considered animal shapes to be the medium term of a particular kind of syllogism. Since we can observe specific relations between the shapes of animals and their moral character (braveness, laziness, generosity, etc.), then if we notice specific analogies of shapes between humans and animals we will be able to conclude that such humans have similar moral traits. The author claimed that the special medium for physiognomy was the face: "Clearest of all are those that appear in the most favourable position. The most favourable part for examination is the region round the eyes, forehead, head, and face."[25]

Pseudo-Aristotle's structuring opposition was centered on moral qualities such as brave-coward, shameless-temperate, and high-spirited-low-spirited, which were in turn connected to a general and supposedly self-evident notion of sexual difference. Women were more evil, less brave, less strong, more gentle, more skilled in rearing children. They had a "smaller head, narrower face, and a more slender neck . . . softer, moister flesh."[26] For example, the lion was the closest animal to the "pure" male type – "gentle, just, and affectionate towards his associates" – while the panther was the most female-like – "petty, thieving, and, generally speaking, deceitful."[27]

Giovanni Battista Della Porta's widely read and greatly influential *De humana physiognomonia*, first published in Latin in 1586, then soon translated in several European vernaculars, took up all the pseudo-Aristotelian themes and deepened them. Della Porta's attitude highlights the fact that physiognomists were becoming more and more straightforward in linking external signs and internal character through the medium of humoral complexions. Not only did he focus almost entirely on the face and build his whole enterprise on zoological comparisons but he also included in the science of physiognomy the fleeting expressions of feelings, albeit not in a systematic fashion. Della Porta began his book by defining physiognomy right away as "a science that from the permanent signs of the body – and from the accidents that change these signs – understands the natural inclinations of the soul." The author also formalized the proper way of reasoning (Figure 3.2): "Let A be strength, B to have big limbs, and C the Lion. All animals

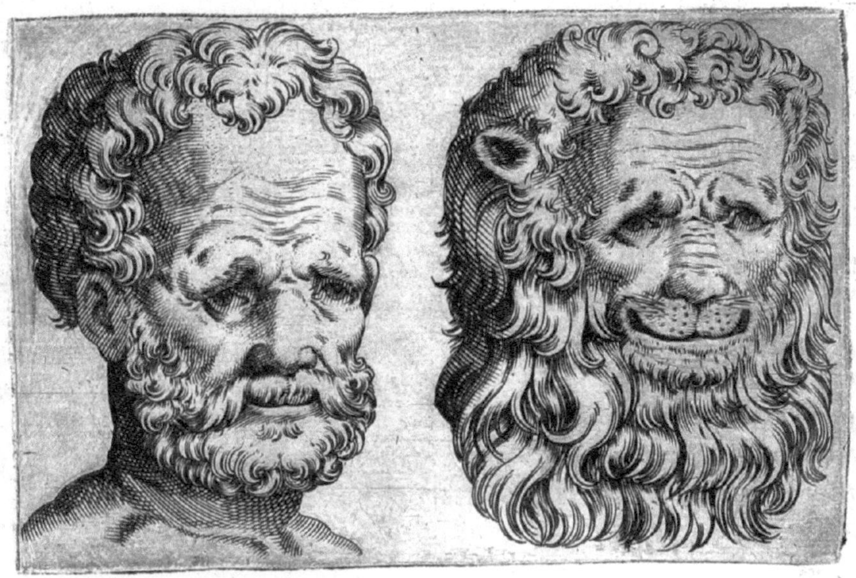

FIGURE 3.2 Giovanni Battista Della Porta, *De humana physiognomonia libri IIII* (1586): a lionlike man.

Source: Courtesy of the Wellcome Collection

with big limbs are strong; all lions and some other animals have big limbs; all lions and some other animals are strong."[28]

Della Porta's book showcases a conception of the human face that came from physiognomy but spread beyond its disciplinary boundaries. In this way, Della Porta's book throws some light on the general cultural conception of the human body, which in turn shifted the "norms of seeing" from the body toward the face.[29] The face was like a dynamic text made of fixed traits and mobile features that were readable through specific techniques of interpretation that only trained natural philosophers could acquire. All physiognomic enterprise had to start from the face, because

> it is the most noble part of the body, the seat of the senses and of the most important part of man, because here sight, hearing, smell, and taste are placed close to one another . . . and if I meet a man I see his face first, which is not true of the chest and the other parts . . . [in the face] we find the most important part of the soul and the gift of intelligence.[30]

The face was not only the most visible part of the body but also "the true witness of our conscience, and it is uncertain, changing, and diverse." The surface of the face and its movements were

> that which reveal as well as that which cover the soul. Therefore it is reasonable to judge a man from his face, unless when the movements of his soul have cooled down. . . . The face is the mirror of the mind because it shows the secrets of the soul through the eyes. Physicians say that the whole body sends its blood and spirits to the face, because the face is the most noble part of the body; therefore, the passions of the whole body and the soul are made evident in the face.[31]

Della Porta pushed the physiognomic way of reasoning to its limits by linking it not only to a moralized version of the Hippocratic-Galenic theory of humoral complexions but also to the classical notion of beauty. Della Porta mentioned the Hippocratic definition of beauty as the best temperament and the perfection of the proper action of each of the parts of the body. This view, he recalled, was opposed to the "philosophical" definition of beauty associated with Plato, according to which beauty was the beauty of the soul, given that the proportion between the parts of the soul reflected the proportion between the parts of the body. Della Porta argued that Galen combined the two definitions.

> One of Physiognomy's axioms, old and shared by all, is that the right disposition of the parts of the body shows a right disposition of the conduct; it is indeed said that those who are monsters in the body are monsters in the soul as well. Beauty is a well-measured disposition of the parts of the body which is model and image of that of the soul.

There was a clear correspondence between the inner and the outer parts of the body: "nature made the body upon the model of the soul."[32] True beauty of the face was "harmonious agreement of the parts."[33] On the other hand,

> those who have an ugly face have a ugly soul too. . . . If someone wants to know the natural cause of this state of affairs, that is because the lack of temperance of the humors in the body makes the parts of the body badly shaped; and the lack of humoral balance causes vices and bad conduct.[34]

A beautiful face was a moral face, as well as a healthy face.

Physiognomy took a normative stance with respect to the ideal male facial shape. Moreover, masculinity had a lot to do with noses. Masculine noses par excellence were thought to be aquiline noses, indicating *gravitas*, authority, and *decorum*. The nose had "a certain royal and noble quality," and it revealed not only the beauty of a soul but also the authority of a person. This is testified by "the Persians who loved to see an aquiline nose in their kings, and by the Jews, who excluded from priesthood those who had an ugly nose or missed a nose altogether."[35] And these government tasks were by definition male tasks, and more precisely upper-class male ones. Most of the physiognomic descriptions of the noses referred to men because, despite the supposed universal character of physiognomic interpretation, it was by far more important in a male-dominated public culture to judge the character of men than that of women. Pseudo-Aristotle established a canon, repeated by physiognomers and physicians throughout the sixteenth century.

> Those that have thick extremities to the nostrils are lazy; witness cattle. Those that have a thickening at the end of the nose are insensitive; witness the boar. Those that have a sharp nose-tip, but a flat one, are magnanimous; witness the lions. Those that have a thin nose-tip are bird-like; but when it is somewhat hooked and rises straight from the forehead they are shameless; witness ravens; but those who have an aquiline nose with a marked separation from the forehead are magnanimous; witness the eagle. Those who have a hollow nose, rounded where it rises from the forehead, and the rounded part standing above, are salacious; witness cocks. But the snub-nosed are also salacious; witness deer. Those whose nostrils are spread are passionate; this refers to the affection which occurs in the temper.[36]

The connection between noses and masculinity also circulated in the most explicit form possible. Della Porta wrote in his physiognomy: "The nose corresponds to the penis, since if one has it thick and long, or thin and long, or short, we can say the same of his penis; in the same way, nostrils correspond to the testicles."[37] Tagliacozzi was not as explicit, but he too made a reference to the fact that irregular noses could be the "object of sly derision."[38]

Tagliacozzi was well aware of the developments of the physiognomic tradition. He recalled that physiognomists, "metoposcopists" (readers of the forefronts) like Girolamo Cardano (1501–1576),[39] natural historians, and astrologers all recognized the deep interdependence of the soul and the body and the mutual transmission of their respective actions and passions. Tagliacozzi particularly insisted on two important pseudo-Aristotelian arguments in favor of physiognomy. One was the existence of a sympathy (*consensus*) between the soul and the body, so that the body could influence the soul. The other was the validity of the reverse principle, namely the fact that the appearance of the body could be modified by the passions of the soul. In other words, he embraced the view that "there is a kind of science that, with the aid of accurate conjecture, can infer the impulses of the mind from the form of the body."[40]

In a more philosophical tone, the Bolognese surgeon went on to explain that each body needed a "specific form" – a technical Aristotelian term to define the soul – and that they were so closely linked that one could easily move from knowing one element to knowing the other. Tagliacozzi clarified that he was dealing not with *mores* in the sense of costumes as they were refined by virtue or vice but with what the Greeks had called the "passions of the soul (*animi passiones*)": anger, love, hate, hope, joy, and so forth. In modern terms, the field of physiognomy would be anthropology, not ethics. Tagliacozzi prudently warned his readers that the soul and the body were indeed separate entities. He argued for free will, a divine gift: "Because the mind or will of man is God-given, it is by far superior to the weak and lowly body, and our power of judgment is so separate and free that it cannot be subject to any corporeal restraints."[41] Yes, it was true that the body offered to the expert gaze signs of the soul, but the exercise of free will was quite another matter. In this respect, Tagliacozzi showed his acute awareness of one of the most thorny issues accompanying the whole history of physiognomy as a learned discipline.

Dignity and infamy

Besides physiognomy, the philosophical, the humanist, and the medico-anatomical traditions gave plenty of arguments to sixteenth-century medical writers discussing the excellence of the human face. Aristotle, in *Parts of Animals*, had stated that

> in man, the portion of the body between the head and the neck is called the *Prosōpon* (Face), a name derived, no doubt, from the function it performs. Man, the only animal that stands upright, is the only one that looks straight before him or sends forth his voice straight before him.[42]

And the Stagirite went on to claim that the higher parts of the body were more noble than the lower parts, because the parts that in the human body were placed in a higher position pointed to the heavens.[43] Cicero's *On the Nature of Gods*, one of the most beloved books by fifteenth- and sixteenth-century humanists, repeated this very same theme of humans standing on their feet with the head, face, reason, and the senses projected toward knowledge of the higher and most noble parts of the world and the heavens.[44] Finally, the early fourteenth-century classic anatomical textbook by Mondino de Liuzzi (c. 1270–1326) gave the idea a medical twist. The anatomist added to the standard praise of the face that the head was upwards also because it was warm and made of a light, airy substance.[45]

It is interesting to notice the merging of traditional medical and physiognomic arguments in the cultural valorization of the face made by Tagliacozzi. In straightforward Galenic fashion, he argued that human body parts had three aims: protecting life (brain, heart, liver); defeating individual death through generation (testicles, the uterus, and the *pudenda*); and, finally – the function of the face – allowing for a better life. The "honor" of the face could be inferred at first sight by its place in the topography of the body. Tagliacozzi praised the divine order of the body that put the genitals and the face at a great distance, because otherwise the genitals would have enslaved the face and even the brain. But luckily "wise Nature" decreed that the face should occupy a higher place, and the genitals had to be placed below, as in animals.[46]

The face was the most excellent part also because "we can discern from the face the temperament of both the entire body and the mind itself": just "as in a painting (*ac in tabula*)" on the face one could see the signs of the temperament, both of the body and of the brain. The skin of the face was thin and elastic and thus it showed the nature and the essence of the humors of the body. A rose-colored face was sign of a warm and moist temperament; a yellow face of warm and dry people; black, dark, and livid signaled the melancholic; a pale and white appearance indicated cold and moist complexions.[47] Moreover, the face offered signs (*indicia*) of many illnesses. Referring to the famous "Hippocratic face," Tagliacozzi regarded the examination of the face as a universal practice and especially useful in devising prognoses. If the face was "different," namely not "according to its nature," one could be sure there was something wrong.

Tagliacozzi endorsed Cardano's threefold explanation of the diagnostic centrality of the face. Looking closely at patients' faces was of key importance because faces were composed of many parts, each of which was sensitive to injuries and illness, and registered in their appearance the action of disease. In the second place, the skin of the face was thin, and therefore it easily revealed the inner underlying bodily processes. Finally, the brain was so close to the face that when people were struck by impressions of pain, joy, and so forth, then the face suddenly, and accordingly, changed.[48] The argument easily slipped from technical medical descriptions to general considerations on human nature. In fact, Girolamo Cardano served as a model in more general philosophical terms too. In his 1551 European bestseller *De subtilitate*, the Milanese scientist had declared that the face was the seat of three "miracles (*miracula*)" or miraculous facts: first, that there could not exist two identical faces in the whole world; second, that on the face we could see the most praised beauty and the most abhorred ugliness;

and, finally, that on the human face we could read one individual's emotional states as rapidly as they change.[49]

From the most humble war surgeon to the most famous and learned physicians, medical practitioners repeated the theme of the nobility and dignity of the human face, often praised in connection with the head.[50] Even the empiric Leonardo Fioravanti, albeit in an ironic manner that cut short on the humanist-style rhetoric of his more learned colleagues, wrote that "the head is the most prominent thing all living creatures have. The truth of this can be seen in that a man with no foot, no penis, no testicles, no arm, no nose and no ears can live; but with no head no one can live."[51]

The importance of the face went well beyond medicine. Cardinal Gabriele Paleotti (1522–1597) in his famous Counter-Reformation-style art treatise argued that, among other things, portraits could count as a physiognomic proof in matters of inheritance.[52] In a similar vein, Tagliacozzi recalled that on the face appeared the signs of a person's parents in the clearest possible way, and that this could help solving inheritance issues: "the features of fathers are seen in sons, surely the truest evidence of the legitimacy of offspring." The surgeon also marveled at the seemingly infinite variety and singularity of individual faces, and he noticed that each one of them was formed by very specific small parts in order to be distinguished from all the others.[53]

Late medieval and Renaissance literature often presented the topics of the theft of identity, impostors, and people not able to recognize themselves by their faces.[54] The first sixteenth-century narrators of the story of Martin Guerre constantly referred to the fact that finding two (almost) identical faces was indeed a "prodigious" or "marvelous" fact.[55] Penal codes judged with much severity wounds inflicted on the face causing permanent disfigurement. The 1458 Bolognese criminal statutes – valid, with integrations, through the whole early modern period – stated that blows to the face were among those serious crimes that had to be denounced by the city's officials, without waiting for the damaged party to make a complaint.[56] Wounds and mutilations inflicted on the face not only were more seriously punishable but could also trigger a specular retribution. For example, the code stated that "the punishment for those who inflict wounds on the face with bloodshed, and damage the eyes with a forbidden weapon is 100 Bolognese lire." If the guilty party could not pay within one month, he must be banished, or his eyes must be cast out in turn.[57]

At the symbolic level, the punishment for those who attacked and "wounded" the image of Christ, the Virgin, and the Saints was heavier if the perpetrators vandalized their faces.[58] One of the city government's public decrees that integrated the statutes, published in 1575, specified that disfiguring wounds were to be treated more severely than other kinds of wounds and could even be punished by corporal punishments at the discretion of the judge.[59] The 1585 decrees on public order were even more explicit: "Given that it is a most heinous crime to disfigure the human face, which has been created similar to God's image," those who committed it were condemned to pay 200 golden scudi and were subject to five years of prison and corporal punishments at the discretion of the judge.[60]

A long-standing theological medieval tradition based on passages from the Leviticus and Thomas Aquinas concerned the suspicious status of mutilated bodies. The context for these ideas was provided by medieval theological debates about the resurrection of the body, generally supported not by a mind-body dualism but rather by

> a sense of self as a psychosomatic unity. The idea of person was not a conception of soul escaping body or soul using body; it was a concept of self in which physicality was integrally bound to sensation, emotion, reasoning, identity – and therefore finally to whatever one means by salvation. . . . Person was not person without body, and body was the carrier of the expression . . . of what we today call individuality.[61]

Bodily continuity was the central idea of personhood, an idea that was sometimes at odds with Aristotelian doctrine but supported by a great number of pious and popular practices in the Christian Middle Ages.[62]

Leviticus, 21:17–20, reads:

> Whosoever he be of thy seed in their generations that hath any blemish, let him not approach to offer the bread of his God. For whatsoever man he be that hath a blemish, he shall not approach: a blind man, or a lame, of he that hath a flat nose, or any thing superfluous, or a man that is brokenfooted, or brokenhanded, or crookback, or a dwarf, or that hath a blemish in his eye, or be scurvy, or be scabbed, or hath his stones broken.

This passage has often been read as the foundation of the doctrine of *Irregularitas*, which prohibited the ordaining of priests to the wounded and the disfigured. This interpretation is correct and supported by canon law, even though, as shown by Irina Metzler, this passage has always been overemphasized and should be relativized. For example, canon law provided for cases of dispensation for the deformed who wanted to access priesthood, as in the 1234 *Liber extra*, a collection of canon laws by Gregory IX, which banned access to higher order for disfigured candidates, but prescribed nothing of the sort for the lower orders, and overall provided for cases for dispensations.[63] The decrees of the Council of Trent generally mentioned the "religiosity" and *gravitas* of ways of behaving, speaking, and moving of clerics but never explicitly mentioned mutilations or disfigurement. Section XXIII of the Tridentine decrees on the requisites and education of the clergy spoke in general of their physical appearance and the lack of physical defects but did not go into further details, a circumstance that could be read as suggesting that it was generally understood that disfigured men could not hold clerical offices.[64]

Theology also left down-to-earth traces. For example, Aquinas, when speaking of regulation of marriage according to canon law, considered facial mutilations, specifically nose mutilations, a good enough reason to end an engagement.

In the *Summa Theologiae*, concerning the circumstances under which the holy vow of marriage could be broken, he wrote that

> if before the wedding one of the engaged parties fall seriously ill with a debilitating illness, such as a paralysis or epilepsy; or if one of the parties become disfigured after they have their nose or eyes cut off; or if their illness puts the good of the offspring in danger, as for example with leprosy; then the two engaged parties can lawfully cancel their mutual engagement in order not to become mutually unpleasant and not to compromise the happy outcome of the marriage.[65]

Theology and the law merged in the emerging discipline of legal medicine. Consulting for a criminal case involving a wound on the face in the 1560s, Sicilian Protomedico Giovanni Filippo Ingrassia (1510–1580) stated clearly that degrees of disfigurement – and the relative severity of the punishment to be administered to the offender – depended on the social condition and status of the wounded man. Ingrassia claimed that not all faces were equal and that there was no such thing as an ugly scar on the face of a poor peasant. On the contrary, disfigurement on the public, political, and constantly visible face of a nobleman, for whom being disfigured meant expulsion form civil and political society, was very serious.[66] In the same period, the criminal court of Venice investigated a case of disguise (*travestimento*) of a peasant, Frangia Cudumini, accused of having impersonated the Venetian governor or Retimo in Crete, where he lived, dressing up with his distinctive red long robe and parading into the town among the jokes and cries of the people and the soldiers. After a long investigation, the Councillor of the criminal court found that the parody had unequivocally failed because the peasant had "an aquiline nose, marked with a black scar on the left and another on the middle of this nose that crosses to the right."[67] In this case too, a badly scarred and irregular nose was a sign of low status, of peasantry.

Ingrassia discussed several degrees of seriousness of facial injuries. One kind included those injuries that damaged the face as an ornament without damaging its more important or vital functions. About this kind of disfigurement he referred to the surgical practice of the Vianeo from Tropea, showing some skepticism about the results but implicitly letting the reader know that he had seen the operation performed:

> Some healer from Tropea who specializes in noses routinely grafts flesh from the arm [onto the nose]; however, the results are far from perfect, for he is not able to remake the skin, and therefore he cannot exquisitely restore the original beauty.[68]

The first systematizer of legal medicine in the West, jurist Paolo Zacchia (1584–1659), discussed Leviticus and Aquinas in his *Quaestiones medico-legales*. Zacchia specifically referred to nose mutilations, recalling all the medical and anatomical knowledge of the times, detailing the nose's functions, and interpreting the biblical passage as referring to physiognomic ideas about deformed noses and bad moral character, rather than to real nose mutilations.[69] On the issue of nose mutilation as an impediment to marriage and engagement, Zacchia interpreted the old canon law in a new way. Zacchia believed that now, after Tagliacozzi's book, it was possible to restore defective noses and so marriage should be celebrated among those patients who have had their noses surgically reconstructed.[70] The mere possibility of remaking lost noses could modify the perception of beauty and honor in significant ways.

Mutilations carried with them a moral suspicion throughout the early modern period. At the level of popular and social perception, cutting off the nose was a kind of punishment associated not only with adultery (especially women's adultery) but also with political treason. This is true of several cultures and historical periods, ranging from ancient Egypt to pre-Colombian America.[71] In the sixteenth century, mutilating faces of the dead enemy after battles was not an uncommon practice.[72] There were known cases of "Turkish" slaves who had been mutilated by cutting off their ears and noses in sixteenth-century Florence,[73] and in general the practice of branding faces and hands of domestic slaves became relatively common in Italy by the later Middle Ages.[74] In medieval Italy, the cutting off of noses was codified as a punishment in the statutes of the northern Italian communes of Belluno (against perjurers and those who benefited from perjury), of Padua (for the same reason), and in the statutes of Corsica (for pimps). Several Venetian women were condemned to have their nose, lip, and eyes cut off in the thirteenth century.[75] Despite the fact that by the sixteenth century corporal punishments appeared to be less common in statutes, and were banished altogether from canon law, as late as 1545, in Venice, a law prescribed that the tongue and nose of thieves had to be cut off so that all the people could immediately recognize them.[76] "A disfigured man was supposed to be a criminal for the majority of the people," as attested by the proverb "beware of the marked ones" (*cave a signatis*).[77] In fourteenth-century Lucca one could ask for a certificate attesting that specific mutilations were due to illness or some other accident and they were not the outcome of a punishment. Those who had been mutilated as a punishment wandered about the countryside begging, or worse stealing and committing other crimes, so that it was a common belief to think that the mutilated were dangerous people.[78]

Despite some exceptions, there was no portrait of the lower classes in the Renaissance. The few portraits of artisans were bitterly criticized by the intellectuals and art theorists of the second half of the sixteenth century.[79] The instruments invented in late medieval and sixteenth-century Europe to document one's identity and to control the movements of suspicious populations – such as gypsies, beggars, and people with plague or coming from places believed to be infected – included no picture and only scantly referred to facial and bodily traits.[80] As it emerges from the famous case of Martin Guerre and Arnaud du Tilh, the peasant witnesses' recorded depositions showed a great deal of doubt concerning skin marks and individual physiognomic features.[81] It might be almost unbelievable for the modern reader, but visualizing the specificity of one's face, and remembering faces, was the preserve of the upper classes. For example, the appearance of the white collar as a fashion item in the second half of the sixteenth century was meant to highlight the facial features of the upper classes.[82] By contrast, the so-called *fedi di sanità*, certificates of good health given and shown at city doors to common people traveling from town to town, very rarely contained physical descriptions of their bearers and more often mentioned the intended itinerary of the traveler.

Very often low-class people were faceless, and they began to have a face only when they got in touch with the criminal justice system or when they were perceived as dangerous for the social and political order. A Bolognese 1580 ordinance against a certain Baldassarre, a wanted criminal, instructed the overseers of one of the city doors in the following terms.

> You will have to be alert and ready to report if a Baldassarre from Rivarolo Villa di Pozzura near Genoa, also called Sanvignonio, the son of a smith, shows up at this door. He is of middle stature, 34-year old, with sparse black beard, thin, a dark-colored face as if he had the plague, a few teeth and not in good shape, and a watery eye. In case you see him you will not let him in," and then call the authorities to arrest him.[83]

Having a face, in the sense of both having a certain symmetry, beauty, and grace and being a distinct and specific individual, was a matter of social class.

Gendered faces

Sixteenth-century beauty was divided along gender lines. Female beauty could not be confused with male beauty. Physiognomists, physicians, and surgeons all made clear that observing human faces carried with it the ability to distinguish between the sexes. Some particulars of the face were specifically male, such as the nose and the beard. Male and female beauty were conceived as different, and the distinction between natural and artificial beauty was key to understanding such difference. The natural-artificial divide was both gendered and moralized; it revolved around the opposing structures of male-female, moral-immoral, true-false.

As we have seen, beauty was located in the higher parts of the body, intellectually and spiritually more elevated. Such a conception brought about a certain ambiguity and a more and more marked protest against the artificial means of enhancing or faking beauty. Makeup and cosmetics, while enjoying wide diffusion among male and female members of the upper and the middle classes, became the symbol of the artificial. In the discourses of the learned, beauty enhancers deceived the eye and fooled the soul. Cosmetics in particular came to be associated with women's moral faults. Among the upper classes, the ideal female beauty consisted of a pale complexion, red lips (the key colors were always red and white, roses, and milk), and a gentle and obedient attitude. All these features were considered "natural" in women. This ideal of female beauty was both sacred and profane. A sixteenth-century edition of a famous book of sermons by fifteenth-century Dominican preacher Gabriele da Barletta (d. after 1480) stated that the Virgin Mary's face was of perfect complexion: "as medical writers say: that color which is composed by red and white is the best."[84] The ideal of male beauty, on the contrary, was characterized by strength, marked traits of the face (the animal model for men was the lion), and a warrior-like attitude. Montserrat Cabré has written that in the Middle Ages the socio-symbolic order assigned women to appearances and men to the public world.[85] This consideration can be extended to the early modern period.

More specifically, in the sixteenth century male beauty was modeled upon the figures of the knight and the soldier: strength, a fear-inducing appearance, braveness, and a certain austerity and *gravitas*. Force characterized men, and gentleness characterized women. Sexual difference, in the form of different humoral balance, contributed to female beauty, and complexional weakness became an attribute of female beauty. In other words, female weakness and social subordination were translated into physical beauty. For this reason male beauty had to be different from female beauty. Men could not be associated with submission. For that same reasons only the upper classes could be beautiful.[86]

In pre-modern times cosmetics was conceived as both an aesthetic and a medical business. This became particularly evident in the books of secrets.[87] Late medieval cosmetics met with a taste for polychromies and a certain new attention toward facial expressions. Already in the *Trotula* collection the face and the hands were the most important locations for cosmetics.[88] Many vernacular treatises of the sixteenth century addressed this question of the true beauty in a similar way.[89]

One passage from the *Cortegiano* by Baldassarre Castiglione (1478–1529) deserves attention, for it embodies the whole moral problem of the natural versus the artificial and its gendered dimension. This passage also recalls the terms of a theme that will be repeated an infinite number of times in the sixteenth century, all the more so after the Reformations had cast a new suspicion on the arts of dissimulation.

> Women are always very eager to be – and when they cannot be, at least to seem – beautiful. So when nature is somehow at fault in this regard, they try to piece it out by artifice. . . . Do you not see how much more grace a lady has who paints (if at all) so sparingly and so little, that whoever sees her is in doubt whether she be painted or not; than another lady so plastered that she seems to have put a mask upon her face and dares not laugh for fear of cracking it. . . . Again, how much more pleasing than all others is one (I mean not ill-favoured) who is plainly seen to have nothing on her face, although it be neither very white nor very red, but by nature a

> little pale and sometimes tinged with an honest flush from shame or other accident, – with hair artlessly unadorned and hardly confined, her gestures simple and free, without showing care or wish to be beautiful! This is that nonchalant simplicity most pleasing to the eyes and minds of men, who are ever fearful of being deceived by art.[90]

Women's natural tendency toward deception and artificiality was conceived as a tendency to alter those natural traits of the face that would have made them beautiful of a simple beauty.

On the other hand, sixteenth-century descriptions of the male body were much drier. Moreover, words like "force," "size," and "stature" are morally charged, and it is hard to disentangle their physical from their moral meaning. The male body was the object of different concerns, mostly "functional" or "utilitarian" ones, before being the object of aesthetic appreciation. Physical appearance had a moral meaning in itself. The best qualities of a male body were strength and power, which were inseparable from dexterity. However, in the sixteenth century, doubts arose about male standards of beauty.[91] First of all, humanists sometimes expressed distrust at male strength as a sign of brutality or savageness. In the second place, youth, or better adolescence, became an object of aesthetic and also of erotic appreciation under the influence of humanist discoveries of the classics.[92] This contradiction signals the existence of two conceptions of male beauty: a beauty of war and a beauty of civility.[93]

At the same time, and especially in Italy, where *Cinquecento* writers of all genres were all too conscious of the loss of political liberty and autonomy of their homelands, excessive use of cosmetics or attention to artificial means of enhancing beauty on the part of males became the object of accusations of effeminacy, subordination, loss of masculine honor, appearance, and moral strength.[94] Tommaso Garzoni lamented that one could see

> the most vile prostitutes and the most shameless catamites who curl their hair like women go about all anointed and scented, and not emperors and kings, who have always done so . . . [these prostitutes and catamites] scent their soft cheeks with a thousand perfumes . . . with perpetual infamy and dishonor of these vituperative times.[95]

Stefano Della Casa (1503–1566) in his *Galateo* warned readers that men should not adorn themselves as women do

> for his adornments will be one thing, himself another; I see many men who have their hair and beards all curled with a hot iron, and have their faces, necks, and hands so shiny smooth and soft that it would be unsuitable for any young wench, even for a tart anxious to bring her wares to market and to sell them at a higher price.[96]

Sixteenth-century readers must have had in mind the description of the effeminate courtier by Baldassar Castiglione. Contrary to having a graceful but manly appearance, this type was "soft and effeminate," all concerned with curling his hair and plucking his eyebrows. These men "gloss their faces with all those arts employed by the most wanton and unchaste women in the world"; they also adopted womanly ways of walking, gesturing, and speaking and "should be treated not as good women, but as public harlots, and driven not merely from the courts of great lords but from the society of honest men."[97]

Della Porta included a description of the "effeminate type" in his book on physiognomy. The effeminate had adopted the habit of artificially caring for his body and face, abandoning the natural dignity and strength typical of male beauty.

> I saw one of them in Naples – he wrote – with sparse or no [facial] hair at all, little mouth, delicate and straight eyelashes, shameful eyes as women's eyes are, weak and subtle voice, white and trembling neck, biting his lips; to sum it up, with the body and gestures of a woman. He was willing to spend time at home . . . and as a woman he minded the kitchen business; he shunned men and engaged in conversation with women, and going to bed with them he behaved more womanly than women themselves; he thought like a woman and he talked about himself in the female person . . .; and the worst was that he bore the nefarious Venus worse than women do.[98]

"Popular" writer Giulio Cesare Croce (1550–1609) was chronologically and geographically closer to Gaspare Tagliacozzi. In a satirical pamphlet written in the form of a letter addressed by Narcissus to the "most beautiful, attractive and perfumed youth of the city" in 1590, Croce-Narcissus presented himself as the defender of beauty and love, an ally of Venus, and wanted to give the young noblemen of Bologna suggestions to defend and advance the "true" beauty. Narcissus, after having stigmatized the effeminate type who spent too much time with mirrors and makeup before going out – "just like women do" – suggested people gifted with natural beauty to "put nothing on their faces . . . to show everyone their beauty." Men who cared normally about their beauty must simply cover their defects and show off their strengths and most beautiful parts. Moreover, "all those who are under our flag" – Narcissus went on – must go once or twice a week to the barber shop and spend "an hour or two there" to have a haircut, be shaved, be washed, and have their hair and skin imperfections polished.[99] This is what natural beauty was all about. It had nothing to do with artificially enhancing one's figure.

Two parts of the face were particularly important in terms of sexual difference and perceptions of masculine personhood: noses and beards.[100] These parts of the body were the object of intense scrutiny in the sixteenth century, both in medicine and in literature.

Tagliacozzi devoted three entire chapters to praise the nose from all possible points of view. He praised the shape and special position of the nose, as well as its role in making a face beautiful:

> Although each part of the face has its own distinction and grace and is positioned with delightful symmetry . . . the nose has a unique property. If it harmonizes with the other parts, it graces the face to the outmost. If, however, is misshapen, crooked, flat, or disfigured by injury (*distortus, pravus, simus, vulnere notatus*), it destroys the integrity of the appearance.[101]

Tagliacozzi then quickly moved to reporting stories of noses that had been cut off in order to preserve chastity and to scare away rapists and seducers. Among them, the story of seventh-century Saint Ebba is perhaps the most significant. Ebba was the Abbess of the Scottish monastery of Coldingham and had cut off her nose and that of her sisters in order to horrify the invader Danes and prevent their lust. Tagliacozzi commented:

> For if the nose is amputated at his apex, the sinuses and recesses of the internal parts lie exposed and huge gaps and dark caverns (*hiatus & cavernae*) are visible; this is surely a horrendous (*horrendum*) and abominable sight.[102]

The surgeon remarked that in this particular case the mutilation was not "shameful" but virtuous, thus revealing that such mutilations were indeed ordinarily considered shameful and underlining the reaction of horror toward one of the features of the "grotesque body." The horrid character of this grotesque face was given by the openness of the external body toward its internal dark recesses. As noticed by Mikhail Bakhtin, the grotesque was characterized by an "unfinished" character of the body, as opposed to the "geometrical closure" of the classical body.[103]

All anatomy and surgery books of the time included detailed descriptions of faces and their parts, as showed, for example, in this diagram by Volcher Coiter (Figure 3.3) and by Giulio Cesare Aranzi's booklet on anatomical *observationes*, which focused almost exclusively on two body parts: female generative organs and heads.[104] Tagliacozzi followed the Galenic tradition, which considered the nose as the link between sensations (smell) and the brain, the seat of the senses. The Bolognese also listed the "usefulnesses" of the nose. First of all, the nose is an important organ of respiration; it has the function of filtering and purifying the air that goes into the lungs through the trachea, thanks to the communication between the nose and the palate. With the help of the nose the human voice is made more clear and speech more distinct. Finally, the nose has "the capacity for rescuing us from the vicious onslaughts of disease, end even from the jaws of death itself," for example when it gives its "friendly help" to the other organs for the expulsion of the catarrh.[105] The nose had the essential function of being a passageway, an organ that regulated the relations between the internal and the external environments.

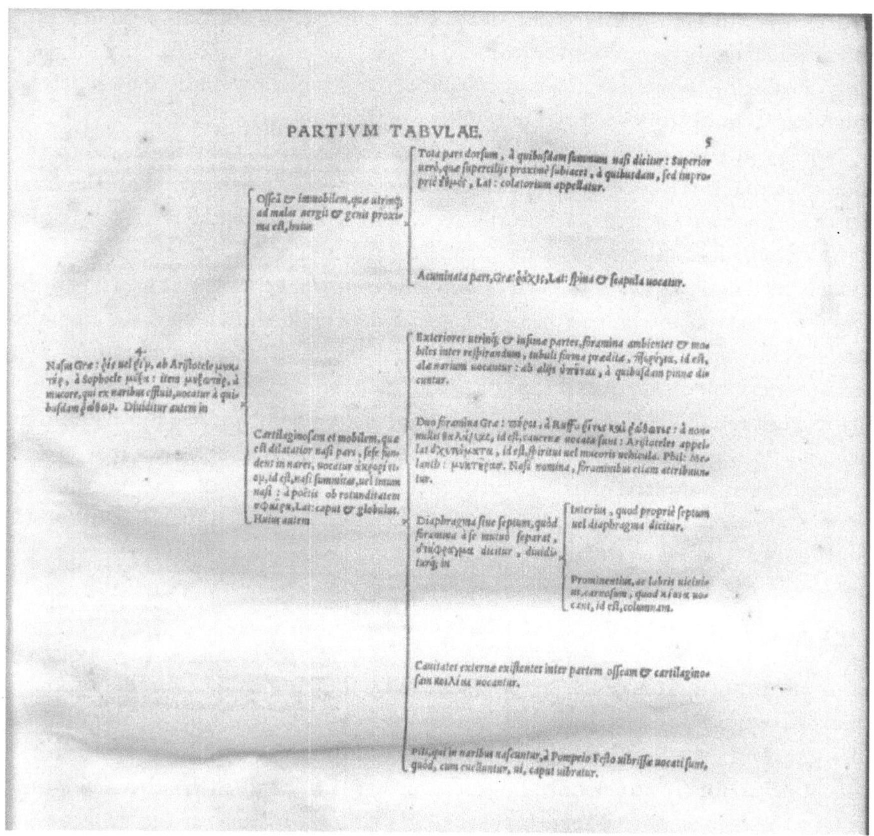
PARTIVM TABVLAE.

FIGURE 3.3 Volcher Coiter, *Externarum et internarum principalium humani corporis partium tabulae* (Nuremberg: in officina Theodorici Gerlatzeni, 1572): table of the parts of the human nose.

Missing noses could elicit horrified reactions; they could mean a lack of masculine attributes; and they could suggest shameful circumstances. Patricia Skinner raised some doubts about the actual popular diffusion of this symbolic connection between the male genitals and the nose in the Middle Ages, but plenty of evidence points toward this direction. It might be that this association formed later.[106] In any case, the association has nothing to do with psychoanalytic theory, as it makes little sense to transfer early twentieth-century Viennese concerns to sixteenth-century Italy.[107] Rather, if one thinks historically, the grounds for this symbolism seem to be provided by the fact that lack of noses was perceived either as a feminizing feature or in any case as a mark of subordination, two characteristics diametrically opposed to upper-class masculinity. Moreover, noses – and especially aquiline noses – were regarded as features of an authoritative masculinity and a virile appearance. Noses and faces did not serve the only purpose of distinguishing men from women but also functioned as marks of social class, to separate certain kinds of men from other kinds of men. The prototypical ignorant and savage peasant-mountaineer, the social type who came to town only for begging or offering their raw labor force, had been described by Giulio Cesare Croce as having "a hooked nose, tip-tilted, with very large nostrils."[108]

Noses figured prominently in the culture of the face. They mattered to the issue of sexual difference in the early modern culture. The extremely influential thesis of Thomas Laqueur, according to whom from ancient Greece up to the eighteenth century there was only one medical and social "one-sex" model that conceived female as the less perfect and reversed image of the male, has been heavily criticized in the past two decades. It has been shown that the one-sex model followed a limited and precise textual tradition and that medieval and early modern medical conceptions of sexual difference were complex and multifarious, not reducible to one overarching model.[109] The insistence on the human face and on some of its particular parts, like the nose, further shows that sexual difference was not just a matter of anatomy and physiology – in other words, not just a matter of medical culture – but a much wider issue, involving different kinds of perceptions of the body.

Face and self

Contrary to historians of the self influenced by the Foucauldean model of sharp breaks, I would argue that in the history of Western personhood, there is no emergence of "the" self or "the" individual but only the emergence of historically specific forms of personhood, more or less similar to each other. The history of the face in the sixteenth century is neither a history of the progressive development of the individual through history nor only a matter of how expressions and self-control have been molded by specific social conditions. Rather, it is a history about the following issue: what kind of men and women and which social class were entitled to have a face and a self? What had they to do, as men or women, in order to be so entitled?

Norbert Elias' thesis on the process of civilization as a process of self-restraint maintains some validity when stripped of its teleological and Euro-centric characteristics.[110] Building on Elias, French historians Courtine and Haroche have showed that in the early modern period manuals of rhetoric, treatises of physiognomy, and textbooks of manners and the art of conversation constantly repeated that the face was the cornerstone of self-perception, of the sense of the other, of the rituals of civil society, and of the forms of political life.[111] In the second half of the sixteenth century, writers started to claim that individuals expressed themselves mainly through their faces. According to Courtine and Haroche, this novelty was connected to the process of privatization of life of the early modern period. The early modern notion of the individual was closely tied to the expression of his or her face, as a bodily translation of one person's inner self. In this way, the history of the face becomes a history of "the emergence of expression" as a sign of individual identity.[112]

This thesis has some value. For example, by the middle of the sixteenth century, clergyman and courtier Giovanni Della Casa, while discussing witticism and humor, could advise his readers not to say obscene words or make vile and dishonorable gestures "as distorting one's face and eyes or gesticulating like a dope, for no one should debase himself in order to amuse the others."[113]

Valentin Groebner has studied practices of identification through reading the skin of people (scars, birthmarks, etc.) from the late Middle Ages to the sixteenth century and has argued that prior to the sixteenth century the body was "opaque." Groebner has also traced the development of the concept of complexion, temperament, or humoral balance, from Galenic theory to its fundamental shift in the sixteenth century. In this period, complexion became the formula for "personality" and migrated from the internal balance of bodily elements to the outside of the body, thus transformed into a congenital category.[114] In this process, the links between the surface of the body and the inner physical and moral makeup of the individual became tighter.

In his 1938 classic essay on the notion of personhood, French anthropologist Marcel Mauss showed how the notion of the person was linked to that of the face. Mauss sketched the trajectory that from the Greek meanings of "persona" (mask) and "face" – attached to the practical use of ritual, tragic, and funerary masks – moved into Roman law to indicate those citizens who fully enjoyed the rights of citizenship (as opposed to slaves). Finally, the notion of person moved into the realm of ethics and a metaphysic of individuality with the emergence of Stoic moral philosophy and the full deployment of Christianity.[115] According to Mauss' schematic history of personhood, the radical novelty of the emergence of the modern notion of person understood as an individual psychological entity – or, in other words, the "self" – was introduced in the late seventeenth century, under the influence of Descartes and Locke.[116]

Fernando Vidal and Caroline Walker Bynum have persuasively argued that the modern self emerged around the same time through a process of disembodiment that marked a radical departure from previously accepted notions of Aristotelian unity of body and soul.[117] Katharine Park argued that in the sixteenth century, the century of anatomy, the relationships between the external and the inner parts of the body, and between the body and the soul, were still close enough, but the human body acquired a certain depth: over the course of the century "the drama of moisture and heat started to give way to an experience of personhood rooted in anatomical terms."[118]

Portraiture offers some insights into the relationships between faces and selves. The visual genre of the portrait bloomed in the Renaissance, evolving from a kind of matter-of-fact description of physiognomy to incorporate more and more symbolic and complex elements indicating the social standing of the subjects. Sixteenth-century portraits in particular abounded with symbols of status, family, and class, because physical and facial traits were only one aspect of the complex network of elements composing selfhood.[119] During the *Cinquecento*, portraits began to circulate outside of the circles of noblemen, noblewomen, lords, clerics, and kings and to be requested from middle-class people too. Caroline Murphy has showed how in the second half of the sixteenth century "scholars at Europe's courts and Universities became increasingly curious not only about distant (or dead) colleagues' ideas and innovations, but also about their physiognomics, manners, gestures, all qualities that could bring erudition to life." Scholars themselves began to assemble quite substantial collections of pictures of those they admired, the most famous and important being Paolo Giovio's *Elogia virorum illustrium*.[120] Even Cardinal Gabriele Paleotti praised the habit of portraying the ancient and contemporary virtuous men as providing moral examples for the bystanders. The Bolognese artistic community in the late sixteenth century profited from the new interest in the scholar's portrait, and a "cult of portraiture of the illustrious" developed.[121]

In late sixteenth-century Bologna – one of the places where the genre of caricature was born – a daring painter such as Bartolomeo Passerotti portrayed young noblemen with perfectly soft skin and intact features. One particular portraiture shows a young gentleman touching his sword and holding a classical statuette of the Greek-like classic image of the body, symbolizing arms and letters as the two key activities of a good son of aristocracy (Figure 3.4). On the other hand, in his caricatures of the lower classes and of people of different skin color or "race," Passerotti could play with forms and even disfigure faces (Figure 3.5).[122] Lower-class men were positioned below the rank at which portraits were painted. Their faces could be represented but not in portraits.

It would not be correct to say that the face coincided with the self. As shown by sixteenth-century portraits, the face was just one element among others that gave plastic representation to the self, along with clothing, behavior, accessories, and so forth. Historians of portraiture have described one feature that can be extended to sixteenth-century culture of the face and reconstructive surgery. Representations – or restorations – of the face and body are always in tension between the two poles. On the one hand, they should capture the individuality of human beings; on the other hand, they should capture the universality of human nature.[123] In sixteenth-century culture the face became more and more described in precise anatomical terms. The human face became a tapestry in which the individuality of the self could be read through a network of analogies between its moral and its physical elements. The face became the surface from which lines departed horizontally and vertically, linking together moral character and expression, social role, physical appearance, and beauty. At the same time, these correspondences lost part of their relevance for the theological, religious, and metaphysical identity of the self, while the reference to its social life progressively took the center of the stage. The face was connected to personhood, and the more intense the perception of details of the face was, the more specific was the perception of someone's individuality. The face is one stage in the historical process of the localization of the self away from the psychological-physical unity toward the brain.

In an essay on allegories of nature in the Renaissance, Katharine Park has traced a shift from the medieval personification of nature (clothed, speaking,

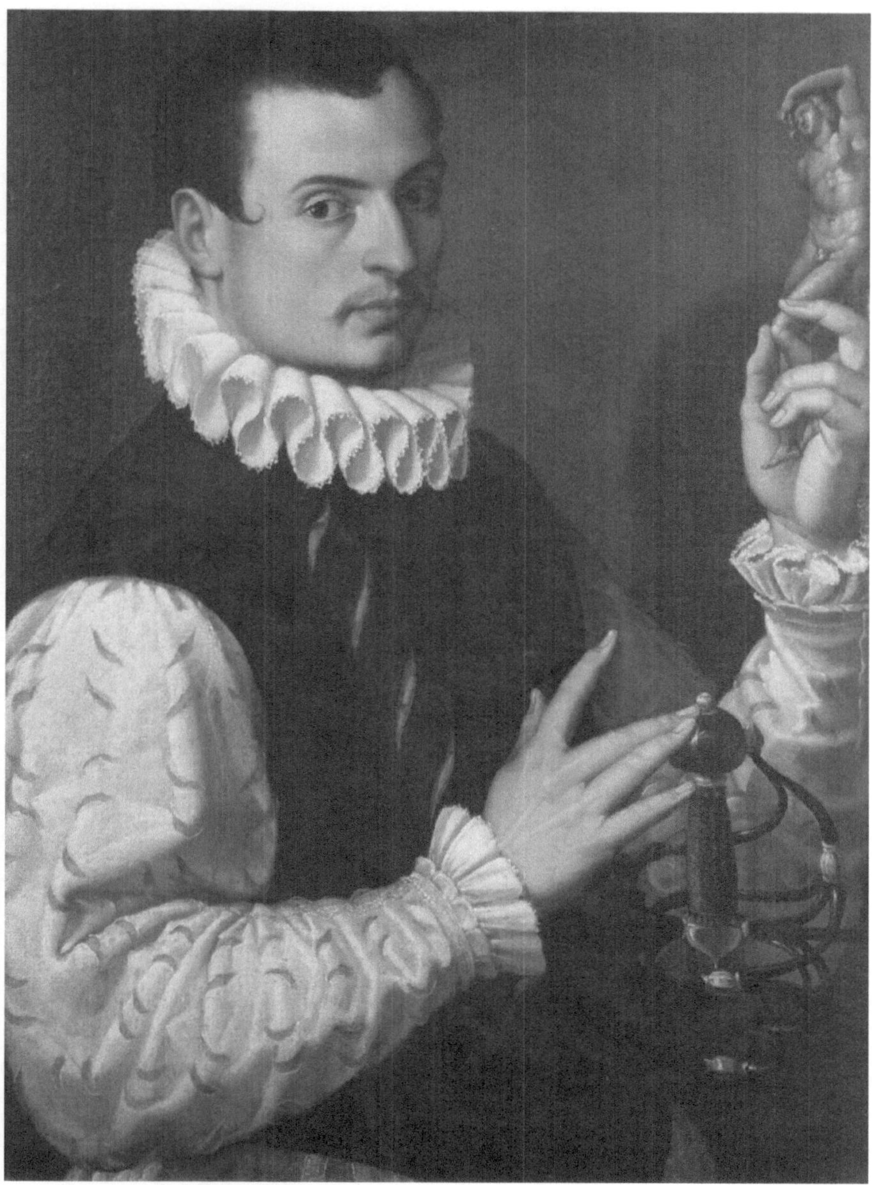

FIGURE 3.4 Bartolomeo Passerotti, *Portrait of a young man* (late sixteenth century). University of Newcastle-upon-Tyne, Hatton Gallery.

Source: ©Tyne & Wear Archives & Museums/Bridgeman Images.

majestic) to the Renaissance and early modern one (naked, with many breasts, enigmatic, and opaque). This shift was connected with changing philosophical understandings of the order and authority of nature. The new personification of nature stood for fertility, creativity, and an optimistic view of the bountifulness

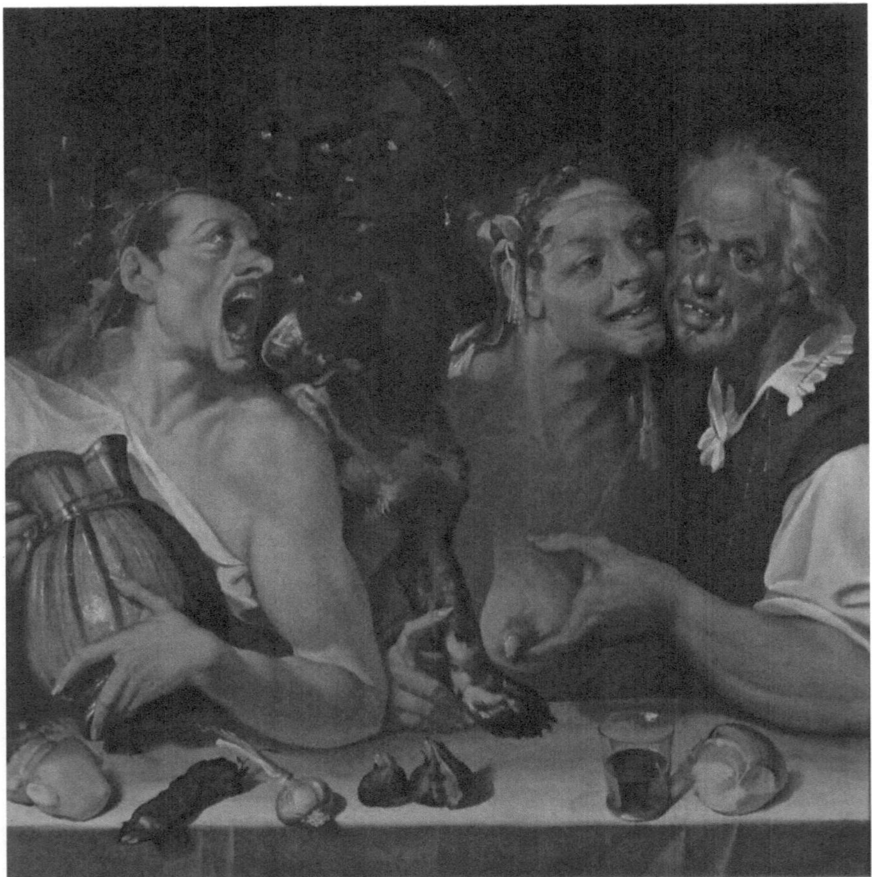

FIGURE 3.5 Bartolomeo Passerotti, *L'allegra compagnia* (late sixteenth century). Private collection (public domain).

of nature, "a regime of plenty." Nakedness symbolized nature's closeness to God's creation and her being untouched and not polluted by human artifice.[124] At the same time, sixteenth-century nature was increasingly represented as "*pre-*moral," namely indifferent to human costumes. Park argued that during that century nature's "functions . . . were set apart from and opposed to the human activities of nurture, domestication, and moral education . . . and her functions were represented in purely physical terms."[125] In turn, this process of separation of the natural and the artificial led to the fact that more and more philosophers, naturalists, and theologians engaged in the enterprise of developing ever more refined skills to interpret her and to "speak on her behalf."[126]

The gendered human face was caught in this double process too. Subject to norms prescribing its natural appearance, the face was at the same time the surface on which the social order was reflected, the moral character could be read by the specialists of nature, and the artificial could be debunked. The contradiction between the emphasis on the natural and the increased attention to the care of the appearance of the face is only apparent. As in a sort of process of cultural *sprezzatura* – the art of masking art – selected artificial means could be used to keep appearances as natural as possible. The sixteenth-century culture of the face, which was in itself an elite culture, became more and more attentive to the distinction of social roles and more and more aware that being a person meant playing different roles. As written by Natalie Zemon Davis: "the greatest obstacle to self-definition was not embeddedness but powerlessness and poverty."[127]

Notes

1 Tagliacozzi, *De curtorum*, p. 10 (1:6–7).
2 Ibid., p. 11 (1:7).
3 Ibid.
4 Ibid.
5 Erwin Panofsky, "The History of the Theory of Human Proportions as a Reflection of the History of Styles," in Erwin Panofsky, ed. *Meaning in the Visual Arts: Papers in and on Art History* (Garden City: Anchor Books, 1955), pp. 55–109, 56.
6 Plato, *Timaeus, Critias, Cleitophon, Menexenus, Epistles*, tr. G. Bury (Cambridge: Harvard University Press, 1929) (*Timaeus* V, 31c), p. 59: "And the fairest of bonds is that which most perfectly unites into one both itself and the things which it binds together; and to effect this in the fairest manner is the natural property of proportion."
7 For example, Vesalius explicitly mentioned it in his quest to represent the normal human body in his *De humani corporis fabrica*; see Nancy Siraisi, "Vesalius and Human Diversity in De Humani Corporis Fabrica," *Journal of the Warburg and Courtauld Institutes* 57 (1994): 60–88.
8 Panofsky, "The History of the Theory," p. 68, note 19; Patrizia Castelli, *L'estetica del Rinascimento* (Bologna: Il mulino, 2005), p. 35; Michael Baxandall, *Painting and Experience in Fifteenth Century Italy: A Primer in the Social History of Pictorial Style*, 2nd ed. (Oxford: Clarendon Press, 1988), pp. 86–93.
9 Umberto Eco, *Storia della bellezza* (Milan: Bompiani, 2004), p. 87.
10 Castelli, *L'estetica*, pp. 35–44; Georges Vigarello, *Histoire de la beauté: Le corps et l'art d'embellir de la Renaissance à nos jours* (Paris: Points, 2014), pp. 39–43.
11 Panofsky, "The History of the Theory," pp. 89–90. Platonist philosopher Marsilio Ficino (1433–1499) defined beauty as "a certain proportion between all the parts, or a real proportion and commensuration, with some new color (*una certa posizione di tutti i membri, o veramente commensuratione e proporzione, con qualche novità di colori*)"; quoted by Castelli, *L'estetica*, p. 46. Artist and polymath Albrecht *Dürer (1471–1528)* in his book on the symmetry of human bodies (published in 1528 and translated into Italian in 1591 as *Della proprtione delli corpi umani*) employed the same concepts of proportion and symmetry. See Ibid., pp. 46–47.
12 Pomponio Gaurico, *De sculptura* [1504], ed. Paolo Cutolo (Naples: Edizioni Scientifiche Italiane, 1999), pp. 152–153.
13 Ibid., pp. 156–157. Panofksy has argued that this way of measuring bodily proportions came from Byzantine art theory much more than from classical art: see Panofsky, "The History of the Theory," pp. 75–76.
14 Gaurico, *De sculptura*, pp. 158–159.
15 Tagliacozzi, *De curtorum*, p. 149 (2:31).
16 Cesare Ripa, *Iconologia*, ed. Sonia Maffei (Turin: Einaudi, 2012), pp. 61–62: "Si dipinge la Bellezza con la testa ascosa fra le nuvole, perché non è cosa della quale più difficilmente si possa parlare con mortal lingua, e che meno si possa conoscere con l'intelletto

umano, quanto la bellezza, la quale, nelle cose create, non è altro, metaforicamente parlando, che un splendore che deriva dalla luce della faccia di Dio, come definiscono i Platonici . . . per dimostrare che ogni bellezza consiste in misure e proporzioni, le quali s'aggiustano col tempo e col luogo. Il luogo determina la bellezza nella disposizione delle Provincie, delle Città, de' Templi, delle Piazze, dell'uomo, e di tutte le cose soggette all'occhio, come colori ben distinti, e con proporzionata quantità e misura, e con altre cose simili; col tempo si determinano l'armonie, i suoni, le voci, l'orazioni, gli abbattimenti, et altre cose, le quali con misura aggiustandosi, dilettano e sono meritamente chiamate belle."

17 For the academic tradition of physiognomy, see Jole Agrimi, *Ingeniosa scientia nature. Studi sulla fisiognomica medievale* (Florence: Sismel/Edizioni del Galluzzo, 2002); Joseph Ziegler, "Philosophers and Physicians on the Scientific Validity of Latin Physiognomy, 1200–1500," *Early Science and Medicine* 12, 3 (2007): 285–312. For its "hermetic" side, see Martin Porter, *Windows of the Soul: Physiognomy In European Culture 1470–1780* (Oxford: Oxford University Press, 2005).

18 With the phrase "culture of the face" I do not mean to imply that the face had a culture or was important only in the Renaissance, or only in Italy. My idea is to describe this particular and historically determined culture of the face.

19 Malagola, *Statuti*, vol. 1, pp. 274–275.

20 From the early eleventh century on, Avicenna and other Arabic-writing natural philosophers tried to include physiognomy within the realm of the sciences alongside with medicine and astrology. Arabic texts by Rhazes, and above all the *Secretum secretorum*, were translated into Latin in the early thirteenth century. Natural philosopher Michael Scotus (1175-c.1232) in his 1230 *Liber physionomiae*, drawing largely on Arabic material, was the first to call physiognomy a *scientia naturae*, which was the first step toward the "scholasticization" of this body of knowledge. Scotus was followed by Albertus Magnus (c.1200–1280), Roger Bacon (c.1219–1292), and later by Pietro d'Abano (1257–1316), who all made use of physiognomic ways of knowing and wrote about it. Medieval authors took pains to distinguish physiognomy from chiromancy and the divinatory arts and to connect it with the science of interpreting the stars, astrology, understood in a nondeterministic way. See Agrimi, Ingeniosa scientia nature; Ziegler, "Philosophers and Physicians."

21 The text of the pseudo-Aristotelian physiognomic book, a Latin version of an anonymous Arabic text, circulated in Western Europe since the thirteenth century and was included in the sixteenth-century editions of Aristotle's complete works, including those by Manuzio and Oporinus. Aristotle discussed physiognomy and the method of the physiognomic syllogism in his books on logic (*First Analytics*, II, 70b, 1–38).

22 Pseudo-Aristotle, *Physiognomics*, in Aristotle, *Minor Works*, tr. W.S. Hett (Cambridge: Harvard University Press, 1936), p. 85.

23 Pseudo-Aristotle, *Physiognomics*, p. 105.

24 Federici Vescovini, "L'individuale," pp. 65–66.

25 Ibid., p. 137.

26 Ibid., pp. 109–111.

27 Ibid., p. 113.

28 Giovanni Battista Della Porta, *Della fisionomia dell'uomo libri sei*, 2 vols. (Naples-Rome: Edizioni Scientifiche Italiane, 2013), vol. 2, pp. 96–98: "una scienza che impara da' segni che sono fissi nel corpo, et accidenti che trasmutano i segni, investigar i costumi naturali dell'animo . . . Sia A la fortezza, aver l'estremità grande B, il leone C. Ogni animale che ha l'estremità grandi è forte; ogni leone et alcuni animali hanno l'estremità grandi; duqnue ogni leone ed alcuni animali sono forti." The first Latin edition dates 1586; the first vernacular edition 1598. On this work and for a rich bibliography, see Bruno Basile, "'Riflessi dell'anima.'" La fisiognomica prima e dopo Della Porta," in Marco Santoro, ed. *La "mirabile" natura. Magia e scienza in Giovan Battista Della Porta (1615–2015)* (Pisa: Serra 2016), pp. 57–70.

29 For the notion of the sixteenth-century norms of seeing the body and of locating beauty on the face, see Vigarello, *Histoire de la beauté*, pp. 20–23. On the function of the illustrations in Della Porta's book as a guiding norm for portraits, see Alfonso Paolella, "L'autore delle illustrazioni delle *Fisiognomiche* di Della Porta e la ritrattistica. Esperienze filologiche," in *La "mirabile" natura*, pp. 81–94.

30 Della Porta, *Della fisionomia*, pp. 99–100: "come parte nobilissima di tutto il corpo, stanza de' sensi e nella quale abita la principal parte dell'anima, perché quivi la vista, l'udito, l'odorato et il gusto abitano ristretti . . . et, incontrandomi un uomo, subito si vede la faccia, il che non avviene al petto e all'altre parti . . . [nella faccia] starà la principal parte dell'anima et in quella il dono dell'intelligenza."

31 Ibid., pp. 163–164: "testimone dimostratore della nostra conscienzia, il quale è incerto, incostante e vario . . . è suo [dell'animo] simulatore e dissimulatore, onde non è fuor di ragione in ogni ora poter giudicare dal volto, fuorché quando sarà raffreddato dai movimenti e passion dell'animo . . . Il volto è infatti spechio della mente, perché, stando taciti gli occhi, ancor si manifesta i secreti dell'animo. Dicono i medici che tutto il corpo manda il suo sangue e spiriti alla faccia, per essere membro più notabile di tutto il corpo; onde le passion di tutto il corpo e dell'animo si conoscono nella faccia."

32 Ibid., p. 464: "E un assioma vecchio et approvato da tutti quelli che fan professione di Fisionomia, che la convenevol disposizione delle parti del corpo dimostra ancora una convenevol disposizione di costumi; e si suol dire proverbialmente che chi è mostro nel corpo è ancor mostro nell'anima. La bellezza è una misurata disposizione de' membri del corpo, che è modello et imagine di quella dell'anima . . . la natura ha fabricato il corpo conforme a gli effetti dell'animo."

33 Ibid., p. 467: "una armoniosa e concordevol concordanza di parti."

34 Ibid., pp. 473–474: "li brutti di faccia sono bruttissimi di animo . . . e se alcuno volesse cercarne la cagion naturale perché i brutti sono cattivi e i belli buoni, a distemperanza de gli uomori nel corpo e mal composti, rendendo le parti del corpo mal composte e la distemperanza de gli umori cagionano i vizii et i mali costumi."

35 Tagliacozzi, *De curtorum*, pp. 25–26 (1:18).

36 Pseudo-Aristotle, *Physiognomics*, p. 121.

37 Della Porta, *Della fisionomia*, p. 146: "Il naso risponde alla verga ché, avendolo alcuno lungo e grosso, overo acuto e grosso o breve, il medesimo si giudica di quella; così le nari rispondono ai testicoli." Famous writers such as Giulio Cesare Croce and the Neapolitan Giovanni Battista Marino (1569–1625) – for example, in *Il padre Naso* (1626) – played with the shared meanings of the nose and the penis. For example, Marino clearly intended to suggest a direct analogy between the *inflated nose and the erected penis* in *La samprognia*, when he described the God of fertility Priapos, noted for his endurance in sexual intercourse and the huge dimensions of his penis, as the "strong herd of the field and the vine" who "with naked head, smoky face, lit as fire, with an enflated nose and red light eyes, while admiring such beauty, brandished his sickle (*robusto custode/del campo e della vigna . . . ignudo la testa/fumante il volto e più che vampa acceso/col naso enfiato e con le luci rosse/mentre tanta beltà quivi mirava/la sua falce vibrava*)." See Giovan Battista Marino, *La samprognia* (Venice: presso Gio. Pietro Bigonci, 1575), p. 122.

38 Tagliacozzi, *De curtorum*, p. 6 (1:4).

39 Tagliacozzi's teacher at Bologna, Cardano built an interpretative art of reading moles and forefronts.

40 Tagliacozzi, *De curtorum*, p. 13 (1:9).

41 Ibid.

42 Aristotle, *Parts of Animals*, tr. A.L. Peck (Cambridge: Harvard University Press, 1937), pp. 216–217 (662b).

43 See Patrizia Magli, "The Face and the Soul," in Michael Feher, ed. *Fragments for a History of the Human Body*, 3 vols. (New York: Zone Books, 1989), vol. 2, pp. 86–129, 94.

44 Cicero, *On the Nature of Gods*, tr. H. Rackham (Cambridge: Harvard University Press, 1933), pp. 257–259 (2.56.140–141).

45 Mondino de' Liuzzi, *Anotomia*, ed. Piero P. Gorgi and Gian Franco Pasini (Bologna: Istituto per la Storia dell'Università di Bologna, 1992), pp. 100–103. On the theme of the erect posture of humanity, see Marjorie O'Rourke Boyle, *Senses of Touch: Human Dignity and Deformity from Michelangelo to Calvin* (Leiden: Brill, 1998).
46 Tagliacozzi, *De curtorum*, pp. 18–19 (1:13).
47 Ibid., p. 19 (1:13).
48 Ibid., pp. 19–21 (1:14–15).
49 Girolamo Cardano, "De subtilitate," in Girolamo Cardano, ed. *Opera Omnia* (Lyon: Jean Antoine Huguetan et Marc Antione Ravaud, 1663), vol. 3, p. 559. See Alessandro Simili, *Girolamo Cardano lettore e medico a Bologna* (Bologna: Azzoguidi, 1969), pp. 56–61; Nancy Siraisi, *The clock and the mirror: Girolamo Cardano and Renaissance medicine* (Princeton: Princeton University Press, 1997), p. 137.
50 Praises of the head and the face can be read in as diverse authors as military surgeon Griolamo Crasso, in Ambroise Paré's anatomy, and in authoritative and learned Schenck von Grafenberg. See Girolamo Crasso, *Diario empirico. Nel quale si dimostra il modo di curare ogni sorte di ferita nel corpo humano* (Venice: appresso gli heredi di Francesco Rampazzetto, 1577), fol. 15r; Paré, *Oeuvres*, vol. 1, pp. 203–204; Johannes Schenck von Grafenberg, *Observationum medicarum rariorum libri VII* (Frankfurt: E. Paltheniana, 1665), book I, p. 1.
51 Leonardo Fioravanti, *La Cirugia* (Venice: appresso gli heredi di Melchior Sessa, 1570), fol. 147r: "E' la testa la principal cosa, che habbino tutte le creature viventi. E che ciò sia vero, si vede, che un humo senza piede, senza il membro, & li testicoli, senza le braccia, & senza il naso, & le orecchie, può vivere: ma senza la testa, nessuna creatura può vivere."
52 Gabriele Paleotti, *Discorso intorno alle immagini sacre e profane* (Bologna: per Alessandro Benacci, 1582), II, fol. 157r: portraits are useful "quando per occasione di liti in parte lontana, bisognasse provare la somiglianza tra padre e figliuoli." Other functions of the portrait included presenting the image of future brides and grooms. The absence of portraits as an obstacle to identification emerges in the case of Martin Guerre too: see Natalie Zemon Davies, *The Return of Martin Guerre* (Cambridge: Harvard University Press, 1983), p. 43.
53 Tagliacozzi, *De curtorum*, p. 10 (1:7).
54 See Valentin Groebner, *Who Are You? Identification, Deception, and Surveillance in Early Modern Europe* (New York: Zone Books, 2007), pp. 17–29.
55 Zemon Davis, *The Return of Martin Guerre*, pp. 104–122.
56 *Statuta civilia et criminalia civitatis Bononiae* (Bologna: Pisarri, 1735–1736), vol. 1, p. 426 (*Rubrica LVI*). On the justice system in early modern Bologna, see Marco Cavina, "I luoghi della giustizia," in *Storia di Bologna*, vol. 3.1, pp. 367–411.
57 *Statuta civilia et criminalia*, vol. 1, p. 480.
58 Ibid., pp. 480–482.
59 ASB, Assunteria di Sanità, 1.
60 BUB 770, Ghiselli, *Memorie*, vol. 18 (1585–1590), fol. 22–23.
61 Caroline Walker Bynum, *The Resurrection of the Body in Western Christianity* (New York: Columbia University Press, 1995), p. 11.
62 Caroline Walker Bynum, "Material Continuity, Personal Survival, and the Resurrection of the Body: A Scholastic Discussion in Its Medieval and Modern Contexts," in Caroline Walker Bynum, ed. *Fragmentation and Redemption: Essays on Gender and the Human Body in Medieval Religion* (New York: Zone Books, 1992), pp. 239–297.
63 Irina Metzler, *Disability in Medieval Europe: Thinking about Physical Impairment during the High Middle Ages, C. 1100–1400* (New York: Routledge, 2006), pp. 40–41. See also Henri-Jacques Stiker, *A History of Disability*, tr. William Sayers (Ann Arbor: The University of Michigan Press, 1999), pp. 23–37. For an excellent discussion of the relationships between the history of disfigurements and disability studies, see Patricia Skinner, *Living with Disfigurement in Early Medieval Europe* (New York: Palgrave Macmillan, 2017), pp. 1–39.

64 See *The Canons and Decrees of the Council of Trent*, ed. Theodore Alois Buckley (London: George Routlege & Co., 1852), session XXII, pp. 149–150; Angelo Turchini, "La nascita del sacerdozio come professione," in Paolo Prodi, ed. *Disciplina dell'anima, disciplina del corpo e dsiciplina della società tra medioevo ed età moderna* (Bologna: Il mulino, 1994), pp. 225–256; Carlo Fantappié, "La professionalizzazione del sacerdozio cattolico nell'età moderna," in Egle Becchi and Monica Ferrari, eds. *Formare alle professioni. Sacerdoti, principi, educatori* (Turin: Codice, 2009), pp. 39–69. The interpretation of this passage from Leviticus is hotly debated by an intersection of disability studies and Bible studies; see, for example, Jennifer Anne Cox, "Disability as Enacted Parable," *Journal of Religion, Disability & Health* 15, 3 (2011): 241–253, with the relative bibliography.

65 Thomas Aquinas, *Summa theologiae* (Bologna: Edizioni Studio Domenicano 1984), vol. 31, p. 69 (Suppl., q. 43, a. 3): "si, ante contractatum matrimonium, aliquam gravem infirmitatem incurrat alter eorum inter quos sunt contracta sponsalia, quae ipsum debilitet nimis, ut epilepsia aut paralysis; aut eum deformet, ut a *abscissio nasi* vel orbitas oculorum aut aliquid huiusmodi; aut quae sunt contra bonum prolis, utpote lepra . . . possunt sponsalia dirimere, ne sibi invicem displiceant, et matrimonium sic contractum malum exitum sortiatur."

66 Giovanni Filippo Ingrassia, *Methodus dandi relationes pro mutilates, torquendis, aut a tortura excusandis*, ed. G. Curcio (Catania: Romeo Prampolini, 1939), p. 70: "ita in rustico, ignobilique homine non existens turpis cicatrix, in nobili tamen, si non speciem mutat, gradum tamen turpitudinis auget." Ingrassia, 67: "od deformitatem hominum consortium fugiant." On early modern legal medicine, see Alessandro Pastore, *Il medico in tribunale: la perizia medica nella procedura penale d'antico regime (secoli XVI–XVIII)* (Bellinzona: Casagrande, 1998), pp. 25–61.

67 The case has been narrated by Bronwen Wilson, *The World in Venice: Print, the City, and Early Modern Identity* (Toronto: University of Toronto Press, 2005), p. 126.

68 Ingrassia, *Methodus dandi relationes*, pp. 74–75. This passage is overlooked by all the histories of plastic surgery I have consulted: "nasarius quidam Tropiensis medicus ex bracchii carne illam instaurare solet; imperfecte tamen, cum pellis refici nequeat, ideoque nec pristina pulcritudo exquisite renovari."

69 Paolo Zacchia, *Quaestiones medico-legales* [first edition 1621–1635] (Nurenberg: Johannes Georg Lochner, 1726), Tom. I, Lib. V, Tit. III, Qaest. IV, p. 411. On Zacchia as the founder of modern legal medicine, see Alessandro Pastore and Giovanni Rossi, ed., *Paolo Zacchia: Alle origini della medicina legale: 1584–1659* (Milano: Franco Angeli, 2008).

70 Zacchia, *Quaestiones medico-legales*, p. 412.

71 For an overview, see Giorgio Sperati, "Amputation of the Nose Throughout History," *Acta otorhinolaryngologica Italica* 29, 1 (2009): 44–50. For example, both Roman law and the *lex Visigothorum* (XII, 3, 4) prescribed mutilation as a punishment for adultery: the former provided for castration of men and *cutting off of the nostrils of women* – men were deprived of their virility and women of their beauty. See *Bruno Dumézil,* "Faire honte dans les sources normatives du haut Moyen Age (V-VIIe siecle)," in Bénédicte Sère and Jörg Wettlaufer, eds. *Shame Between Punishment and Penance/La honte entre peine et penitence* (Florence: SISMEL/Edizioni del Galluzzo, 2013), pp. *49–64,* 52. On disfiguring and cutting off noses as punishment for adultery and political crimes, see Valentin Groebner, *Defaced: The Visual Culture of Violence in the Late Middle Ages* (New York: Zone Books, 2004), pp. 67–86; Monga, "Odeporica e medicina"; Patricia Skinner, "The Gendered Nose and Its Lack: 'Medieval' Nose-Cutting and Its Modern Manifestations," *Journal of Women's History* 26, 1 (2014): 45–67. *Carolingian law* prescribed that members of conspiracies and "secret societies" should cut each other's hair and/or nose: see Antonio Pertile, *Storia del diritto italiano dalla caduta dell'Impero romano alla codificazione*, 5 vols. (Bologna: Forni, 1965), vol. 5, pp. 341–342. During the crusades of the eleventh and twelfth centuries, rhinotomy was a codified punishment in Frankish Jerusalem for adulterous women and soldiers guilty of treason: see Piers D. Mitchell,

Medicine in the Crusades: Welfare, Wounds and the Medieval Surgeon (Cambridge: Cambridge University Press, 2004), pp. 128–129.

72 John Gagné, "Counting the Dead: Traditions of Enumeration and the Italian Wars," *Renaissance Quarterly* 67, 3 (2014): 791–840, p. 84.

73 Finucci, *The Prince's Body*, p. 86.

74 Groebner, *Who Are You?*, pp. 108–111.

75 Pertile, *Storia del diritto*, vol. 5, pp. 252–254.

76 Ibid., pp. 256–257.

77 This sentence was widespread in the sixteenth century, both in Latin and in the European vernaculars. In Italian, it is often present in literature, for example in Torquato Tasso and Carlo Dossi; see Renzo Tosi, *Dizionario delle sentenze latine e greche* (Milan: BUR, 2017) number 829, p. 601.

78 Pertile, *Storia del diritto*, vol. 5, p. 374.

79 On this point, see Enrico Castelnuovo, *Ritratto e società in Italia* (Turin: Einaudi, 2015), pp. 82–88.

80 Groebner, *Who Are You?*, pp. 171–221.

81 Davies, *The Return of Martin Guerre*, pp. 62–72.

82 See Cavallo, *Artisans of the Body*, pp. 54–55.

83 ASB, Assunteria di Sanità, Recapiti, n. 1, busta 1580, fol. 7v-8r: "Starete con ogni esquisita vigilanza avertito, se a cotesta Porta capitasse un Bald.ra del luoco da Rivarolo Villa di Pozzura sul Genoese aliquando nominatur Bald.ra Sanvignonio detto il figlio del spadaro d'anni 34 in codesta statura giusta, poca barba e nera, magro di vita, di colore scuro in faccia, che par' appestato, pochi denti et non molto buoni, et con l'occhi destro che gli lagrima, nel qual caso non mancarete farlo restare fuori dalla Porta."

84 Gabriele da Barletta, *Sermonum celeberrimi* (Venice: ex officina Ioan. Bapt. Somaschi, 1571), vol. 1, p. 173: "ut dicunt auctores medicinae: quod ille color qui est compositus ex rubeo, et albo, est optimus;" quoted by Baxandall, *Painting and Experience*, p. 57. On the relationships between beauty, art, color, and cosmetics, see Romana Sammern, "Red, White and Black: Colors of Beauty, Tints of Health and Cosmetic Materials in Early Modern English Art Writing," *Early Science and Medicine* 20, 4–6 (2015): 397–427; Patricia Berrahou Phillippy, *Painting Women: Cosmetics, Canvases, and Early Modern Culture* (Baltimore: Johns Hopkins University Press, 2006).

85 Monsterrat Cabré, "Beautiful Bodies," in Linda Kalof, ed. *A Cultural History of the Human Body in the Middle Ages* (Oxford: Berg, 2010), pp. 127–148, 146–147.

86 Vigarello, *Histoire de la beauté*, pp. 27–38.

87 See William Eamon, *Science and the Secrets of Nature: Books of Secrets in Medieval and Early Modern Culture* (Princeton: Princeton University Press, 1994), pp. 234–266.

88 On the Trotula textual tradition, see Monica Green, "Introduction," in *The Trotula: A Medieval Compendium of Women's Medicine* (Philadelphia: University of Pennsylvania Press, 2001), pp. 1–67.

89 On Renaissance cosmetics for women, see Michelle Laughran, "Oltre la pelle. I cometici e il loro uso," in Carlo Marco Belfanti and Fabio Giusberti, eds. *Storia d'Italia. Annali vol. 19: La moda* (Turin: Einaudi, 2003), pp. 43–82; Joyce De Vries, *Caterina Sforza and the Arts of Appearance* (Aldershot: Ashgate, 2010); Evelyn Welch, "Art on the Edge: Hair, Hats, and Hands in Renaissance Italy," *Renaissance Studies* 23, 3 (2009): 241–268; Paola Tinagli, *Women in Italian Renaissance Art: Gender, Representation and Identity* (Manchester: Manchester University Press, 1997), pp. 84–120.

90 Baldassar Castiglione, *The Book of the Courtier*, tr. Leonard E. Opdyke (New York: Scribner's, 1903), p. 55 (I, 40): "Gran desiderio tengono universalmente tutte le donne di essere e, quando sser non possono, almen di parer belle; dove la natura in qualche parte in questo è mancata, esse si sforzano di supplir con l'artificio . . . Non vi accorgete voi, quanto più di grazia tenga una donna, la qual, se pur si acconcia, lo fa così parcamente e così poco, che chi la vede sta in dubbio s'ella è concia o no, che un'altra, empiastrata tanto, che paia aversi posto alla faccia una maschera, e non osi ridere per

non farsela crepare . . . Quanto più poi di tutte piace una, dico, non brutta, che si conosca chiaramente non aver cosa alcuna in su la faccia, benché non sia così bianca né così rossa, ma col suo color nativo pallidetta e talor per vergogna o per altro accidente tinta d'un ingenuo rossore, coi capelli a caso inomati e mal composti e coi gesti simplici e naturali, senza mostrar industria ne studio d'esser bella? Questa è quella sprezzata purità gratissima agli occhi e agli animi umani, i quali sempre temono essere dall'arte ingannati." On the moral condemnation of women qua users of cosmetics in sixteenth-century Italy, see also Meredith Ray, *Daughters of Alchemy: Women and Scientific Culture in Early Modern Italy* (Cambridge: Harvard University Press, 2015), pp. 62–72; Boyle, *Senses of Touch*, pp. 124–127.

91 Cavallo, *Artisans of the Body*, p. 3.

92 See also Michael Rocke, *Forbidden Friendships: Homosexuality and Male Culture in Renaissance Florence* (Oxford: Oxford University Press, 1996), pp. 227–236.

93 Gabriel-André Perouse, "La Renaissance et la beauté masculine," in *Le corps à la Renaissance*, pp. 61–76. In Chapter 6 I will go back to this point in examining plastic surgery patients, whose identity was constructed in print by Tagliacozzi and other learned surgeons as military gentlemen who were also concerned by the new culture of appearances.

94 On gender politics and the courtiers' life, see Stephen Kolsky, *Courts and Courtiers in Renaissance Northern Italy* (Aldershot: Ashgate, 2003); Amedeo Quondam, *Forma del vivere. L'etica del gentiluomo e i moralisti italiani* (Bologna: Il mulino, 2010); Gerry Milligan, "The Politics of Effeminacy in *Il Cortegiano*," *Italica* 83, 3/4 (2006): 345–366; Ian Frederick Moulton, "Castiglione: Love, Power, and Masculinity," in Gerry Milligan and Jane Tylus, eds. *The Poetics of Masculinity in Early Modern Italy and Spain* (Toronto: Centre for Reformation and Renaissance Studies, 2010), pp. 119–142.

95 Garzoni, *La piazza*, vol. 2, p. 995: "non regi e imperatori andar, come già andavano anticamente, onti, e profumati, ma le vilissime meretrici, et i sfrontati ganimedi, che increspano le chiome a guise di femine . . . et spargono le morbide guancie di mille profumi . . . con perpetua infamia et disonore di questo secolo vituperoso."

96 Della Casa, *Galateo, or the Rules of Polite Behavior* [1558], ed. M.F. Rusnak (Chicago: The University of Chicago Press, 2013), p. 70 (chapter xxxviii): "acciò che l'ornamento non sia uno e la persona un altro; come io veggo fare ad alcuni, che hanno i capelli e la barba inanellati col ferro caldo, e 'l viso e la gola e le mani cotanto strebbiate e cotanto stropicciate che si disdirebbe ad ogni femminetta, anzi ad ogni meretrice, quale ha più fretta di spacciare la sua mercatanzia e di venderla a più caro prezzo."

97 Castiglione, *The Book of the Courtier*, p. 29 (I.19).

98 Della Porta, *Della fisionomia*, p. 501: "io ne viddi uno in Napoli di pochi peli in barba o quasi niuno, di piccola bocca, di ciglia delicate e dritte, di occhio vergognoso, come donna; la voce debile e sottile non poteva soffrir molta fatica; di collo non fermo, di color bianco, che si moderva le labra et insomma con corpo e gesti di femina. Volentieri stave in casa . . . come donna attendeva alla cucina et alla conocchia; fuggiva gli omini e conversava con le femine volentieri e, giacendo con loro, era più femina che l'istesse femine; ragionava come femina e si dava l'articolo femineo sempre . . . et il peggio era, che peggior d'una femina sopportava la nefanda Venere."

99 Giulio Cesare Croce, *Lettera mandata da Narciso alli più belli, vaghi, et profumati giovani di questa città* (Bologna: per Vittorio Benassi, 1590) (pages are not numbered).

100 On Renaissance beards and masculinity, see Douglas Biow, "The Beard in Sixteenth-Century Italy," in Julia J. Hairston and Walter Stephens, eds. *The Body in Early Modern Italy* (Baltimore: Johns Hopkins University Press, 2010), pp. 176–195; Jean-Marie Le Gall, *Un idéal masculin. Barbes et moustaches, xv–xviii siècles* (Paris: Payot & Rivages, 2011).

101 Tagliacozzi, *De curtorum*, p. 25 (1:17). Throughout the chapter, there is, once again, more than an echo of Galen, who wrote, for example: "Beauty is disregarded in the nose, lips, and other parts, because [in them] the beauty of their usefulness far surpasses the pleasure aroused by their appearances. But if a little bit of the lip or the alae of the

nose were cut off, it is not easy to express how ugly it would make the whole face." See Galen, *On the Usefulness of the Parts of the Body*, 2 vols., tr. Margaret Tallmadge May (Ithaca: Cornell University Press, 1968), vol. 2, p. 530 (*De usu partium* 11.II.153).

102 Tagliacozzi, *De curtorum*, p. 25 (1:18). For a contextualization of this story, see Skinner, *Living with Disfigurement*, pp. 103–132.

103 Mikhail Bakhtin, *Rabelais and His World*, tr. Hélène Iswosky (Bloomington: Indiana University Press, 1984), pp. 25–26; Skinner, *Living with Disfigurement*, pp. 44–52.

104 Giulio Cesare Aranzi, *Anatomicarum observationum liber, ac de tumoribus secundum locos affectos liber* (Venice: apud Iacobum Brechtanum, 1587).

105 Tagliacozzi, *De curtorum*, pp. 25–32 (1:17–22).

106 Skinner, "The Gendered Nose," pp. 51–52.

107 For an anachronistic psychoanalytic reading of sixteenth-century noses, see Finucci, *The Prince's Body*, p. 90.

108 Giulio Cesare Croce, *Le sottilissime astuzie di Bertoldo. Le piacevoli e ridicolose simplicità di Bertoldino col Dialogus Salomonis et Marcolphi e il suo primo volgarizzamento a stampa*, ed. Piero Camporesi (Turin: Einaudi, 1978), p. 7: "il naso adunco e righignato all'insù, con le nari larghissime."

109 Thomas Laquer, *Making Sex: Body and Gender from the Greeks to Freud* (Cambridge: Harvard University Press, 1990). Criticism of this model has been strong and it is expanding; see, for example, Joan Cadden, *The Meanings of Sex Difference in the Middle Ages: Medicine, Science, and Culture* (Cambridge: Cambridge University Press, 1993); Gianna Pomata, "Menstruating Men: Similarity and Difference of the Sexes in Early Modern Medicine," in Valeria Finucci and Kevin Brownlee, eds. *Generation and Degeneration: Tropes of Reproduction in Early Modern Europe* (Durham: Duke University Press, 2001), pp. 109–152; Michael Stolberg, "A Woman Down to Her Bones: The Anatomy of Sexual Difference in Early Modern Medicine," *Isis* 94 (2003): 274–299; Katharine Park, *Secrets of Women: Gender, Generation, and the Origins of Human Dissection* (New York: Zone Books, 2006); Patricia Simons, *The Sex of Men in Premodern Europe: A Cultural History* (Cambridge: Cambridge University Press, 2011); Helen King, *The One-sex Body on Trial: The Classical and Early Modern Evidence* (Farnham: Ashgate, 2013).

110 Norbert Elias, *The History of Manners*, tr. Edmund Jephcott (New York: Urizen Books). For convincing criticism of several aspects of Elias' thesis, see Stuart Carroll, *Blood and Violence in Early Modern France* (Oxford: Oxford University Press, 2006), pp. 1–28; and the comprehensive Jeroen Frans Jozef Duindam, *Myths of Power: Norbert Elias and the Early Modern European Court* (Amsterdam: Amsterdam University Press, 1994).

111 Katharine Park has also individuated self-discipline of the body as one key aspect of Renaissance cultures of the body: see Katharine Park, "Was There a Renaissance Body?" in Allen J Grieco, Michael Rocke, and Fiorella Superbi Gioffredi, eds. *The Italian Renaissance in the Twentieth Century* (Florence: Leo S. Olschki, 2002), pp. 321–335.

112 Jean-Jacques Courtine and Claudine Haroche, *Histoire du visage: exprimer et taire ses emotions (xvi-début xix siècle)* (Paris: Payot & Rivages, 1988), pp. 23–34; Judith Wechsler, *A Human Comedy: Physiognomy and Caricature in Nineteenth-Century Paris* (Chicago: The University of Chicago Press, 1982), pp. 15–16, described a structural distiction between physiognomics and pathognomics that roughly corresponds to Courtine and Haroche's chronological one.

113 Della Casa, *Galateo*, p. 47 (chapter xx): "storcendo il viso e contraffacendosi, che niuno dee, per piacere altrui, avvilire se medesimo."

114 Groebner, *Who Are You?*, pp. 117–148.

115 Marcel Mauss, "A Category of the Human Mind: The Notion of Person, the Notion of Self," in Michael Carrithers, Steven Collins, and Steven Lukes, eds. *The Category of the Person: Anthropology, Philosophy, History* (Cambridge: Cambridge University Press, 1985), pp. 1–25.

116 Mauss, "A Category of the Human Mind," pp. 21–22.

117 Fernando Vidal, "Brains, Bodies, Selves, and Science: Anthropologies of Identity and the Resurrection of the Body," *Critical Inquiry* 28, 4 (2002): 930–974; Bynum, "Material Continuity, Personal Survival."

118 Park, *Secrets of Women*, pp. 261–262.

119 I do not even begin to compile a bibliography on Renaissance portraiture; most relevant for the present research are Hans Belting, *Facce. Una storia del volto*, tr. Cristina Baldacci and Pietro Conte (Rome: Carocci, 2014), pp. 151–168; Sandra Cheng, "The Cult of the Monstrous: Caricature, Physiognomy, and Monsters in Early Modern Italy," *Preternature: Critical and Historical Studies on the Preternatural* 1, 2 (2012): 197–231; Castelnuovo, *Ritratto e società*; Peter Burke, "The Presentation of Self in the Renaissance Portrait," in Peter Burke, ed. *The Historical Anthropology of Early Modern Italy: Essays on Perception and Communication* (Cambridge: Cambridge University Press, 1987), pp. 150–167. On representations of blackness in late Renaissance Europe, see Kate Lowe, "The Stereotyping of Black Africans in Renaissance Europe," in Kate Lowe and T.F. Earle, ed. *Black Africans in Renaissance Europe* (Cambridge: Cambridge University Press, 2005), pp. 17–47; Kate Lowe, "The Black Diaspora in Europe in the Fifteenth and Sixteenth Centuries, with Special Reference to German-Speaking Areas," in Mischa Honeck, Martin Klimke, and Anne Kuhlmann, eds. *Germany and the Black Diaspora: Points of Contact 1250–1914* (New York, Oxford: Berghahn Books, 2013), pp. 38–56. For useful summaries of discussions of race in early modern Europe, see Rebecca Earle, *The Body of the Conquistador: Food, Race, and the Colonial Experience in Spanish America* (Cambridge: Cambridge University Press, 2012), pp. 187–215; Cristina Malcomson, *Studies of Skin Color in the Early Royal Society: Boyle, Cavendish, Swift* (London: Routledge, 2016), pp. 1–27. On the importance of costumes and physiognomies as markers of identity and articulation of differences among peoples, see Wilson, *The World in Venice*, pp. 70–132, 186–254.

120 Murphy, *Lavinia Fontana*, pp. 50–51.

121 Ibid., p. 58.

122 On Passerotti's caricatures and grotesque works, see Angela Ghirardi, *Bartolomeo Passerotti, pittore, 1529–1592: Catalogo generale* (Rimini: Luisè, 1990), pp. 63–75, 225–229. Important and diverse sixteenth-century intellectuals like Paleotti, Pietro Aretino, and the art theorist Giovanni Paolo Lomazzo lamented that in their times even lower-class people, such as artisans, could aspire to have their images immortalized and that they actually found painters ready to paint their portraits: see Castelnuovo, *Ritratto e società*, pp. 84–85.

123 See Bernard Berenson, "The Effigy and the Portrait," *Aesthetics and History in the Visual Arts* (Pantheon: New York, 1948), pp. 190–200.

124 Katharine Park, "Nature in Person: Medieval and Renaissance Allegories and Emblems," in Lorraine Daston and Fernando Vidal, eds. *The Moral Authority of Nature* (Chicago: The University of Chicago Press, 2003), pp. 50–73, 60–62.

125 Ibid., p. 68.

126 Ibid., p. 73.

127 Natalie Zemon Davis, "Boundaries and the Sense of Self in Sixteenth-Century France," in Thomas Heller, Morton Sosna, and David Wellbery, eds. *Reconstructing Individualism: Autonomy, Individuality, and the Self in Western Thought* (Stanford: Stanford University Press, 1986), pp. 53–63, 53. For a recent summary of the complex stakes of a history of the face as the site and vector of identity, expression, and representation, see Jean-Claude Schmitt, "For a History of the Face : Physiognomy, Pathognomy, Theory of Expression," *Kritische Berichte* 40, 1 (2012): 7–20; for a map of irregular faces according to class, gender, and race see Patrizia Bettella, "The Marked Body as Otherness in Renaissance Italian Culture," in Linda Kalof and William Bynum, eds. *A Cultural History of the Human Body in the Renaissance* (Oxford: Berg, 2010), pp. 149–181.

4

HEALTH AND APPEARANCE

An intense debate developed around Galenic notions of health and beauty in the second half of the sixteenth century among prominent surgeons and physicians. But the care of appearance occupied pride of place in the writings of humbler practitioners like professors of secrets and barber-surgeons. Taking into account these different traditions, this chapter describes Tagliacozzi's way of conceptualizing the distinction between "true" and "false" beauty. For Tagliacozzi, this distinction was gendered in itself. Moreover, for him just like for barbers and professors of secrets, there was a certain contiguity – sometimes even overlapping – between health and appearance.[1] The closeness between these two areas was represented by the concept of *politezza*, which ran across professional distinctions between barber-surgeons and learned surgeons.

Different practitioners of the body had different views on the relationships between the care of health and appearance, but a close link between these two endeavors was constant across the whole spectrum of professional categories. By the second half of the sixteenth century, Italian learned surgeons debated the nature of beauty and health through learned discussions of Galen and other humanistic sources. They all maintained a gendered distinction between restoring beauty and health and enhancing beauty, but at the same time they all thought that a learned and legitimate branch of cosmetics existed, opposed to what they called *mangonica*, *comptorica*, or *fucatoria*. This latter side of cosmetics was for them to be assimilated to artificially enhancing beauty; this beauty was therefore considered false because it was separate from health and it was associated to the social types of the vain woman, the effeminate man, and the slave dealer embellishing his "product." Tagliacozzi tried to make these boundaries even more rigid by tracing a distinction between cosmetics and reconstructive surgery. Professors of secrets like Fioravanti were much less subtle in theoretical distinctions and elaborated a vast array of cosmetic remedies that did not pay much attention to distinctions between health and beauty. Finally, barber-surgeons' goal was a form of care of the face that they thought was essential for the sake of men's *politezza*, the physical and moral virtue of having an orderly appearance. On the other hand, barber-surgeons did not hesitate to jump into the debates on health and beauty, and they claimed that their art was part of surgery or of the legitimate branch of cosmetics. Overall, the concept of *politezza*, which at least in the context of health care was distinctly referring to men, brought together all these categories – if not in theory, at least in practice.

True and false beauty

As we have seen, one of the most popular tropes of the culture of the face was the opposition between the natural beauty of the human features and the artificial means employed by some – mostly women and effeminates – to enhance or to bring about beauty. This opposition could be translated in a rather precise way in medical terms.

Tagliacozzi was the one who brought the topics of cosmetics and medical beauty in deeper touch with the overall culture of the face of his times. Despite the fact that in practice the borders between cosmetics and surgery, between health and appearance, were very fluid, four conceptual oppositions structure Tagliacozzi's text: (1) artificial enhancement of nature versus restoration of natural forms; (2) mere beauty versus beauty that derives from perfection of actions and functions; (3) morally deceiving beauty versus natural beauty as a sign of man's dignity; (4) medicine and surgery versus cosmetics.

Learned surgeons and physicians, mostly in the medical centers of Bologna and Padua, took up a few passages from Galen and integrated them with contemporary notions of beauty in order to discuss the opposition between false beauty and true beauty. For them, making a distinction between the arts of frivolous cosmetics and the serious and legitimate medical practice of cosmetics was both an epistemological and a socio-political gesture of demarcation. Serious physicians wanted to respond to the challenges of the contemporary culture of beauty and the face without falling in the moral gray zone – often a black zone, to abuse the metaphor – of the artificial, the deceptive, and the adulterous. The whole culture of the face described in the previous chapter supported these physicians' view of a fundamental, if problematic, moral difference between medical beauty and "degenerate" beauty. At the same time, these learned doctors made use of the culture of the professors of secrets, filled their books with recipes for treating imperfections of the face, and gave much more space to facial appearance in their books than their medieval counterparts.

As Mariacarla Gadebusch-Bondio has argued, this medical debate, which was unfortunately silent on the thoughts of patients, reveals that patients called upon the surgeons for psychological and aesthetic reasons, not always because the functionality of their face was compromised. Surgeons had to translate these issues into technical and medical ones.[2] Spots on the skin, pustules, swellings, and warts on the face were of course a different thing from serious injuries and facial mutilation, but they belonged to the same culture of the face.

Galen discussed the relations between beauty and health in several passages of his works, but he dealt more extensively with this issue in the *Letter to Thrasiboulos*. The general question tackled here was whether "healthiness" belonged to medicine or gymnastics. The physician of Pergamon defined health in a quite "modern" way as being able to perform everyday tasks: "a state in which the performance of activities undergoes no hindrance, and is not susceptible to impairment, is health 'in condition'." However, this state was different from a "good condition," which was "the position of a kind of excellence of the functions."[3] The theme of true versus false beauty, or appearance versus nature, immediately followed. For Galen, who echoed Plato (*Gorgias* 465b), the "art of cosmetic adornment" was to be listed among the "perverted arts," together with the art of creating an athletic condition that was considered "unnatural" because the body became too much performing. Now,

> the perverted arts provide an apparent good in each area with which they are concerned, whereas the arts proper provide that which genuinely exists in that area. We should further consider that, if what is generally known as the cosmetic art is productive of a false kind of beauty, it must be regarded as a perverted art, a form of flattery. There must be some other art responsible for the creation of genuine, true beauty, which consists in excellence of complexion and flesh, and good proportion of the parts – qualities which obtain in the case of natural good condition.[4]

Health was nothing but the capability of each part of the body to exercise its proper function.

> Surely everyone would agree in not wanting any part unable to perform its function – eyes unable to see, for example, a nose unable to smell, legs unable to walk. . . . In fact, none of the things we require is required in an imperfect state . . . In needing any of these things we also need them in their perfect form [*teleios*, performing its goal properly]. . . . If, then, we require not an imperfect performance of functions but a perfect one, we shall not require an imperfect constitution of the body with which we perform these functions.[5]

In turn, "good condition" (*euexia*), a state achieved through gymnastics, was the perfect form of the state called "health." Therefore, there could be no good condition without health.

At this point, Galen displayed his almost proverbial teleological way of reasoning: everything that existed had a goal, which corresponded to "the good of that thing according to its nature." Now, the body, as it existed, had its goal too, which was a unified goal (therefore, we cannot separate and subdivide its goals), and we cannot separate the productive from the preservative art of the healthy body.

> There is a common misconception that the good of the body is divided into health, strength, and beauty, and that one may posit a productive and a preservative art for each of these. This . . . must be refuted . . . beauty is made up of good complexion, good flesh, good proportion, and certain other factors; why should it not be the case, similarly, that the good of the body is made up of health, strength, and beauty?[6]

It is clear that health was the good of the body itself: "the causes of true health in a body will be no different from those of strength or beauty" and "if something is going to make our body strong or beautiful it will automatically also make it healthy."[7] The natural function of the body – upon which beauty, strength, and health depended – proceeded from the constitution of the body, as "beauty is a necessary consequence of the former set of conditions, ugliness of the latter." All these things went hand in hand.[8]

The best definition of the higher good of the body was perfection of the functions; next, it was the good condition described as health; and finally, beauty followed as a necessary consequence. But Galen forcefully argued that this threefold distinction was somehow artificial, because all the three goods were one in practice. The point is that there was no (legitimate) art which produced beauty that did not produce, at the same time, function and health. When a physician or a surgeon produced a healthy state, restored it, or preserved it, "functioning or beauty . . . would follow of necessity, even if the practitioner did not want them to."[9] The logical conclusion of all this was that "cosmetic" medicine (*ars exornatoria*) restored beauty, while *ars comptoria* adulterated faces and deceived the bystanders: "The goal of the *comptoria* art is to bring about a kind of artificial beauty. The decorative part of medicine, which agrees with nature, preserves everything in the body, and from this follows a natural beauty."[10]

Cosmetic concerns of patients and surgeons were very much alive in the later Middle Ages. Arabic encyclopedias were explicit on the care of appearances.[11] Avicenna's fen on cosmetics became the model for treatises on "decoratione." Avicenna ignored distinctions between health and beauty, appearance and significance. Instead, he dealt with hair care, skin color, serious skin afflictions and issues of appearance (perspiration, body odor, etc.), obesity, and cracked nails. Avicenna blended cosmetics and therapeutics, and Latin authors did not raise again the question of health and beauty before the fourteenth century. For example, both the Salernitan collection De ornatu mulierum and the Regimen by Aldobrandino da Siena (d. 1287) mixed hygiene and cosmetics and always targeted women on these topics. Luke Demaitre has argued that the transition from the country courts to the urban life pushed physicians toward matters of appearance and, at the same time, that this increased interest on the part of the clientele made the Galenic issue resurface.

Medieval medical texts presented an increased interest in superficial marks, especially on the face. Bernard de Gordon (c.1270–1330) praised the excellence of the face in terms we are already familiar with and included a series of cosmetic dyes and ointments for women's faces, prefaced by the caveat that all this was "acceptable if it is applied for the sake of men."[12] Henri de Mondeville devoted three chapters of his surgery book to the *decoratio* of men. He introduced this art with lots of warnings: *decoratio* could be contrary to God and justice and it could be done for deception and fraud, but Mondeville also made a concession to realism in acknowledging that these practices were very profitable among wealthy ladies.[13] Likewise, the great systematizer of medieval surgery Guy de Chauliac took up the Galenic distinction between medical and popular cosmetics and wrote that

> the dispositions that appear on the face can be natural or preternatural. The natural ones require preservation if they are beautiful, and decoration if they are ugly, for example preserving whiteness or making the face whiter and redder if necessary. Those [dispositions] which are preternatural require correction, like pustules, spots, and excessive hair – this is what Galen meant when . . . he stressed the difference between cosmetic and decorative parts of medicine. . . . Indeed decorative treatment is legitimate, while cosmetic treatment is not, and it is not honest either, just like Galen said.[14]

Those who used makeup just for their own pleasure were to be denied treatment, while women who wished to be more beautiful for their husbands could legitimately seek the physician's help.

Late medieval surgeons had a relatively good conscience about caring for beauty. With respect to sixteenth-century surgeons and physicians, medieval medical writers felt much less need to provide theoretical justification for "decorative" remedies and to articulate elaborate discussions about the subtleties of the theories of beauty. On the other hand, both theoretical discussion on the statute of cosmetics with respect to medicine and the space devoted to practical issues of the face greatly increased in the sixteenth century, supported by a specific culture of the face. Moreover, by the second half of the sixteenth century, an increasing preoccupation with the hygiene of the body sometimes blurred the distinction between medical prevention (washing hands, combing the hair, cleaning the pores of the skin, blowing noses) and cosmetics.[15]

The first physician who discussed these Galenic topics in the sixteenth century was Gabriele Falloppio, professor of medicine in Padua, in his 1566 booklet titled *De decoratione*. The book already contained all the topics discussed by other learned surgeons and physicians in the following decades. Moreover, Falloppio was a teacher and friend of Mercuriale in Padua and thus can be placed at the beginning of the Paduan-Bolognese debates on beauty and medicine.[16]

In the preface, Falloppio argued that there were two ways of treating

> the art of the good: preserving the present, and restoring the desired. . . . Since medicine is an art, it must necessarily have an end, which is the perfection of its subject, that is, the perfection of the human body . . . [which is given by] its strength and its potential for action . . . and it is this integrity of the body, and how often it can execute its actions in a perfect way.[17]

If the body was the organ of the soul, Falloppio went on, and if its goal was action, then the highest perfection of the body was its force and strength in performing actions. Therefore, the goal of medicine was to preserve the body's strength, namely the highest goal of the body. Health, in turn, could be defined as the virtue, or perfection, of the body. Falloppio added to the Galenic features of strength, health, and beauty a fourth one, more Aristotelian: habit, in the sense of a habit of performing excellence of function. "We must not neglect those who say that beauty is the *summum bonum* of the body; indeed, it concerns everyone, not just women but men too, not just the young, but the old too; and it is a virtue, therefore it is good for the body." The good only appeared to be fragmented, but it was one

> the result of health, a good habit of the body, beauty, and strength in actions. So we can say that health and good habit are causes of beauty and strength in performing the body's actions; beauty and strength are effects and fruits of those causes. If we consider together causes and effects, we see that the good is one.

The *summum bonum* and the goal of medicine were an "aggregation of four virtues: health, strength, beauty, and habitus." This is why beauty was a legitimate concern for medicine.[18]

But Falloppio warned his readers: beauty was double.

> One is colored, counterfeit, false, and for these reasons it must be called non-natural or preternatural . . . and this one pertains to slave dealers, prostitutes, and it is lewd and artificial; in fact it destroys natural conditions, and it brings about the worst features through art, that which is desired by the old, the young, and women. [Through this art] women destroy their charm, old people lose their importance, the young let go of their virility. The other kind of beauty is called natural, and it must pertain to anyone; those who lack it are ugly.[19]

The former beauty was associated not just with women but also with men who had lost their virility; the latter beauty was a "natural composition and symmetrical connection among the parts of the body." Fake colors and fake softness of the parts were not part of natural beauty, which only concerned "the substance, color, quantity, place, figure, and conformation of the parts."[20] In other words, classical beauty and medical beauty were a perfect match for each other. Therefore, there were two ways of restoring beauty: the "curative" and the "decorative." Beauty could be restored in two ways, just as it could be lost in two ways: either when the part lost its health or when an accident happened. When the physician dealt with restoring the beauty lost in an accident, that was "curative" medicine; when he treated the beauty "per se," it was "called cosmetics, or *ornatoria*, or *decoratoria*." Of course, there was a further difference between the *comptoria* and *ornatoria* arts, because the *comptoria* "destroys nature and adds things that are not to be found in nature," while the *decoratoria* "always looks to the things that are according to nature in one single man as in the whole human species, in this single part as in the whole body."[21] We could not find a more straightforward example of the moralization of the natural and the stigmatization of the artificial, at the same time intrinsically conceived in gendered terms.

Girolamo Mercuriale not only discussed these very same topics more in depth and in a more erudite way in his 1585 *De decoratione* but also was so impressed by Tagliacozzi's technique that he published a long letter by him in the second edition (1587) of this work.[22] Mercuriale was undoubtedly the most influential figure in this debate on "learned cosmetics" and a real go-between because he befriended Tagliacozzi and he was the teacher of Giovanni Tommaso Minadoi. In particular, Mercuriale devoted a great deal of space to imperfections of the face in his *De decoratione*, and years before the debate bloomed he had already approached the topic of medicine and cosmetics in his 1572 book – based on students' notes – on skin diseases, *De morbis cutaneis et omnia corporis humani excrementa tractatus*.

This latter work was divided into five chapters. The first was devoted to the skin diseases of the head; the second dealt with the skin diseases that affected the whole body (including leprosy); the third was titled "on excerements," but it was almost entirely devoted to urine; the fourth treated excrements of the belly; and finally the fifth dealt with sweat, tears, spit, mucus, and ear wax. Clearly, there was a good deal of overlaps between the work of professors of secrets, barber-surgeons, and Mercuriale's book. Besides the use of Latin, the difference was that Mercuriale discussed at length the causes of these phenomena according to the official and learned medical theoretical tradition, while the empirics' books had a much more practical approach.

At the beginning of *De decoratione*, Mercuriale asked whether skin problems were part of medicine or of the *comptoria* art. He discussed a serious issue: because it was not clear whether the skin performed any action – and diseases were obstacles to actions – were the problems of the skin of the head and the face proper diseases or just damages to beauty? Mercuriale argued that the skin did not perform any "common" actions but only "specific" actions, namely actions that were not relevant for the whole body but only for single parts of it. For example, the skin helped the nourishment of the veins by assimilating, uniting, and distributing them. Many scholars believed that these skin diseases were to be called "illnesses affecting beauty (*morbos in pulchritudine*)," but Mercuriale disagreed. He argued that Galen never mentioned such diseases and that beauty was just a synonym for health, because it was present only in healthy bodies. As Plato said, "ugliness is nothing but a dissonance between things that are connected to each other; likewise, illness is a dissonance; therefore, ugliness is an illness, and beauty is health." Beauty was, for Mercuriale, nothing but the effect, the fruit of health, and therefore the distinction between health and beauty was purely superficial. It was accurate for him to claim that

> the art of medicine can deal with both beauty and ugliness, but not in themselves or directly: in fact, only indirectly. Indeed, a physician deals in the first place with health and sickness, but since, as Galen said, beauty is the fruit of health, and deformity is produced by sickness in the same way, then as Galen has written, it follows that the art of medicine deals with beauty and ugliness.[23]

Learned physicians wanted at the same time to write about appearances and to write about them in a way that would distinguish them from lowly practitioners and writers.

The heavily exploited theme of the two kinds of beauty was treated by Tagliacozzi with specific references to social life:

> one [kind of beauty] is true and inborn (*natiuum*), and harmonizes with the ideal nature and proportions of the body (*corporis constitutione & temperie*), because, according to Hippocrates, we can judge it by bodily actions. This kind of beauty does not declare itself in whiteness of complexion, effeminacy, smoothness of skin, or any other such niceties. The second kind of beauty is neither true (*verum*) nor natural but is counterfeit, impure, and spurious (*adulterina & arte accrescita*); it is of use to dealers who wish to make a profit (*mangonibus*) and to the effeminate men who are overly concerned about their appearances.[24]

There were, to be more precise, three kinds of beauty: the real one, or Hippocratic, mixing together the aesthetic of the classical body and the functionalist, medical Galenic definition of beauty; the second kind, which "comes about through Nature's generosity and careful fashioning," sometimes obscured by the parts' important function; and finally "artificial beauty that apes Nature (*naturae simia*) in order to allure and entice."[25] This kind of artificiality was conceived less in ontological than in social and moral terms: rather than troubling the order of nature, it induced men, like the effect of a *trompe l'oeil*, to take as natural that which was artificial. Tagliacozzi went on explaining that common sense suggested that "the face is the first thing we notice; it immediately engages the eye, whether pleasantly or unpleasantly. The female face attracts men's eyes, allures them, conquers reason, and sows the first seeds of love."[26] Tagliacozzi's approach was in a way not only sociological but even proto-anthropological, as he mentioned two norms of criminal law: a prohibition against writing on the faces of the condemned, while allowing it on the hands and legs, because the face was the expression of beauty, and the fact that when different parts of the body were buried in different places, the primary site of remembering and mourning was where the head was buried.

Later in Book I, Tagliacozzi directly asked to what "category of preternatural afflictions . . . my procedure should be assigned?"[27] Galen distinguished two kinds of disease: "One kind occurs as a result of a superabundance of one or another bodily part, while the other stems from a deficiency." If some part had been mutilated or it was imperfect from birth, then one could speak of a natural deficiency (or abundance, in the opposite case). "The mutilation of nose, lips, and ears does belong to the category of deficiency" and thus was part of therapeutic medicine (*ad curatricem medicinam*). This kind of medicine restored the lost health of each single part of the body.

> Indeed, if we consider how ignoble and repulsive mutilation of the lips, ears, and nose can be, we might think that my procedure belongs not to the most praiseworthy part of medicine but is merely a question of cosmetics. Mutilated or missing parts confer so much shame and ugliness (*foeditas, turpitudo, aspectus pravitas*) on the appearance that all the nobility and elegance of the face is lost. If these parts are restored, the original grace and beauty of the face returns.

It is not without some reason that someone could say that this restoration procedure concerned not curative medicine but cosmetics (*ad comptoriam pertinere*). But this, Tagliacozzi emphatically stated, was wrong.

> The cosmetic art provides what Nature has denied – a healthy appearance, an attractive coiffure, and any number of other niceties – while my procedure restores what Nature has given and chance has taken away. The aim of this procedure is not to please the eye (*non ut oculos delectent*) but rather to benefit mind and soul (*sed ut animae operanti emolumento sint*). This end is accomplished by admirable means and not through the use of ignoble and sordid artifice; the latter practice befits whoremongers and the like but not good physicians and followers of the great Hippocrates. In fact, the main purpose of this procedure is not the restoration of the original beauty of the face in itself, but rather the rehabilitation of the part in question. Its beauty lies in the faultless performance of the functions (*actiones*) decreed it by Nature. This beauty is not artificial, spurious, or unworthy; rather, it is true and authentic. . . . These are the reasons for placing my procedure in the realm of curative and no other. I would not disagree, however, with the claim that this operation does, in fact, restore the original beauty of the face.[28]

It is with some badly dissimulated pride that Tagliacozzi described himself as an artist in that he gave back beauty to the human face.

The care of appearance

Learned surgeons knew that they could not dismiss a vast clientele of both men and women looking for aesthetic treatments. For example, Giulio Cesare Aranzi, discussing warts in his *De tumoribus*, made clear that the main inconvenience of warts was aesthetic. He added that sometimes, when patients became too insistent, it was okay to put the surgeon's reputation at risk to embellish one's face, "especially if they are women who desire to enhance the beauty of their faces: sometimes it is allowed to push them away; in fact, exhausted by such requests, we consider the idea of almost unwillingly performing the procedure."[29]

It is remarkable that sixteenth-century medicine and surgery books devoted much more attention than their earlier counterparts to the face and its "diseases," thus blurring the distinction between health and appearance. Sixteenth-century lists of issues, vices, and imperfections concerning the face were much longer than their medieval counterparts.[30] For example, Giovanni Andrea Dalla Croce's list of affections that troubled the face was much longer than those one could find in medieval surgery books. Almost the entire first book was devoted to affections that could disfigure or simply make the face ugly:

> [U]lcers, blood aposteme (*abscessi, essiture, foroncoli, panarizzi, carboni maligni, antraci*), choleric aposteme (*erisipele, herpeti, pruni, formiche, vesiche, inflassioni, sfaceli, gangrene*), flegmatic aposteme (*edemi, nodi, scrofole, absessi, glandule*), melancholic aposteme (*cancri, scirri, aneurismi, echimomi, varici*), swellings (*polipi, mori, porrifici, porri, verruche, calli, sesto dito*).[31]

Moreover, by the early sixteenth century cosmetics became more prominent because more skin surface was showed off in the face and in the neckline.

Leonardo Fioravanti's *Compendio di tutti i secreti rationali* can be read as an example of the scope of the market of cosmetics; at the same time, the recipes in this book are a perfect testimony of what has recently been called "household science" and "recipe knowledge."[32] In the "Discourse on make up with many necessary information (*Discorso sopra la materia de belletti con molti avvertimenti necessarii*)," the seller of cosmetic secrets wrote that

> there are many several material things that women use to adorn themselves and to make themselves beautiful, of which I will speak at length; indeed, this topic is no less important than medicine and surgery, because women desire so much these things, that they would suffer through any kind of torture (*supplicio*) to appear more beautiful than they are. Many times they use substances and remedies that accomplish the opposite and severely harm not just the face" but their whole body.

Fioravanti intended to warn women from using dangerous cosmetics, and he expressed the ardent desire for women to "say good things" about him and, so to speak, to spread the word, because he loved women and makeup was "a noble and beautiful thing to use."[33]

Fioravanti was of course advertising his skills and products as a makeup artist and merchant, so his tone was not moralistic at all. The list of his secrets included how to remove spots and other marks for the women's face; how to make a plaster to remove facial hair ("Many women have their face excessively hairy, that which is very ugly to see, because it disfigures a beautiful face"); general depilation of men and women; how to darken hair, eyelids, and beards; hair coloring ("When grey or white hair start to appear on a man's or woman's head and face, and they want to darken them in order to appear younger, this is what they have to do"); how to turn a white beard into a beautiful blonde one; the offer to reproduce two variations of blondeness for women: the Neapolitan fashion and the Venetian fashion; how to paint women's eyelids black (French or Spanish fashion); several recipes on how to make women's lips more red; special "waters" to wash, clean up, and whiten women's face; how to prepare waters that cancelled or hid the marks and scars of the pox (*varolo*), burnings, and so forth; oils that did clean and whiten the face; and many others.[34]

Men were far from abstaining from using cosmetics, but enhancing beauty remained described as an eminently female concern. Fioravanti described the "features women want in order to look beautiful" as follows:

> The first quality a woman wants is to be rich, in order not to be despised. The second is to be generous, so that she will be loved. The third is to be honest, so that she will not be blamed. The fourth is to be young, so that she will be strong and robust. The fifth is to be merry . . . [these conditions] are the best sort of make-up a woman can find and use; and if the above mentioned qualities cannot be attained, women might want to whiten their face, hands and chest, so here is what she should do.[35]

Ambroise Paré wrote too of cosmetic recipes but less light-heartedly than Fioravanti. He talked about a wig for those who had lost their hair; of some feathered wigs for women who had gray hair and did not want to be considered old but kept

> deceiving men . . . and in order to appear higher than they really are they wear heels like the Spanish and Italian women. They [women] do many other things to deceive men, but I don't want to describe them, since I do not want to wrong them.[36]

Della Porta's *Magia Naturalis* included many cosmetic secrets but – echoing Guy de Chauliac – felt the need to specify that such recipes were acceptable for women only insofar they used them in order for "the wife to be fancied by her husband."[37]

Two early modern manuals for barber-surgeons, written in vernacular by professionals who might be called "learned barber-surgeons," give us a rather accurate description of their self-presentation and of how they viewed their professional task of caring for people's appearance. Pietro Paolo Magni's (c. 1525–1586) vernacular manual of phlebotomy (1584) provides the first example. The book was organized around the categories of bloodletting and cauterization, with bloodletting occupying the greatest portion of it. The emphasis was on the veins, which were described, as in anatomy books, from head to toe. The barber-surgeon's view of the body was indeed decidedly vein-centered and surface-based.

Magni focused on bloodletting in the first place and warned the reader that many people were wrong in performing the operations pertaining to bloodletting, because "this art is indeed a dangerous art, and it is part of that branch of Medicine called Surgery." This was showed by the illustrious physicians who were also surgeons, but "in our times this part [of medicine] is fallen into the hands of non-experts, who practice it in an improper and unworthy way."[38] So this book was also addressed to scholars. Magni was echoing the argument of learned sixteenth-century surgeons and anatomists, who all complained that surgery, such an important art, had fallen prey to the ignorance of the empirics.[39]

For Magni, the good barber-surgeon had to be pious, have a "good sight (*buona vista*)," be quick, be "clean" (*polito*), be sober with wine, be of honest habits, and be modest and affable. Barbers visited all sorts of people and treated all sorts of body parts of both men and women, and often they happened to hear many secrets, gossip, joys, and sorrows, but above all "they can kill women and men with their lancets and razors." Therefore, the barber's hand must be "light (*leggiera*)," and "he will always be more praised if he is quick rather than slow." *Politezza*, the art of being precise and swift with the razor, was one of the best qualities for a barber. Barbers had to be affable because "most of the times with their words and kind ways they convince patients to let themselves be treated."[40]

Barbers had also to be careful and judicious in all the other operations – washing the head, cutting hair, shaving beards, and honoring the face of the person they shaved. They had to take into account the status of their clients "because most of the time the beard will make the man appear handsome or ugly, so they must be very able to handle the razors . . . and careful that their hands will not bother the patient."[41] Health and aesthetics were overlapping tasks for barbers.

Tiberio Malfi's *Il barbiere* built on sixteenth-century manuals but added an even more learned self-presentation of the profession, especially by emphasizing anatomical instruction and by declaring that he had sought the help of masters of anatomy to make his art "more authoritative."[42] The textbook was divided into three parts, dealing respectively with "ornaments" and the general precepts of the barber's art; the anatomy of the veins, arteries, muscles, and nerves; the practical use of leeches, scarifications, cupping glasses, cautery, vesicatories, and how to open up living animals.

In the dedication to the reader, Malfi linked the art of barbers to the "Decorator's art" and to "Medicine," stating that it was equally useful to them. Then he complained that so few of its practitioners had written on it. In Book I,

Malfi clearly included the barbers' art within the body of medicine and argued that, besides Hippocrates and Galen, very few exceptional men were able to embrace the whole body of medicine in all of its parts. He then argued that there were several ways to distinguish the parts of medicine, one of them being the distinction between dietetics, pharmacy, and surgery. But another distinction was that between curative, conservative, and preservative; some physicians added the *Evettica* (the art of reinforcing bodies), *gerocomica* (the art of caring for the old), and the art of governing little children. Some other added the *Decoratoria*, which was different and separate from the *Fucatoria*, the art of makeup (*belletti*).[43] Malfi and Severino were clearly aware of the learned debates on medicine and beauty.

But for Malfi the most important distinction was twofold: "Physic in the hands of philosophers," and "Surgery in the hands of simple operators." Malfi was also perfectly aware of the history of surgery and referred to Guy de Chauliac in tracing this separation back to Rolando, Ruggiero, and "the four masters" of surgery who had so greatly advanced the field. An even most important separation medicine had to suffer was that between barbers and bloodletters, after which "Barbers were assigned two parts of medicine: the *Decoratoria*, which we mentioned above, and one part of Surgery."[44]

Malfi also had an explanation for the reason why many barbers practiced surgery, and it had to do with urgency, necessity, timeliness, and professional urban geography.

> The other part of medicine – he wrote – is called surgery, and it was mainly practiced by physicians but later it passed (if not the whole of it, at least some of its parts) into the hands of barbers. . . . Surgery treats wounds and evils that happen suddenly, that present an immediate threat to patients, either for the bad effects of air or for the loss of blood, or, again, for the extreme pain, and surgeons must always be ready and never have to wait to operate; regularly, physicians are not to be found in their homes (since they are often busy away from their homes, and they do not have workshops) and therefore barbers took their place [to treat these urgent evils] since they are always ready in their workshops.[45]

But there was another, deeper and, so to speak, cultural reason why barbers took over surgical tasks:

> [B]esides necessity, the other reason [why barbers took over surgical tasks] was the affinity or closeness between operations which have to do with the same subject, because barbers deal with the lack of beauty and cleanliness (*politezza*), and therefore little by little it became easy for barbers to perform those operations which treat dissolutions of continuity [injuries] that disfigure and ruin beauty, all of which operations are surgery's task.[46]

This was a rather striking declaration of the continuity between the care of injuries and the care of beauty and cleanliness, and the field of intervention of barbers and surgeons was indicated as that which was placed in between *salute* and *politezza*.

While Malfi was aware of the fact that barber-surgeons were part of the artisanal class, nonetheless, given the special status of the object of their care, they deserved better consideration. He thus emphasized the intrinsic dignity of the object of barbers' art: the human body and especially its face. Among all the arts and crafts, only the barbers' art "has for subject, as its privilege and special prerogative, the treatment of man by means of the sense of touch, and it is indeed all about this, and the correction of nature's imperfections."[47] Finally, the surgical part of the barber's art was also good for men, because it soothed pain, eased anxiety, sometimes saved men from death, and preserved their health.[48]

There is no better summary of the standard barbers' self-description than the one given by Tommaso Garzoni.

> Their [barbers'] art is clean and polite, since its aim and goal is the body's good appearance, that which is brought about by shaving, washing, cutting, and rubbing the people who ask for their services. And it can be practiced with very little money, because it needs only a washbasin, a couple of razors, a lancet, a hairgrip, a comb, a scalpel . . . two pairs of cloths, a sponge, a brazier with some carbon, a bucket of lye [caustic soda], and a little bit of water of roses to put on the patients' face – these tools make up the whole lot of the barbers' architecture. Barbers also let blood from the sick and apply cupping glasses, they dress wounds, bandage, pull out rotten teeth and similar things, and therefore their art . . . is subaltern to the science of medicine. . . . A dexter hand and good eyesight are the most desired qualities in a barber.[49]

Politezza, one of the goals of the barbers' art, namely the care of the superfluities and excrements of the body (hair, bad humors, bad blood, sweat, nails), was at the same time the *politezza* of the social body, and barbers were taking care of an orderly body that belonged to a well-ordered social world. *Politezza* could indicate clean and beautiful figures and refined manners, civility, and ability to appear in public and to deal with others in a civil manner. In other words, *politezza* was a hygienic, aesthetic, and political virtue at the same time.[50]

Now, this concept of *politezza* was used by a lay observer of Tagliacozzi's work. In a passage I have quoted in Chapter 2, the chronicler Francesco Galliani wrote in his note on the death of Tagliacozzi:

> Today 7 November [1599] the excellent physician Gaspare Tagliacozzi passed away, the most famous physician of our age in the art of surgery, who used to make noses, lips, and ears to those who had lost them because of they had been wounded or other things, and he used to make them with so good a *politezza* that he almost overtook nature.[51]

The word *politezza* is very important here, because, as we have seen, it was the term barber-surgeons used in their self-definition and that was used to qualify their art. Tagliacozzi was identified as the one person who cared for the *politezza* of the noble class.

Trading zones

This association of beauty, *politezza*, and reconstructive surgery probably intensified in the seventeenth century. Ovidio Montalbani (1601–1671), a key character in the cultural life of Bologna in the first half of the seventeenth century, has left a testimony of the highly nuanced relationships between different practitioners of the body.[52] In 1670 he published a history of the city's guilds, titled *L'honore de Collegi dell'arti della città di Bologna. Brieve trattato Fisicopolitico e Legale Storico*, in which he reflected on the situation of the arts and crafts starting from the mid-sixteenth century. In the chapter devoted to the barbers' guild, ranked only at the 21st place in the hierarchy of the 27 guilds, Montalbani mentioned several themes in a rather haphazard manner, reflecting the confusion of categories and the continuity among practitioners of the body, as well as between the care of health and the care of *politezza*. Right at the beginning, barbers were linked to the practice of cosmetics and surgery and described as dependent upon the power of the College of Medicine: "The guild of barbers mainly practice cosmetic medicine, and many parts of surgery, as a liberal concession of the College of Physicians of this city."[53] Among the most important of the barbers' tasks there was phlebotomy, the art of drawing blood by applying leeches and by cutting the veins, an activity that was straightforwardly defined "surgical medicine" (*medicina chirurgica*). Immediately after that, Montalbani claimed that barbers or, better, barber-surgeons, should study the Latin works of the late sixteenth and early seventeenth centuries written by learned surgeons and physicians, such as Marco Antonio Olmi's *Physiologia barbae umanae*, "in order to learn about the facts concerning virility, and especially the art of embellishing human bodies (*per intendere gli accidenti della Virilità . . . e massimamente l'abbellimento del corpo umano*)"; and Scipione Mercurio's *La Comare*, an obstetric manual from which barber-surgeons could learn many useful things on childbirth. Most interestingly, Montalbani said that barber-surgeons must place themselves

> under the guidance of the most excellent *Dottori Arcicirurgi*, who do know that most admired, and world-famous, art of remaking many body parts which have been lost, about which one of our Collegiate physicians of the past century, Gaspare Tagliacozzi, has published the most admirable volume *de Curtorum Chirurgia, pro insitionem* [sic].[54]

Barbers practice the art of "*mangonizzare*, that is to embellish and clean up men's hair and beards of all their excrements and external superfluities," something which "must not aim at a vicious end, but only at improving the patients' health, always keeping as far as possible from womanly enhancements of beauty, an endeavour which, in contrast, must be left in the hands of maids, who unfortunately are experts in this malicious art."[55] Barber-surgeons, just like learned surgeons, had to attend to people's health, not to enhance their beauty, like women asked and female make-up experts did. Going down the list of the barbers' activities, Montalbani recalled that in ancient Rome they used to be bath and thermal spa attendants and that this tradition had been revived in his times, as barbers worked as public and private steam-bath attendants "in order to clean up the body for the sake of health (*a fine di procurar le mondezze del corpo in ordine alla sanità*)." To sum everything up, Montalbani described the barber-surgeons' goal as "procuring the pure cleanliness of human bodies (*procurante la pura mondezza de' corpi humani*)," which was indeed a goal worth of the greatest honor and respect.[56]

I only want to highlight here a few things in Montalbani's passage. First is the confusion of language referring to the practitioners of the body ("arci-surgeon," "barber," "surgeon"). Second, that cosmetics and surgery were placed on a continuum or at least within the same professional culture. Third, that works of learned surgery and medicine were suggested to barbers as important sources of information for their surgical-aesthetic concerns. Fourth, the ways gender distinctions were translated into medical discourse on the differences between cosmetics and medicine. And finally, the function of cleaning and policing the human body was almost ubiquitous in barber-surgeons' and surgeons' self-definition. Both professional categories took much pride in it because it indicated that the subject of their art was the human body and its public, visible, presence.

In her study of the health-care system in Bologna, Gianna Pomata described a double model of perception of illnesses in early modern medicine: one based on the obstruction and evacuation of the body and the other based on the control of humors and organs through diet. These two models refer to two professional figures: "healers" and "protectors" (the latter being represented by Collegiate physicians in their role of Protomedici). The relationship between patient and healer was horizontal and conceptually linked to self-therapy; the patient-protector relationship was instead vertical and implied dependence upon a higher authority. "In the long run – Pomata wrote – the vertical model of healing won over the horizontal model."[57] More generally, patients wanted treatments to be effective, while medical authorities wanted them to be orthodox.

Pomata argued that barber-surgeons were caught between these two fires. On the one hand, patients regarded barbers as "healers"; on the other hand, medical authorities always tried to regulate and control the barbers' practice. "Barber-surgeons were, so to speak, doubly vulnerable: they could lose their fee not only if a patient was unsatisfied with therapy but also, even in case of successful treatment, if they had not abided by the Protomedici's rule." Pomata argued that this was one of the main reasons for the decline of the cure agreement in the seventeenth century: barber-surgeons tried to get rid of the agreement model to lower the pressure on their performances.[58] In this way, the liminal position of barber-surgeons played a crucial role in the transformation of the medical profession and the decline of the juridical form of the "agreement for a cure" – the form of a contract between patient and healer in which the former paid the latter only when and if he or she felt cured – by the late sixteenth century and in the "waning of a view of medicine which allowed for self-diagnosis and self-therapy." This change was linked to the pressure that patients were exerting on barber-surgeons from below and the pressure medical authorities were exerting from above. On the one hand, barber-surgeons were required to practice under a physician's supervision and not simply upon patients' request; on the other hand, their business depended upon a view of healing and the body widely based on self-perception and self-diagnosis. For example, people who were feeling sick asked barber-surgeons to draw blood, without consulting a physician, thus pressing barber-surgeons to act outside of the boundaries of the law. Many barber-surgeons found themselves in this difficult position. Indeed, there had always been a link in the early modern world between barbers and "the tradition of self-therapy," in which knowledge and skills were perceived as something that could be evaluated by the patients themselves, not only by medical practitioners.[59] I would add to this picture the fact that barber-surgeons were often the first health-care professionals the sick got in touch with and that as such they could also act as mediators and go-betweens, putting in contact patients with other figures of healers, including the physicians.

My use of the phrase "practitioners of the body" to refer to all kinds of surgeons is somehow anachronistic, because the actors would have always kept in mind the difference between a graduate physician and a barber-surgeon. But this use of the phrase meets the goal of underlining the continuity, in terms of skills and technical competence, between the most advanced empiric surgeons and graduate surgeons. When understood as different kinds within one and the same category of practitioners of the body, surgeons do not clearly fit this dichotomy between healers and protectors. Among barber-surgeons and physicians there was a relationship not only of subordination and unrest but also of collaboration and division of labor. The relationships between empiric surgeons and graduate surgeons could be described in terms of "trading zones," as sites in which a two-way exchange – not always peaceful, often conflictual – of knowledge and skills took place.[60] This will become particularly evident in the next chapter, which focuses on specific reconstructive techniques that were the realm of empiric surgeons, graduate surgeons, and all sorts of natural historians, gardeners, and farmers.

Notes

1 I translate *politezza* with "appearance" in the title of the chapter, but I shall often use the Italian in the text to remind the reader that the word *politezza* is truly polisemic and that I have found no adequate English tranlsation.

2 Gadebusch-Bondio, "I pericoli della bellezza 'mangonica'," p. 428; and Gadebusch-Bondio, *Medizinische Ästhetik*, pp. 84–125.

3 Galen, *Letter to Thrasiboulos* in Selected Writings, tr. Peter Singer (Oxford: Oxford University Press, 1997), pp. 57–58 (815–816).

4 Galen, *Letter to Thrasiboulos*, p. 60 (820–822).

5 Ibid., p. 61 (823).

6 Ibid., pp. 63–64 (827–829).

7 Ibid., p. 64 (829).

8 Ibid., p. 65 (831).

9 Ibid., p. 66 (834).

10 Galen, "De compositione medicamentorum secundum locos," in Karl Gottlob Kühn, ed. *Opera omnia* (Leipzig: Cnobloch, 1821–1833), vol. 12, p. 434 (337–338): "Comptoriae quidem scopus est, ut pulchritudinem acquisititiam inducat. Exornatoriae vero medicinae partis, ut quicquid secundum natura est, id omne in corpore custodiat, ad quod consequitur etiam naturalis pulchritude." On Galen's teleology and functionalism, see Mark Schiefsky, "Galen's Theleology and Functional Explanation," *Oxford Studies in Ancient Philosophy* 33 (2007): 369–400.

11 See Luke Demaitre, "Skin and the City: Cosmetic Medicine as a Urban Concern," in Brian Nance and Eliza Glaze Florence, eds. *Between Text and Patient: The Medical Enterprise in Medieval & Early Modern Europe* (Florence: SISMEL/Edizioni del Galluzzo, 2011), pp. 97–120.

12 Bernard de Gordon, *Lilium medicine*, 2.2, fol. 28ra-b; quoted by Demaitre, "Skin and the City," p. 108.

13 Mcvaugh, *The Rational Surgery*, pp. 120–126; Demaitre, "Skin and the City," pp. 100–109; Laurence Moulinier-Brogi, "Esthétique et soins du corps dans les traités médicaux latins à la fin du Moyen Âge," *Médiévales* 46 (2004): 55–72.

14 de Chauliac, *Inventarium*, vol. 1, p. 319: "Disposiciones que in facie apparent quedam sunt naturales, quedam preter naturam. Naturales indigent conservacione si pulchre sunt et decoracione si turpes, velut esset albedinem custodire et albiorem facere et rubicondiorem si licitum fuerit. Que vero preter naturam indigent correcione, velut est pustulacio et maculacio et superpilacio, et hoc intendebat Galienus dicere . . . quando ponebat differenciam inter comaticam et decorativam partem medicine . . . Nam licet decorativa curacio sit licita, comatica vero non est licita nisi gracia honestatis, unde Galienus ubi supra."

15 On this point, see Sandra Cavallo and Tessa Storey, *Healthy Living in Late Renaissance Italy* (Oxford: Oxford University Press, 2013), p. 267.

16 Giuseppe Ongaro and Elda Martellozzo Forin, "Girolamo Mercuriale e lo studio di Padova," in Alessandro Arcangeli and Vivian Nutton, eds. *Girolamo Mercuriale: medicina e cultura nell'Europa del Cinquecento* (Florence: Olschki, 2008), pp. 29–50, 30–31.

17 Gabriele Falloppio, "De decoratione," in Gabriele Falloppio, ed. *Opuscula* (Padua: apud Lucam Bertellum, 1566), fol. 34r-v. "ars de bono, vel praesens conservando vel desideratum restituendo . . . Cur medicina ars sit, necessarium est habere unum finem, qui sit perfectio subiecti, circa quod versatur: quod est perfectio corporis humani . . . robur & vim ad actiones obeundas . . . ista integritas corporis, quoties potest integras actiones perficere."

18 Ibid., fol. 34v-35r: "Ultimo non desuere qui dixere pulchritudinem esse bonum corporis summum. cum haec ab omnibus affectetur, non solum foeminis, sed maribus: non modo iuvenibus, sed senibus, cumque etiam virtus sit, ideo est summum bounum & perfectio . . . aggregatum ex his est ex sanitate, bono habitu, pulchritudine, & robore actionum videamus an res ita se habeat. accipiamus sanitatem, & bonum habitum, hi sunt causa pulchritudinis, & roboris in actionibus; pulchritudo & robor sunt fructus, sunt effectus itarum causarum. si coniugamus causas, & fructus, unum erit bonum . . . ex quatuor virtutum aggregato, quae sunt sanitas, robur, pulchritudo, & habitus."

19 Ibid., fol. 35r-v: "altera fucata, adulterina, ficta, & non vera, quae non naturalis, vel praeter naturalis dicenda . . . & hanc appellamus mangonicam, vel comptoriam, & haec meretricia, vel cynedica dicitur; nam destruit conditiones naturae, ut artis aliquot pessimas conditiones inducat; quam si affectant senes, iuvenes, & mulieres. Mulier destruit

venustatem: senes gravitatem amittunt: iuvenes virilitatem perdunt. Altera pulchritudo naturalis dicitur, quam unusquisque affectare debet: & qui non affectat, turpis est . . ."

20 Ibid., fol. 35v: "compositionem, & connexionem naturalem, ac symmetriam partium inter se . . . substantiam colorem, quantitatem, situm, figuram, & conformationem partium."

21 Ibid., fol. 36r: "comptoria destruit naturam, & addit quod non est in natura. Decoratoria semper respicit id, quod est secundum naturam in isto homine, vel in tota specie, velim in hac, velim in illa parte."

22 Mercuriale, *De decoratione liber*. On Mercuriale's teaching and practice in Bologna, see Alessandro Simili, *Gerolamo Mercuriale lettore e medico a Bologna. Nota II: Il soggiorno e gli insegnamenti* (Bologna: Azzoguidi, 1966).

23 Girolamo Mercuriale, "De decoratione liber," in Girolamo Mercuriale, ed. *De morbis cutaneis* (Venice: apud Iuntam, 1601), pp. 2–3: "turpitudinem nisi aliud esse, quam dissonantiam rerum cognatarum; sed morbus est huiusmodi dissonantia: ergo turpitudo est morbus, & consequenter pulchritudo erit sanitas . . . Artem medicam posse versari etiam circa turpitudinem, & pulchritudinem, sed non primario, neque per se: verum consequenter solum. nam versatur medicus primo, & per se circa sanitatem, & aegritudinem, sed quia ex sanitate pulchritudo tanquam fructus quidam nascitur, ut dicitur Galenus, ex aegritudine deformitas; hinc est, quod scribit Galenus medicum, & artem medicam versari circa pulchritudinem, & turpitudinem." On these works by Mercuriale, see Sabrina Veneziani, "Le lezioni dermatologiche di Girolamo Mercuriale"; and Enrico Peruzzi, "La concezione della bellezza nel *De decoratione*," in *Girolamo Mercuriale*, pp. 203–215, 247–256, respectively. On ugliness in early modern European culture, see Naomi Baker, *Plain Ugly: The Unattractive Body in Early Modern Culture* (Oxford: Oxford University Press, 2010).

24 Tagliacozzi, *De curtorum*, p. 15 (1:10–11), translation modified. Other faces, dark faces of other peoples – mainly the threatening armies of "Turks" and the enslaved "Turks" – were indeed part of the culture of the face. Besides this reference to practices of embellishing the slaves' faces, I have mentioned earlier that there are known cases of owners mutilating Turkish slaves, cases of branding slaves in early modern Italy, and that caricature and disfiguring portraits circulated of black people. Raffaella Sarti has been able to collect reliable information only about 32 "Turkish" slaves in Bologna between 1572 and 1708, but their presence was more numerous, given that figures concerning the Muslim slave population in sixteenth- and seventeenth-century Italy have been estimated to be between 40,000 and 50,000 individuals and given that converts also lived in Italy, sometimes in a state of semi-slavery; see Raffaella Sarti, "Bolognesi schiavi dei 'Turchi' e 'Turchi' schiavi dei Bolognesi tra Cinque e Settecento: alterità etnico-religiosa e riduzione in schiavitù," *Quaderni storici* 107, 2 (2001): 437–473, p. 451; Salvatore Bono, *Schiavi musulmani nell'Italia moderna* (Naples: Edizioni Scientifiche Italiane, 1999). Lucette Valensi has showed that Muslim slaves not only came as war prisoners (e.g., after the famous 1571 battle of Lepanto 3,600 war prisoners were traded as slaves in Italy) but were also chased in real sea and land man hunts; see Lucette Valensi, *Ces étrangers familiers. Musulmans en Europe, xvi–xviii siècles* (Paris: Payot, 2012).

25 Tagliacozzi, *De curtorum*, p. 16 (1:11).

26 Ibid., p. 17 (1:12).

27 Ibid., p. 57 (1:41).

28 Ibid., pp. 58–59 (1:43).

29 Giulio Cesare Aranzi, "De tumoribus," in Giulio Cesare Aranzi, ed. *De humano foetu*, p. 177: "praesertim si mulieres fuerint quae decorandae faciei consulant, vix aliquando subterfugere licet; imo precibus fatigati curationem pene inviti aggrede cogimur."

30 Vigarello, *Histoire de la beauté*, pp. 48–49.

31 Dalla Croce, *Cirugia universale, Sommario* (pages are not numbered). This interest in cosmetic remedies for facial unaesthetic spots and issues was widespread. For example, Cristina Bellorini has showed that Cosimo I de' Medici annotated with great care such remedies against spots on the face in the first edition (1544) of Mattioli's commentary

on Dioscorides: see Cristina Bellorini, *The World of Plants in Renaissance Tuscany: Medicine and Botany* (Ashgate: Farnham, 2016), p. 26.

32 Elaine Leong, *Recipes and Everyday Knowledge: Medicine, Science, and the Household in Early Modern England* (Chicago: The University of Chicago Press, 2018), pp. 3–4. On Fioravanti and the culture of the professors of secrets, see Eamon, *Science and the Secrets*, pp. 168–193; William Eamon, *The Professor of Secrets: Mystery, Medicine, and Alchemy in Renaissance Italy* (Washington, DC: National Geographics, 2010), especially pp. 41–56; Piero Camporesi, *Camminare il mondo. Vita e avventure di Leonardo Fioravanti, medico del cinquecento* (Milan: Garzanti, 1997); Ray, *Daughters of Alchemy*, pp. 14–72.

33 Leonardo Fioravanti, *Del compendio dei secreti rationali* [first edition 1564] (Turin: appresso gli heredi del bevilacqua, 1580), fol. 118r-v: "Sono varie, et diverse le cose materiali, con le quali le donne di continuo vanno adoperando per farsi belle, et ornate, delle quali ragionerò a pieno: percioché non è di minor importanza, che si sia la medicina, et la cirugia, perché le donne son tanto vaghe di tal cosa, che non lasciano supplicio nissuno a patire, per parer più belle di quello, che sono, e molte volte operano alcune cose, chef anno spesso contrario effetto, e grandissimo nocumento non solo alla faccia . . ."

34 Ibid., fol. 123r-145v: "Sono molte le donne, le quali hanno la faccia pelosa oltra modo, la qual cosa è molta brutta da vedere: percioché disconcia, et disforma assai una bella faccia . . . Quando ad una donna, o ad un'huomo gli incomincia a venire i pelli canuti, e li vuol far negri per parere più giovane, faccia in questo modo."

35 Ibid., fol. 141v-142r: ". . . piacer a tutti. La prima qualità adunque che vuole havere una donna, è che sia ricca, acciò non venga disprezzata. La seconda qualità è che sia generosa, acciò sia amata. La terza conditione è che sia honesta, acciò non venga biasimata. La quarta conditione è che sia giovane, acciò sia forte, e garglairda. La quinta conditione è che sia allegra . . . questa sarà la miglior sorte di belletti che si possino trovar, né usare, e quando non potessero havere le dette qualità, & si volessero fare bianche la faccia, le mani, et il petto, faccino questa seguente ricetta, & sarà bellissima."

36 Paré, *Oeuvres*, vol. 2, p. 622.

37 Giovanni Battista Della Porta, *Magiae naturalis libri XX* (Naples: Orazio Salviani, 1589), p. 362; quoted by Elena Lazzarini, "Alle origini della chirurgia plastica nei 'libri dei segreti' e nei trattati del XVI Secolo," *Genesis* 10, 1 (2011): 39–62, p. 39.

38 Pietro Paolo Magni, *Discorsi intorno al sanguinar i corpi humani* (Rome: appreso Bartolomeo Bonfadino & Tito Diani, 1584), p. 2: "l'essercitar quest'arte è cosa periculosa, & cavata da quella parte della Medicina, che chiamano Churugia . . . a i tempi nostri questa parte è venuta in mano d'alcuni imperiti, i quali scioccamente e indegnamente l'essercitano."

39 Vesalius' *De fabrica* (1543), in the dedication to Charles V, had given a standard version of the causes of the present corruption of medicine he was aiming at correcting, in that "the technique of surgery fell into neglect and was, as it were, handed over to laymen and people with no knowledge of the disciplines that go to serve the healing art. No more pestilent affliction could possibly have crept upon it." See Andreas Vesalius, *On the Fabric of the Human Body*, 3 vols., tr. William Frank Richardson (San Francisco: Norman Publishing, 1998), vol. 1, p. xlvii.

40 Magni, *Discorsi*, p. 3: "possono con la lancetta, o con il rasoio dar la morte al'huomo, o donna, nel suo operare . . . sia presto: perché sempre sarà più lodevole, ch'esser lento . . . perché il più delle volte con le parole, e gratie loro fanno, che l'infermi, & altri si lascino servire."

41 Ibid., p. 4: "perché il più delle volte barba farrà parer l'huomo bello, e brutto, & anco di forme poi maneggiar bene il rasoio . . . e lor' mani non diano noia al patiente."

42 Maria Conforti has persuasively argued that the work was co-authored by Malfi and the professor of anatomy at the Neapolitan studio and correspondent of William Harvey, Marco Aurelio Severino (1585–1656); see Maria Conforti, "Medicine, History and Religion in Naples in the Seventeenth and Eighteenth Centuries," in Ole Peter Grell and Andrew Cunningham, eds. *Medicine and Religion in Enlightenment Europe* (Aldershot: Ashgate, 2007), pp. 63–78, 67–68.

43 Tiberio Malfi, *Nuova prattica della decoratoria manuale e della sagnia; l'una a barbieri, et l'altra a chirurgici singolarmente necessaria* [first edition 1626] (Naples: appresso Ottavio Beltrano, 1629), pp. 1–3.
44 Ibid., p. 3. The author is here following Vesalius' narrative of the decline of surgery that the anatomist had placed in *De fabrica*'s dedication to Charles V.
45 Ibid., pp. 3–4: "L'altra parte di Medicina, detta Chirurgica, come che principalmente sia essercitata da' medici, pure per alcuni accidenti fu trasferita, e riposte (se non tutta almeno in parte) nelle mani de' medesimi Barbieri . . . Percioché curando la Chirurgica per ordinario ferrite, e mali, che di repente avvengono, e che portano momentaneo paricolo, o per l'offesa dell'aria, o per lo spargimento del sangue, o per gli estremi dolori, onde non patiscono indugio, nè dilation di tempo; & I medici tali non sono, che dimorino in casa (per essere ordinariamente occupati fuori, o per non tenere officina) in luogo loro successero li Barbieri, che parati sempre si trovano assistendo nelle loro officina."
46 Ibid., p. 4: "l'altra ragione, oltre la necessità, fu l'affinità, o diciamo vicinanza dell'operationi nello stesso suggetto, ciò ch'adempendo il Barbiero il mancamento della bellezza, e della politezza, con facile passaggio si riducesse di passo in passo a correggere i difetti della solutione del continuo, che difformava, e guastava essa bellezza, nella quale versa la Chirurgia."
47 Ibid., p. 6: "[l'arte del barbiere ha] per proprio privilegio, e singolare prerogativa, col tatto immediato delle mani lo stesso huomo ha per suggetto, e circa l'istesso tutta si versa, emendando l'imperfettioni della natura."
48 Ibid., p. 7.
49 Garzoni, *La piazza*, vol. 2, pp. 1375–1376: "L'arte di questi è medesimamente netta e polita, avendo per fine e per scopo la politezza del corpo, la qual si causa dal radere, dal tosare, dal lavare, e stropiciar ben bene le persone che fan ricorso a loro. E si mette in essecuzione con pochissima spesa, imperoché un bacile, dui rasoi, una lancetta, un gamaut, una molletta, un pettine . . ., due para di fazzuoli, una spongia, un focone con un poco di carboni, un secchio di lissiva, e una zucchetta d'acqua rosa da sbruffare in faccia, compiscono tutta l'architettura de' barbieri. Servono anco i barbieri per cavar sangue agli amalati e per mettergli le ventose, medicar le ferite, far le stoppate, cavare i denti guasti, e simili altre cose, onde l'arte loro . . . è subalternata per questo alla scienza della medicina . . . La destrezza della mano è desiderata sopra tutto ne' barbieri, così l'occhio bono."
50 Gianna Pomata, "Barbieri e comari," in Giuseppe Adani and Gastone Tamagnini, eds. *Cultura popolare nell'Emilia Romagna. Medicina, erbe, magia* (Milan: Silvana Editoriale, 1981), pp. 161–183, 175; Cavallo and Storey, *Healthy Living*, pp. 257–267.
51 BUB 3839, *Cronica, o sia Diario di Francesco Galliani (1589–1600)*, fol. 83v: "Adì 7 di Novembre [1599] passò di questa vita lo eccellente dottore in Medicina Gaspare Tagliacozzo famosissimo più che alcun altro fosse di nostra età nell'arte della Cirusia, il quale faceva il naso, labra et orecchie a quelli li erano state tagliate per ferite, o altro, e li faceva con tanta politezza, che di poco di più bello crea la natura."
52 Ovidio Montalbani was a professor of philosophy, medicine, and mathematics, Prior, and subsequently archivist of the College of Medicine and Philosophy. He also was a public historian and the compiler of the annual astrological predictions of the Senate: He served as a magistrate, as an officer of the tax fund (the "Gabella Grossa") that funded the salary of the studio lecturers, and finally he became the curator of Aldrovandi's museum of natural history and the editor of his works.
53 Ovidio Montalbani, *L'honore de Collegi dell'arti della città di Bologna. Brieve trattato Fisicopolitico e Legale Storico* (Bologna: Benacci, 1670), p. 90: "L'arte dei barbieri esercita principalmente la Cosmetica Medicina, ed in buona parte la Cirurgia, per concessione liberale del Collegio de' Signori Medici di questa Città."
54 Ibid., p. 91: "a i quali non è ignota l'arte mirabilissima, e famosissima per tutto il Mondo di restituire molti membri affatto perduti, di che uno dei nostri Dottori Medici Bolognesi

Collegiati dell'andato secolo, cioè il Tagliacozzi, ha lasciato in istampa l'ammirabilissimo Volume *de Curtorum Chirurgia, pro insitionem* [*sic*]."

55 Ibid.: "mangonizzare, cioè l'abbellire, e mondare da escrementiti e estrinseche superfluità de i Capegli, e Barbe gli Huomini . . . non dev'esser indirizzato al fine venalicio vitioso, ma solo al migliorare la sanità del mangonizzato, lontanissimo sempre dall'intricarsi ne gli abbellimenti Donneschi, lasciando simile impaccio alle Fantesche pur troppo instrutte in quest'arte dolosa."

56 Ibid., pp. 91–92.

57 Pomata, *Contracting a Cure*, pp. 140–141.

58 Ibid., p. 148.

59 Ibid., pp. 152–153.

60 I use this expression in the meaning Pamela O. Long has given to it, building on the work of Peter Galison: see Pamela O. Long, "Trading Zones in Early Modern Europe," *Isis* 106, 4 (2015): 840–847.

5

GRAFTING HUMANS AND PLANTS

One of the memorials dedicated to Tagliacozzi on the walls of the Archiginnasio presents a rather unique feature: it mentions by name Tagliacozzi's teaching assistant Pompilio Tagliaferri (1559–1639) from Parma.[1] In fact, Tagliaferri was not a simple assistant. He had studied medicine in Padua and graduated in Rome. Probably he acted as a dissector while Tagliacozzi dealt with the most theoretical aspects of the demonstrations, according to a script that, despite the appearances, did not cease to exist in the century of Vesalius.[2] Indeed, in the memorial inscription Tagliacozzi is described as someone who explains human anatomy, and the dedication includes Tagliaferri "on account of his special ability and adroitness in accomplishing [dissections] most skillfully and in most beautifully demonstrating [human anatomy] with the best generosity and diligence."[3] Interestingly enough, this Tagliaferri, who is never mentioned in the official roll of the Bologna studio lecturers, was a professor of botany in Rome for a while and had studied botany along with anatomy. By 1601, he became professor of anatomy and the keeper of the botanical garden at the newly founded University of Parma.[4] A contemporary chronicler of Parma recalled that he was an expert practitioner of obstetrics, that he was marvelously skilled in the art of surgery, and that he performed a wondrous but unspecified treatment in Ferrara on a certain Signora de' Bentivogli. He is also said to have been a virtuoso musician, an expert in recipes and pharmacology, and renowned for composing several botanical manuscripts and herbals, which were all lost after his death.[5] It was an interesting partnership with a botanist for Tagliacozzi, who took one botanical practice, grafting, and transferred it to surgery.

The natural-artificial opposition occupies a central place in an analysis of Renaissance reconstructive surgery, not only with respect to the moral perception of the face and conceptions of beauty but even more so at the level of epistemology and ontology.[6] This surgical procedure was at the same time a way of knowing the human body and a way of approaching a bundle of thorny ontological issues that ultimately challenged, even against Tagliacozzi's intention, the traditional natural-artificial distinction. The reconstructive procedure of the damaged parts of the face was one of the several sites in which the conceptions of nature and art – understood as techne, as man's work on and with nature – underwent a deep crisis in the late sixteenth century. It is well known that the historiographical construct, once called "the Scientific Revolution," is nowhere to be found[7] and that "there is no such thing" in history.[8] I embrace here the alternative conception of slow, nonlinear transformation in practices and concepts that concerned several domains of early modern knowledge. Surgery, agriculture, gardening, and horticulture are examples of those practices that have been for a long time considered marginal, through which a process of blurring of the boundaries took place regarding the most serious and important concepts that are associated with the changes of this period. It is not possible to argue that in early modern Europe there was a precise moment in which, for example, the idea of nature as a personified creative force gave way to the idea of nature as a law-governed, impersonal set of processes or that nature and art ceased all of a sudden to be hierarchically ordered. But it is possible to show that, in practice as well as in theory, the natural-artificial opposition became an issue.

By following the history of a practice – grafting – rather than a discipline – surgery – this chapter approaches Tagliacozzi's text from the point of view of ontology and epistemology. It describes the classical distinction between art and nature that, in its various meanings, constituted the background for several concepts and practices of the sciences of men, plants, and gardens. It discusses the many contradictions and oscillations concerning the natural-artificial opposition that are to be found in Tagliacozzi's book and the respective roles of the human artifex and of nature in this surgery procedure. I argue that these difficulties were linked to the practical example he chose as the main guide for the operation itself: grafting. This chapter also discusses classical and contemporary practices and theories of grafting that were in place by the late sixteenth century, as well as the contexts in which they originated and developed in new vernacular and Latin genres: the rise of natural history, commercial exchanges, novelties from the New World, and the process of taking back the countryside by a leisured noble class. Finally, I clarify the main epistemological and ontological issues in Tagliacozzi's book.

Art and nature

The most important and often repeated conceptualization of the difference between nature and artifice in Renaissance European intellectual circles came from Aristotle's *Physics*. In Book II, the philosopher had claimed that natural products have an innate or internal principle of motion or change, while artificial objects precisely lack such inherent internal principle of change.[9] However, Aristotle introduced a nuanced distinction between two ways in which art worked with respect to nature. Either the arts "carry things further than Nature" or they "imitate Nature": the arts either perfect nature or they simply imitate nature without altering it.[10] The paradigmatic examples of the former kind of "perfective" arts were medicine and agriculture, and it was in the Hippocratic tradition that art first appeared as the "servant of nature."[11]

From the very beginning, the trope of art imitating nature implied an ambiguous relation between the passivity and the activity of human makers, between art as a mirror and art as production. In classical antiquity this relationship implied two features: art was dependent upon nature – it used nature's material; imitated its functions, processes, and appearance; followed its regularities – and ancillary to nature – it cooperated with nature to help it reach its full potential. The idea seems to be rooted in medical thought from the beginning, as it was understood that medical arts imitated bodily functions and processes. Medicine itself was said to copy nature or to aid and support nature's power to heal. At the same time, nature guided humanity to develop the arts.[12] In the Aristotelian-medical sense, to perfect nature did not mean to create an artificial product as perfect as a natural object but rather to help nature display its potential. Galen contrasted the works of nature and art by considering sculpture and painting as purely superficial *mimesis*, which left the inner structure of objects intact. Therefore, by elaborating on the Aristotelian idea of the inner principle of change, Galen made the art versus nature distinction a matter of surface and depth.[13] For Galen, despite the appearances, art could not work on matter and transform it the way nature did.[14]

These first two intertwined meanings – art imitating nature and art perfecting nature – were the most important ones for Tagliacozzi, who entertained a complex conceptual game with them in an effort to justify his procedure in philosophical terms. But other meanings played a role too. Following Close's essay, we find the idea that art is based on experience, or study, of nature, an idea that was indeed very much tied to the trope of art imitating nature. The idea of art and nature proper of the rhetorical tradition is even more interesting: classical Roman rhetoric exercised a deep influence in humanistically trained medical writers, and it blurred the boundaries between the two poles of the artificial and the natural. This was the idea according to which art, conceived as training, skill-building, discipline, practice, could perfect individual nature or talent.[15] This rhetorical conception was closely tied to the idea that art operated by using nature's material, again a variation of the conception of the perfective art that was particularly employed in classical examples on politics and medicine.

It was a classical commonplace to claim that art began in nature, and this idea played a fundamental role in discussions on grafting. Partly for these reasons of logical and ontological derivation of art from nature, art was conceived as inferior to nature by the majority of Renaissance thinkers. This idea of the inferiority of art was linked, in turn, to the idea that nature was a skillful artist.[16] A.J. Close left out of his remarkable list the contribution of ancient and Renaissance engineers, machine-makers, and alchemists, which historians have universally recognized as one of the most decisive sources for the conceptualization of art and nature in the "age of the new."[17] Ancient writers on mechanics introduced the idea of the "conquest" of nature, in that they thought they could make nature behave differently and alter its natural course. This meant that the four natural elements were forced to behave against their natural inclinations.[18] The theme of placing nature under violent investigation, test, and even torture in order to make her confess the truth can also be found in the alchemical tradition. Alchemists introduced a different conceptual relationship between art and nature: art could change the structure and matter of nature and replicate – not just imitate or perfect – nature's processes.[19]

Engineering, natural history in its connection with the "discoveries" of the New World, commerce, the culture of collecting, medicine, and alchemy[20] have all been mentioned in recent historiography of early modern science as working on the slow and nonlinear subversion of the classical art versus nature distinction that is associated with the novelties, and the sense of novelty, so widespread in sixteenth-century scientific culture. Several excellent recent works describe the many ways in which the natural-artificial epistemological and ontological boundaries came to be an issue. Daston and Park have showed that at the conceptual level the natural came to be opposed, or at least compared to, not only to the artificial but also to old and new ontological states: the unnatural, the supernatural, and, above all, the preternatural. The latter was a state given by the rare conjunctions of natural causes that produced strange effects, which were understood as singular exceptions rather than violations of the natural order.[21] Paula Findlen has argued that the importance assumed by the concept of *lusus naturae* allowed scholars and practitioners to highlight "man's ability to match nature's complexity with his own artifice" and suggested that it is in the practices of experimentation and playfulness of natural historians, gardeners, anatomists, surgeons, and natural philosophers that the boundaries between natural and artificial came into question in sixteenth-century science, also under the long-lasting influence of Pliny and of Ovid's *Metamorphoses*.[22]

One of the most celebrated figures of this age of the new was Francis Bacon (1561–1626). Bacon's natural history program suggested to investigate nature under three categories: (1) nature in its unrestrained state (*natura in cursu*); (2) nature in accidental conditions, such as in the production of monsters (*natura errans*); (3) nature as "constrained, moulded, translated, and made it as it were new by art and the hand of man" (*natura vexata*). Bacon's reformation of natural history was of course based on *natura vexata*. The Englishman claimed that "things artificial differ from things natural not in form or essence, but only in the efficient [the agent]."[23] This remarkable passage has been interpreted in different ways. Paolo Rossi has seen in it the influence of a centuries-long tradition of mixed mathematics, engineering, and all sorts of technical cultures of machine-making, which strongly emphasized the ability of art to change the natural course of the phenomena.[24] Daston and Park argued that Bacon was abolishing the distinction between the natural and the artificial under the influence of the culture of collecting and the reports on singular wonders, coupled with the ways of arguing of seventeenth-century gentlemanly culture. In their account, Bacon realized that art and nature mutually imitate each other and that the opposition between art and nature was best overcome by looking at the marvels produced by each.[25] Newman has showed that Bacon was actually citing almost literally common tropes of the alchemical tradition, which were based in turn on a radical interpretation of the broad Aristotelian definition of the perfective arts.[26] In any case, by the late sixteenth century the roots of the ontological and epistemological crises of the natural-artificial distinction were firmly grounded.

Grafting humans

Gaspare Tagliacozzi claimed that his elaborate procedure of skin grafting was modeled upon the ancient art of grafting plants and trees. He had read about it in the sixteenth-century humanistic editions of the Roman writers of *res rusticae*, or agriculture, husbandry, and country lifestyle. The learned surgeon made reference only to this literature, and especially to its most accomplished first-century author, Columella (4–70 CE), and his ten-volume *De re rustica*. However, fascination with grafting and the reach of the practices of playing with branches, trees, and fruits were far broader and reflected contemporary passions for agricultural and horticultural knowledge and practice.

In chapter ten of the first book of *De curtorum*, the Bolognese physician recalled the main stages and principles of his reconstructive procedure. The material – the skin – and its site had to be close, ready, and at hand, if surgeons wanted to successfully connect it to the mutilated part. Once connected to it, the material had to reproduce the shape of the part in order to be similar to its original state. "The material of which I speak is simple skin; before it is joined to the mutilated part, it must be carefully marked out and raised up." The site where this "material" was taken from was, as we know, the anterior part of the upper arm. The skin flap was then joined to the mutilated parts with sutures; several ligatures and bindings were then employed until the skin and the mutilated part "grow together." Once these parts were firmly joined, "the skin is removed from the arm and molded into the shape of the missing part; then, it must be carefully observed and cared for so that it may at least become strong and stable."[27] Tagliacozzi went on: "I have derived the principles of this surgical procedure from agriculture, specifically from the process of grafting."[28]

The surgeon believed that it was important to understand what the ancient classical authors had said about grafting practices in order to clarify his surgical procedure. In this way, he wanted to account for the origins of this practice and its development up to the present, because his goal was "to defend [this practice] from the calumny of those spiteful men who believe that it was born of chance instead of reason."[29] Tagliacozzi was simply saying that this was not the art of an empiric and this was why he took up the learned antique tradition of agriculture and horticulture in the first place. Indeed, the ancients – Tagliacozzi went on – discovered this art with great difficulty, because the procedure was new, but they rationally elaborated on their own experiences.

Tagliacozzi was pushing his interpretation of the "ancients" to its limits, glossing over their insistence on chance. Latin writers such as Pliny and Lucretius both had written that men discovered the art of grafting by pure chance while observing the varieties and wonders of the infinitely creative nature. Pliny (23–79) had argued that "Nature has herself been our instructor; but grafting was taught to us by Chance (*casus*), another tutor and one who gives us perhaps more frequent lessons." In this passage chance figured as a teacher, and a teacher who helped nature's teaching. Pliny also invented an origin story:

> [A] careful farmer, making a fence round his house to protect it, put under the posts a base made of ivy-wood, so as to prevent them from rotting; but the posts when nipped by the bite of the still living ivy created life of their own from another's vitality, and it was found that the trunk of a tree was serving instead of earth.[30]

In a similar vein, about a century earlier, the Roman poet Lucretius (c. 99–55 BCE) had explained that from observation of the natural operations of grafting, man domesticated nature and created a cultivated human landscape. Man imitated the creativity of nature, used its material, and at the same time produced humanized natural products.

> But the pattern of sowing and the beginning of grafting (*insitionis origo*) first came from nature herself the maker of all things, since berries and acorns falling from trees in due time produced swarms of seedlings underneath; and this also gave them the fancy to insert shoots in the branches and to plant new slips in the earth all over the fields. Next one after another they tried ways of cultivating the little plot they loved, and saw wild fruits grow tame in the ground with kind treatment and friendly tillage. Day by day they made the forests climb higher up the mountains and yield the place below to their tilth, that they might have meadows, pools and streams, crops and luxuriant vineyards on hill and plain, and that a grey-green belt of olives might run between to mark the boundaries, stretching forth over hills and dales and plains; just as now you see the whole place mapped out with charming variety, laid out and intersected with sweet fruit-trees and set about with fertile plantations.[31]

However, Columella was Tagliacozzi's polar star. Historians consider Columella the moment of "maturation" of ancient Roman agronomy and husbandry, and his book has often been described as a breakthrough in the history of agriculture, given its systematic nature and its blend of practical and theoretical approaches to farming lands and gardens.[32] The opening of the preface of *De re rustica* shows that Columella endorsed an image of nature as a creative force that gave man abundance and needed only to be helped out and cultivated. Columella wrote that "those politicians" – actually thinkers influenced by the Epicurean idea that nature could age – who complained about the unfruitfulness of the soil, the inclemency of the weather, and the scarcity of crops were all wrong. Indeed,

> it is a sin to suppose that Nature, endowed with perennial fertility by the creator of the universe, is affected with barrenness as though with some disease; and it is unbecoming to a man of good judgment to believe that Earth (*Tellurem*), to whose lot was assigned a divine and everlasting youth, and who is called the common mother of all things – because she has always brought forth all things and is destined to bring them forth continuously – has grown old in mortal fashion.[33]

In his book, Tagliacozzi almost transcribed Columella's passages on grafting, describing the four modes of grafting the classic writer talked about, based on slips, shoots, buds, or vine branches (*furculuum, semen, gemmam*, or *traducem*).[34] Just like a surgeon, the skillful grafter had to be able to use sharp tools, such as a scalpel and a knife, and then he needed to learn how to bind together the grafted parts with special plasters, ointments, and bandages to protect the parts from "wind and heat."[35]

The third method of grafting, based on manipulating buds, was a delicate and difficult procedure, "not suited to every kind of tree" but only to those that had "moist, juicy and strong bark, like the fig-tree; for this both yields a great abundance of milk, and has a stout bark, and so a graft can be very successfully inserted by the following method." It was the most relevant method as far as human skin grafting was concerned. The instructions given by Columella were indeed remarkably similar to Tagliacozzi's procedure.

(1) The farmer must select a young and healthy branch of the tree from which to take a graft, "and you should look out on them for a bud which has a good appearance and gives sure promise of producing a sprout." (2) Farmers must make a mark on it which leaves the bud in the middle of it, "and then make an incision all round it with a sharp knife and remove the bark carefully" in order not to damage the bud. (3) They must choose the healthiest branch of the other tree (the one that must receive the graft). (4) Farmers must then cut out a part of the bark of the same dimension of the graft and strip the bark off. (5) They must make sure that the shoot prepared from the first branch fits the receiving tree "so that it exactly corresponds to the area on the other tree from which the bark has been stripped." (6) They must bind the bud well all round and "daub the joints of the wound and the ties round them with mud, leaving a space, so that the bud may be free and not constricted by the binding." (7) Skilled grafters must cut away the shoot and upper branches of the tree that has received the graft, "so that there may be nothing to which the sap (*succus*) can be drawn off or benefit from the sap to another part rather than the graft." (8) "After the twenty-first day [they must] unbind the scutcheon" – note that the time length of the operation is the same as in human grafting.[36]

Tagliacozzi valued the fact that Columella demonstrated that plants and trees with nothing in common could indeed be grafted together. The surgeon made precise reference to the analogical correspondence between human skin and bark and placed humans within a cosmological continuum including plants and animals.

> A perceptive person will realize that the last two methods [buds with bark attached to branches; and one shoot placed into a cleft on another tree] provide the evidence that led the founders of reconstructive surgery to believe, as I do, that the restoration of mutilated parts could be accomplished in a similar way. . . . The skin of the upper arm (from which the graft is taken) is, after all, very similar in nature to the skin of the parts for which restoration is possible. Moreover, if the bark of one tree can coalesce with the bark of another, as in the case of inoculation, there is no reason to believe that skin, which is analogous to bark (*cutem ipsam, quae cortici respondet*), cannot be firmly and safely joined to other parts of the same body.[37]

There is a complete map of analogies at play in Tagliacozzi's commentary on Columella. Facial mutilations were comparable to the tree cleft; the skin taken from the arm was comparable to the olive branch; the excised skin corresponded to the olive branch once it had been inserted in the fig tree.[38]

Another crucial feature of both procedures concerned the time of the year they had to be carried on. Tagliacozzi recommended practicing human skin grafting in the spring, but he added that, unlike plant grafting, his procedure could also be performed at different times of the year. The reason was that human heat was more constant and powerful than plants' heat.[39] In explaining according to what physiological principles the procedure worked, Tagliacozzi took almost for granted that the success of the procedure was based on the doctrine of "generative heat" of both vegetal and animal bodies. The success of grafting in both humans and plants, he wrote, "depends on the presence of heat." Heat nourished the graft if the procedure was made on plants – and this is why it was more successful if practiced in the spring – and "the first practitioners of skin grafting, mindful of these precepts, wisely emulated nature in their investigations of how amputated or mutilated parts could be restored or reshaped."[40]

Tagliacozzi also took the time to reply to what he considered naïve criticisms. He claimed that his procedure was not a matter of generating new nerves and arteries, which everyone who was learned in medicine knew was impossible; rather, it was either a matter of joining together already existing vessels or of reviving the transplanted veins.[41] This issue was connected to interpreting correctly the Galenic theory of generative heat. For example, the greatly influential Giovanni Andrea Dalla Croce had written:

> When one part of the nose is completely amputated and taken away – especially if it is the cartilage – then you must abandon all hopes to heal it,

> since those parts are made of blood and spermatic parts, which don't grow and don't conglutinate when they are removed. Galen said that it is not impossible that the missing parts, which are generated by blood, can be regenerated, but those that are generated from the semen [i.e., the so-called spermatic parts], cannot really be regenerated.

According to the Galenic tradition, the spermatic parts of the body, generated in utero through a mixture of male and female semen by several successive concoctions of blood, could not be regenerated. Only "fleshy" or "sanguinary" parts were believed to be able to grow again. Spermatic parts were the hard and structuring parts of the body, while fleshy or sanguinary parts were the soft flesh and fat placed in between the spermatic.

> Those who claim that they can regenerate a completely severed nose – Dalla Croce went on – are not even worthy of being heard. There is neither natural artifice nor human artifex that can enjoy such high privilege of being able to attach a nose which has been entirely severed from the face. For this reason, if you find a nose which is wounded and only half dead, do not cut it off and throw it away, since I have seen some of those half-detached noses healed, attached, and restored.[42]

Giovanni Battista Cortesi, Tagliacozzi's pupil, writing in 1625, was careful in addressing the issue and specified that nature could not regenerate the spermatic parts that constitute lips, noses, and ears; instead, he invoked a collaboration between art and nature in regenerating the fleshy parts only.[43]

Farmers and gardeners were not the only artisans to which the graduate surgeon compared himself. No matter how learned surgery was, it was a manual art after all. While discussing the quantity of skin to be chosen for the graft – a rather delicate matter, because a lesser or bigger quantity of skin could really affect the positive outcome of the procedure and damage the patient – Tagliacozzi made use of an interesting sartorial analogy. Just like clothes must fit the body perfectly, so the skin of the graft must fit the mutilation – he wrote.[44] Indeed, this whole discussion is interesting in that Tagliacozzi had to deal with uncertainty and empirical observation but still had to get a rule for action. The problem was that in many cases, once cut off, the skin flap reduced in size. Therefore, surgeons had to study the mutilated part as well as the skin of the upper-arm region in order to understand the causes of this reduction and to be able to predict what the right size of the flap would be. But Tagliacozzi admitted that there was no single and infallible method to know the exact dimension of this reduction in size of the skin graft. Careful and repeated observation was therefore the only method recommended to surgeons if they wanted to overcome this lack of certitude. More specifically, surgeons had to pay attention to the texture of the skin.

Tagliacozzi presented human grafting as a variation on plant grafting, whose history was old and dignified by the great men who were able to extract norms out of a fortunate observation of natural phenomena. Surgeons had to imitate the farmers who imitated nature in their task to perfect natural forces and to second nature's immense creative power. Unfortunately for Tagliacozzi, however, things were not so simple, and the relationship between art and nature turned out to be much more complex. The Bolognese surgeon ended his discussion on Columella and plant grafting by pointing out that his procedure was not supposed to produce new objects. Reconstructive surgery was not interfering with the makeup of the world: a clear sign that he was worried about the implications of the analogy with agriculture. "Skin grafting, on the other hand, does not attempt to create a whole new life; rather, it is concerned with the restoration and renewal of a particular part."[45] But was it really so? And where did this anxiety come from?

Grafting plants

The second half of the sixteenth century witnessed, on a European scale, a wide flourishing of vernacular and Latin works on agriculture, horticulture, botany, and natural history of plants, which targeted, in different ways, the upper classes, the middle-class landowner or renter of land, the scholar, and the peasant.

With respect to agriculture and land cultivation, the late sixteenth century was a period of revolution.[46] Fueled by the reorganization of classical and medieval botany, a new agriculture began to take shape based on continuous rotation, alternation between agriculture and farming, and the beginning of a massive cultivation of forage. In economic terms, the period was characterized by an essential tension between two "systems of agriculture": one which was based on the transformation of work into capital and the other which consisted in the maximization of land exploitation.[47] This period has also been described in terms of "refeudalization," because the urban nobility became more and more interested in the countryside, buying and renting land. Moreover, noblemen cultivated the lifestyle of the country villa, far away from the masses of urban poor begging in the streets, the dangerous miasmas of the city, the pressures from the new centralized states, and the lowly people making a living by practicing the mechanical arts.[48]

By the middle of the sixteenth century, several factors generated a rise in the prices of crops, such as the excess of gold and silver coming from the Spanish ships sailing from the New World, the constant population growth (which was stopped only by the famine of the 1590s), and a renewed intensity of commerce – a consequence of both the abundance of goods and the increase of population. Urbanized northern Italian noblemen were struck by the rise of crop prices and massively decided to invest in land, sometimes even deciding to establish their residence in the countryside. In turn, this socioeconomic process was mutually syntonic with the process of cultural isolation and cultivation of class-specific sentiments of honor that were characteristic of the sixteenth-century noble ideology. As Stefano Guazzo (1530–1593), humanist lawyer at the Gonzaga court of the Monferrato, noted in his famous manual of manners *La Civil Conversatione* (1574), gentlemen were much more happy in the countryside, where they were treated as kings, rather than in the city, where they were simple citizens just like many others.[49]

Parallel to this culture of country lifestyle, a vernacular how-to literature developed by the middle of the century. This literature was more rich in technical detail and targeted not just the landowner or the playful nobleman but also the renter and the manager of the land. The explosion of commerce, a new empiricist sensibility, new systems of patronage that made the court a center of learning, and the opening up of university courses to the teaching of *materia medica* in newly funded botanical gardens were all circumstances that fueled the development of natural history. Natural history, botany, and the arts of agriculture, horticulture, and gardening were closely intertwined, linked by a new sensibility for the representation of nature given by geographical broadening, travels, the rediscovery of the classical sources, and the valorization of direct observation. By the beginning of the sixteenth century, gardens were used as sites of instruction to complement lectures on medicinal plants. Botany became more and more important for agriculture too by the second half of the sixteenth century, while gardens and orchards became the space for experiments that would have been too risky to practice directly in the fields.[50]

Three major features regulated the typology of gardens in sixteenth-century Italy. First, middle-sized gardens produced for the landowner's table; second, vegetable patches were valued as part of the peasants' salary; and finally, suburban and urban market gardens provided for urban populations. Besides field cultivation, gardens and orchards became a regular feature in Renaissance Italian dwellings. Moreover, commercial market gardening developed everywhere just outside the city walls of northern Italian cities. A new class of property managers emerged, who employed peasants in regular ways, especially exploiting the chances offered by these market gardens. For suburban small towns and villages in particular, such gardens became a necessity, and the borders between gardens, vineyards, and orchards became blurred. In this context, gardens had to produce income, not just pleasure. Just as they did in medicine, the languages of beauty and of usefulness blended in the literature on gardening. It is important to underline that, despite divisions of class and labor, peasant gardeners' manual skills – these open-air "invisible technicians" – were a determinant factor in the cultivation of excellent local varieties and exotic plants in the gardens of the wealthy and the natural historians.[51]

From a wider cultural perspective, gardens and orchards symbolized the complex relationships between the natural and the artificial. Mid-sixteenth-century Italian gardens were not just places of peace and serenity – according to the imagery of the *locus amoenus* – but also places where hybridization, monstrosity, and violence were staged.[52] It was specifically in the second half of the sixteenth century that the presence of plants and flowers in Italian gardens increased and a new role for gardeners emerged.[53]

This was a sort of a golden age for Italian gardens. Renaissance art and garden theory required that art imitate nature and that nature offered art the raw materials that had to be shaped into artificial forms. In this context, nature was conceived as a reflection of the cosmic order: imitating nature meant that art must imitate not only nature's appearance and form but also its underlying order. Sixteenth-century literature on agriculture often repeated that "nature produces better fruit if planted and cultivated," and gardens were one of the most prominent places where the categories of art and nature became more porous. In gardens, the relationship between the natural and the artificial was seen not as the victory of one over the other but as a competition among equals, and sometimes as cooperation. The interaction of art and nature, their "conjunction, or incorporation" was ubiquitous in the context of both gardening and agriculture.[54] As John Dixon Hunt has written, gardens are "cultural landscapes," namely "sites where human beings discover and realize whole patterns of belief, authority, and social structure"[55] – and, I would add, patterns of distinction and hybridization between nature and art.

Tagliacozzi's map of analogies between plants and humans came from a long way and had broad cultural resonances. A tight network of analogies and symbolic connections tied together plants and humans in the Renaissance. Aristotle had written that

> just as in animals there are homogeneous limbs, so also in plants. All the composite parts of the plant are like the limbs of the animal; the bark of the plant resembles the skin of the animal in nature, and the fibres correspond to the sinews of the animal. And so on with the rest of its parts.[56]

There existed a strong pre-modern strong tradition that imagined man as *arbor inversa*, a reversed tree, with hair compared to the roots, the chest to the trunk, the leaves to the words, the flowers to the intentions, the branches to force and power, and the bud to the thoughts.[57] In sixteenth-century Italy, Torquato Tasso (1544–1595) saw a deep analogy between the life cycle of men and plants:

> What is truly wondrous is that I find in them, when I look closely, all the accidents and examples of human youth and old age, because plants when are still new and green, have a clean (*polita*) and smooth bark, but when they grow old, their bark gets full of wrinkles, curls up and gets harsh.[58]

The vegetal and the human belonged to a life system of correlated powers, to a mutually integrated system in which the natural and the human communicated and were recognizable through many signs: one was the mirror of the other. In both human and plant anatomy alike the thread of life passed through juices, saps, nourishment, and so forth.[59]

Writers of agricultural treatises agreed on the fact that plants had feelings too. Natural historian Pietro Andrea Mattioli (1501–1578) attributed some kind of religious feeling and sensibility to plants, noticing that they turn toward the sun early in the morning as in prayer.[60] Metaphors of plant life were employed by Henri de Mondeville, as part of a tradition of learned surgery that can be connected directly to sixteenth-century medical education. In general, medieval religious symbolism was marked by the vegetal symbolism for the events of birth, and the intertwining of men and plants was a symbol of generation. The two main metaphorical functions of plants were generation and the flux of vital stuff in the body. However, the parallel between the farmer and the surgeon was lacking in Mondeville and in medieval surgeons, who on the other hand employed very frequently the metaphor of the roots, especially referring to human veins and how they nourish the body.[61]

Sixteenth-century natural history took up this theme in the same terms. Besides the discourse on plant and animal transmutations carried on by Ulisse Aldrovandi in his *Monstrorum Historia*,[62] another example that was surely very much in the mind of Tagliacozzi and the other surgeons was the Bolognese naturalist's *Dendrologia*, a work on plants and trees published posthumously by Ovidio Montalbani in 1668. The book is composed of two volumes. The first one opens with a chapter on "trees in general," then each chapter is devoted to one single plant. All chapters follow the natural historical order, composed by the following elements: name, etymology, denominations, shape, description, cultivation, birthplace, illnesses and remedies, medicinal uses, symbolism, emblematics, fables, moral meanings, and mirabilia.

The first part of the first book is eloquently titled *Dendranatome*, the anatomy of trees. Aldrovandi's arguments were very similar to the summary of similitudes between humans and plants that he had read in Giovanni Battista Della Porta's *Phytognomonica* (1588), a book entirely devoted to "the method for investigating the forces that animate plants though their parts and their way of living, of which they are fixed and mobile signs."[63] There, Della Porta had summarized the main points on such similarity according to the classical sources, from Theophrastus to Pliny to Plato's trope of man as inverted tree. Della Porta had also mapped the benefits humans could gain from these plants by virtue of these similarities, both in health and in sickness, through a close reading of the inner essence of plants as reflected by their external appearance.

Aldrovandi claimed that, like men, trees are either "urban" (*urbani*) or "wild" (*sylvestri*). "All plants, and trees in particular, are most clearly composed by not just similar, but also composed parts; we are persuaded of this fact by demonstrative reason, and we are convinced by anatomy." Aldrovandi explained that in both plants and humans there was an innate generative heat, from which "vegetative actions" proceeded. Like humans, plants had veins as an instrument for nutrition through the passage and transportation of juices. Plants also had non-motory and non-sensory nerves that were robust and steadfast. Just like men, Aldrovandi went on, trees were protected by a sort of skin under which a membraneous substance was to be found, just like human flesh. As far as "the whole conformation of trees (*Arborum totali conformatione*)" was concerned, trees had limbs like humans,

> which can be recognized, whence we call one part of tree head and brain, other parts we often take notes on as feet, arms, fingers, nails, hair, ears, and eyes; and all of them participate of the tree's perfection, as most noble vegetative complements.

And if we go on and make a proper dissection of a tree, we will find

> the hardest bone, flesh, nerves, veins, and muscles . . . and all plants and trees have a dermis and an epidermis, as well as parts of skin which circle them as a protective layer, from which layers all natural faculties come and they perform their tasks through the proper organs, as varied, specific and individual as it can get.[64]

Aldrovandi analytically commented upon an eloquent image (Figure 5.1) and explained the point-by-point analogy between a plant and a human. Moreover, trees could be beautiful and suffer injuries on their surface that could make them ugly.[65] Finally, Aldrovandi listed many occurrences of moral comparisons between men and trees, clearly showing a certain familiarity with Renaissance man-tree tropes.[66]

This anatomical connection between vegetal and human worlds was not just a topic for scholars and for the Latin-reading elite. Widely popular *Idea del Giardino del Mondo* by Tomaso Tomai (d. 1593) – part book of secrets and part popular scientific encyclopedia – made an original comparison between human beard and grass. After repeating the traditional explanation of human beard as dried vapor coming out of the pores of the skin, Tomai had to explain why men had it while children and women did not, and he devoted one entire chapter to this issue. Tomai wrote that human beard gets out of the vapors of the body just as grass grows out of the vapors of the earth, and

> just as grass does grow neither in extremely dry and sandy places, nor in too humid and watery soils, so children and women do not have hair on their faces and bodies because they are so cold that the pores of their skin are closed and vapors cannot get out, or they drown within the softness and humidity of their bodies.[67]

Here, the usual theme of the complexional difference among the sexes took a new turn, in which vegetal and human bodies obeyed, once again, to the same logic.

Grafting is defined today as "the natural or deliberate fusion of plant parts so that vascular continuity is established between them . . . and the resulting

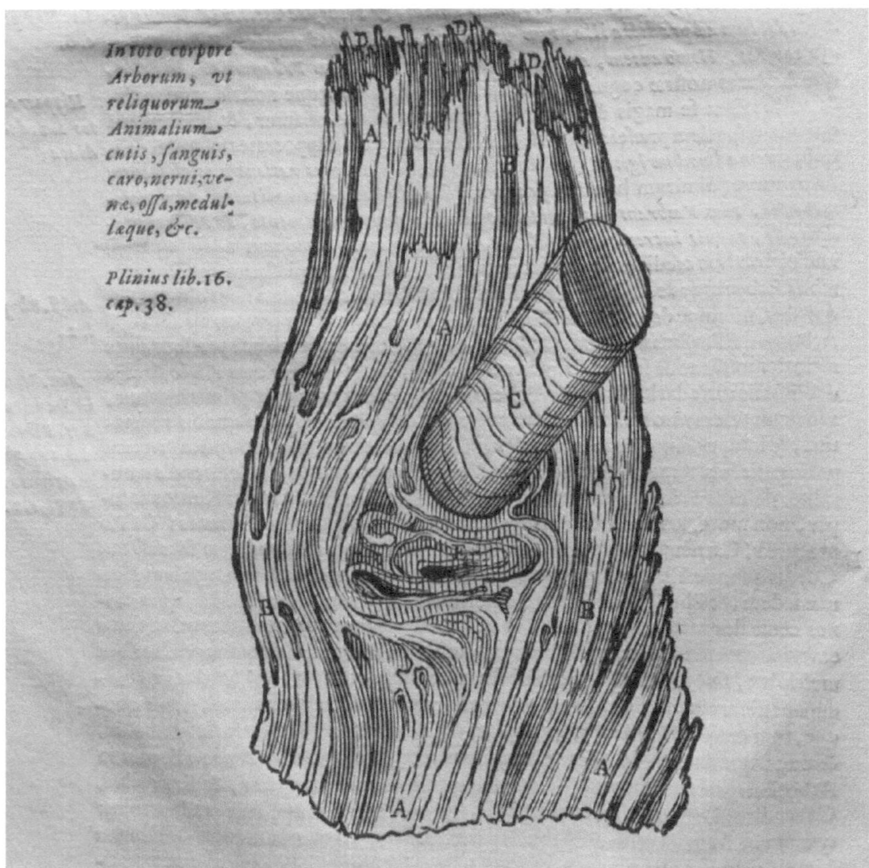

FIGURE 5.1 Ulisse Aldrovandi, *Dendrologiae naturalis* (1667): anatomy of a tree.

genetically composite organism functions as a single plant."[68] Besides the reference to genetic makeup, which points to modern correlate of pre-modern ideas of radical ontological alteration, the first part resonates with early modern interpretations of the practice. Grafting through external offshoots – a technique probably known since the first millennium BCE – is one of the major technologies in the history of agriculture.[69]

By the Middle Ages grafting became one of the favorite examples of advocates of alchemy.[70] In the *Book of Hermes*, a treatise on alchemy which might be a translation from Arabic that existed in several manuscript copies from the thirteenth to the fifteenth century, the author took issue with the opinion according to which humans could not reproduce the products of nature.

> The natural wild tree – the author claimed – and the artificially grafted one are both trees. . . . Nor does art make all these things; rather it helps

> nature to make them. Therefore the assistance of this art does not alter the nature of things. Hence the works of man can be both natural with regard to essence (*secundum essentiam*), and artificial with regard to mode of production (*secundum artificium*).[71]

This passage, a broad interpretation of Aristotle's conception of the perfective arts, became a topos in medieval alchemical literature and shaped early modern debates on technology. Alchemists had always maintained that the creation of grafted plants was no different from the natural birth of plants. Both wild trees and artificially grafted trees were the product of the same natural causes: in one case, the agent was chance; in the other, it was human intervention.

Sixteenth-century alchemists pushed forward the limits of this art-nature ontological equivalence. Unlike physicians, alchemists claimed to use nature not only to heal but also to produce entirely new substances. Unlike farmers and gardeners, who believed they could transform nature through grafting, alchemists claimed they could also accelerate nature's productive process.[72] In any case, few alchemists made the strongest ontological claim that they could produce entirely new objects that had never existed before, and most often they were more cautious in dealing with such a dangerous distinction, also passible of demonological interpretation. For example, in *De la pirotechnia* (1540) metallurgist Vannoccio Biringuccio (c.1489–1540) mentioned certain alchemists who claimed they could make trees and grass grow without their seeds being planted and could give fruits form, color, and odor different from their natural ones.[73] Also very interesting was the distinction between a good and a bad alchemy made by Biringuccio: the good one helped natural processes; the bad one was deceptive, "founded only on appearance" and produced intentional fakes, making things "appear at first sight to be what they are not."[74] It is interesting here to note more than a strong echo of the distinction between vulgar cosmetics and reconstructive surgery.

One of the most significant examples of the literature on the lands, gardens, and country lifestyle for the upper classes is *La villa*, published in 1559 by the Milanese humanist lawyer Bartolomeo Taegio (c. 1520–1573). The book was dedicated to the Emperor Ferdinand I, and the author introduced himself as a devotee of agriculture and the science of stars. The context was the narrative of a dinner party in the country villa of the Milanese gentleman Camillo Porro, where the "gardener (*hortolano*)" told many "secrets" to the guests. Among the many marvelous things discussed in the book with literary prowess as well as scientific rigor, Taegio recalled the habit of playfully shaping fruits, mainly citrons and pumpkins, also mentioned by Biringuccio.

> I am telling you – Taegio had the gardener say – that if you wish to see in pumpkins, in cedars (if you have them) new and strange faces, you should have someone make a crystal jar of the shape you like, and then place them [the fruits] inside these jars when they are still very young, and you will see that the pumpkin will grow up similar to the jar, and the thing should work.[75]

The discussion went on and focused on grafting, in a tone that alternated between technical language and the language of wonder and medicine:

> on this pear tree and on this red blackberry bush you can graft oranges, whose sourness you can sweeten by making a hole in the middle of the trunk, thus channeling out the bad humor, to the point that the fruits are well formed, and then you must dress their wound with lotus; from all this you will see a wondrous effect.[76]

Taegio was fully aware of the fact that nature changed under the repeated, patient, gradual work of men, because in the most beautiful gardens "one clearly sees that nature gives way to industry, and that it changes its way after a patient work."[77] While describing the marvelous garden at the villa of Castellazzo, property of a Senator of Milan who used to flee from the city whenever he could, Taegio penned a striking passage on the creation of a "third nature" through grafting.

> Here are without end the ingenious grafts that show with great wonder to the world the industry of a wise gardener, who by incorporating art with nature brings forth from both a third nature, which causes the fruits to be more flavorful here than elsewhere.[78]

Taegio was not the only one who brought up the theme of a third nature in the sixteenth century. Indeed, there was a widespread conception of grafting and horticulture as an incorporation of art and nature that was productive, which brought about something new in the world by challenging the traditional natural-artificial distinction.[79] Moreover, all these writers were echoing Ovidian themes that were ubiquitous in contemporary culture, shaping iconographic programs of "grotesque" hybridizations of the human and the natural, such as the Holy Wood of Bomarzo near Rome, designed by the architect Pirro Ligorio (1513–1583) in 1547 (Figure 5.2), and the famous paintings by Arcimboldo (1526–1593) in the late sixteenth century (Figure 5.3). Such grotesque iconography, far from being an expression of the unbound fantasy of the artists, was actually part of a culture of scientific collection and a quest into the limits of the natural world.

Natural historians all across Europe shared both a technical competence with the manipulation of plants and a feeling of amazement and wonder toward the hybrid and new products of grafting. Pietro Andrea Mattioli's commentary on Dioscorides mentioned the "natural brotherhood (*naturae germanitas*)" of all plants, to the point that they could transform into each other. Mattioli also recalled that plants and trees could be wild or cultivated and that the wild became cultivated when appropriately transplanted, treated, and grafted in the domestic garden.[80] Dutch naturalist Rembert Dodoens (1517–1585) in his *Histories of Plantes* (1578) noted that early modern gardeners cultivated "several flowering plants . . . into showy varieties not originally found in nature." Dodoens'

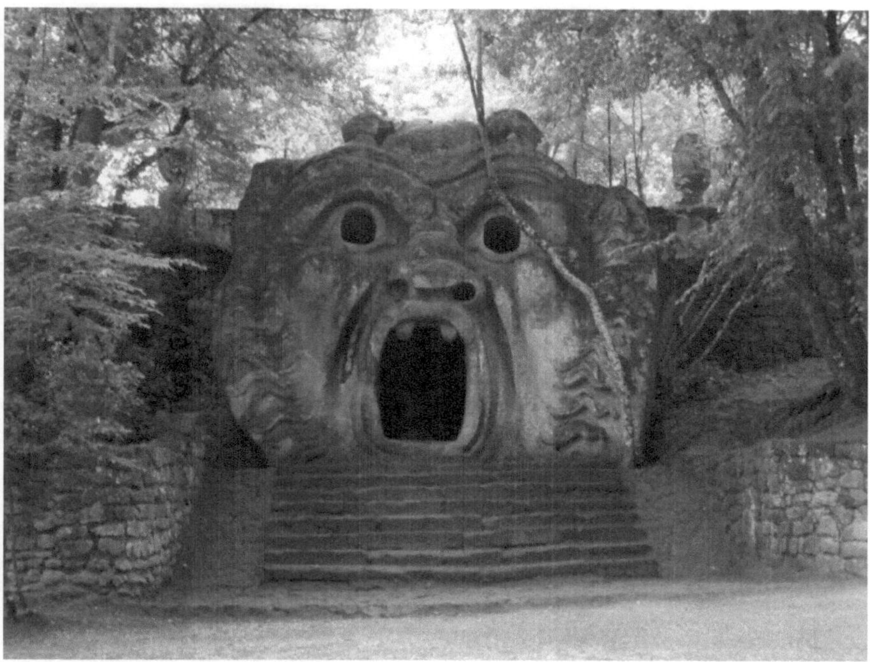

FIGURE 5.2 Pirro Ligorio, *The Holy Wood of Bomarzo* (1546): grotesque (public domain).

carnation is a good example. His "small tulpia" resembles tulips, but "florists were able to cross-breed them to produce the striking varieties avidly collected and painted in seventeenth-century still lives."[81] Aldrovandi's *Dendrologia* also played with the theme of the "learned hand" of the gardener who grafted apple trees, remarking upon the product of grafting techniques as being a "union" of art and nature.[82] Even when not explicitly noticed, a constant challenge to the natural-artificial distinction ran as an undercurrent in the literature on natural history as well as in that on the country lifestyle of the leisured classes. In his most visionary work, the reformer of natural history, Francis Bacon, enthused about grafting in his description of Solomon's gardens:

> We have also large and various orchards and gardens, wherein we do not so much respect beauty, as variety of ground and soil, proper for divers trees and herbs: and some very spacious, where trees and berries are set whereof we make divers kinds of drinks, besides the vineyards. In these we practice likewise all conclusions of grafting and inoculating, as well of wild-trees as fruit-trees, which produced many effects. And we make (by art) in the same orchards and gardens, trees and flowers to come earlier or later than their seasons; and to come up and bear more speedily than by their natural course they do. We make them also by art greater much than their nature;

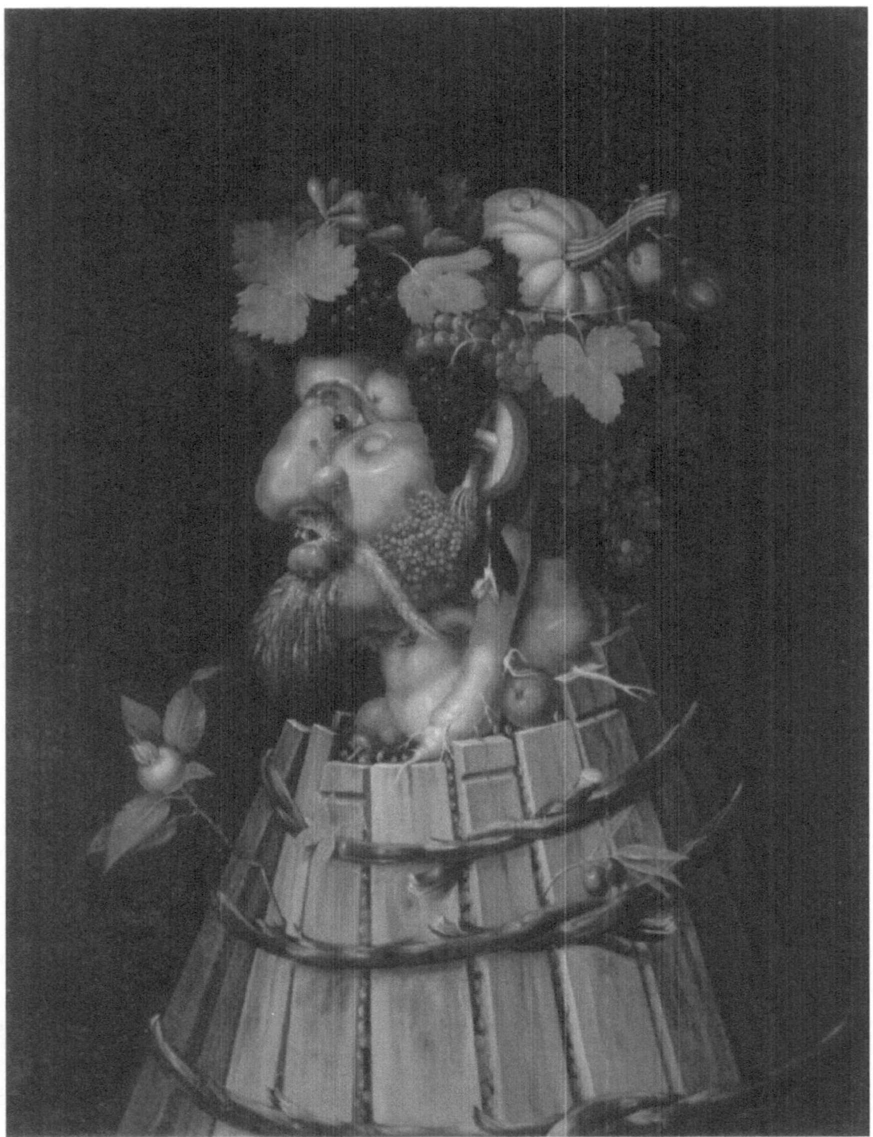

FIGURE 5.3 Arcimboldo, *Autunno* (1573). Paris, Musée du Louvre (public domain).

> and their fruit greater and sweeter and of differing taste, smell, colour, and figure, from their nature. And many of them we so order, as they become of medicinal use. We have also means to make divers plants rise by mixtures of earths without seeds; and likewise to make divers new plants, differing from the vulgar; and to make one tree or plant turn into another.[83]

Even if he does not mention grafting explicitly, Vincenzo Viviani (1662–1703) – the first biographer of Galileo Galilei (1564–1642) – tells how Galileo loved to experiment with plants at his villa of Bellosguardo near Florence, for the sake of both pleasure and knowledge.

> He himself – Viviani wrote – used to prune and bind the vineyards in his villa, and he used to do so with more than ordinary observation, industry, and diligence; and always he liked to farm, which was for him at the same time a pastime and a way of philosophizing about the life and nutrition of plants, about the generative power of seeds, and about all the other admirable operations of the divine maker.[84]

The interest in grafting and in experimenting with plants as two of the godfathers of the seventeenth-century "Scientific Revolution" should be placed in the context of the fascination with the marvels of plant cultivation.

The same fascination, and the same conceptual and ontological uncertainties, can be found in the more technical literature on agronomy. Agostino Gallo (1499–1570), a low-rank nobleman from Brescia who moved to the countryside, published his *Vinti giornate dell'agricoltura e de' piaceri della villa* in 1550, then edited many times with significant additions (the final edition is from 1570). This is arguably the most important work of agronomy of sixteenth-century Italy. The book has clear links with Columella, but a new idea of agriculture emerged from it: more intensive, focused on reduced times of rest for the soil, emphasizing the development of specialized cultivations to answer the demands of the market, and pushing for a move away from foodstuffs for direct consumption and toward foodstuffs for manufacture and transformation. The book has the form of a dialogue. A few noblemen gathered at a villa in Poncarale near Brescia (in Venetian territory), invited by Vincenzo Maggio, who went to visit his friend Giovanni Battista Avogadro to see his lands. The fifth, sixth, and seventh days were devoted to the topic of gardens and orchards.

Gallo mused on why agriculture, "the most noble and necessary art in the world," was not held in higher esteem among princes and noblemen. Among the most beautiful features of agriculture, Gallo listed "seeing abundant crops develop from a seed, big trees develop from a slender trunk, and flavorful fruits from a tender graft":[85] grafting was mentioned from the start as one of the most marvelous accomplishments of the art. The issue of grafting then came up because Vincenzo asked Giovanni Battista whether it was better to plant wild trees or domestic trees, which could be grafted with wild ones at a later stage. Giovanni Battista replied that it was better to graft a wild tree on a domestic one, because "it will produce bigger, tastier, juicier fruits than the other one."[86] Gallo then described the four methods of grafting, with only small changes from the traditional description by Columella, including an illustration of the main procedure and the tools to be employed (Figure 5.4). The technical description was followed by one paragraph titled "in praise of grafting (*elogio dell'incalmare*)." In this passage, the author described all the benefits of the art, with a special emphasis on ontological transformation, the high-class quality

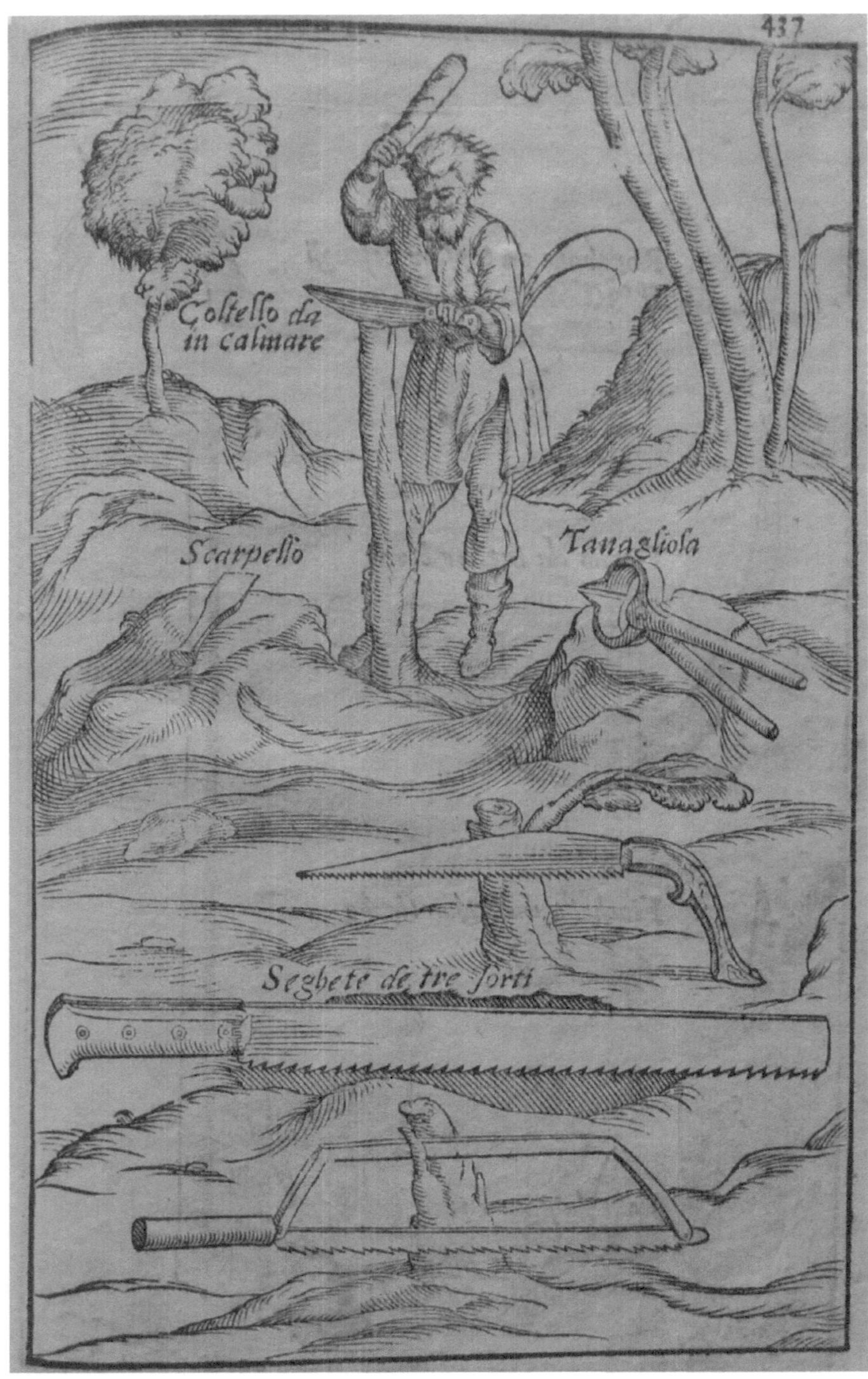

FIGURE 5.4 Agostino Gallo, *Le vinti giornate dell'agricoltura* (1570): tools for grafting.

of the procedures, and the practical purpose of importing new species from the newly discovered faraway lands.

> VIN. Truly, the art of grafting is one of the most beautiful things in agriculture, since one can transform wild trees into domestic ones, the sterile into the fertile ones, the tasteless into the tasty ones, the old into the ripe ones. And not only can one transform one species into the other so that different fruits can be accommodated on one single tree, but we can also bring foreign plants among us, and our plants among the foreigners. GIO. BAT. Who could be so good to explain all the usefulness and the convenient things, and the great joys one can feel while grafting, and in picking up the first fruits with the very same hands that have nourished, cultivated, and grafted them? If I were to tell you how much this glorious art has been celebrated by Princes, Dukes, and the most ancient Lords of this world, I do not know when I would end.[87]

In the same years, Ravenna-born agronomist Marco Bussato (d. around 1600) described himself as a specialist of grafting and claimed that he was able to make a living mastering these techniques for villa gardens.[88] Bussato actually described grafting and the cultivation of fruit trees as one of the two "branches" of agriculture, the other being the cultivation of soil. But while the latter was hard and only provided humans the necessary nutriment for life, "on the opposite, cultivating trees is not hard at all: and then trees which have been well cultivated, and with good judgment, how much beauty, grace, and pleasure do they give to man's sight!"[89] Grafting trees was part of a wider culture of aesthetic pleasure and technical enhancing of natural beings. Bussato's book did not present any specific innovation in the art of grafting, but it was illustrated by 30 good-quality engravings of gardeners at work and gardening instruments (Figure 5.5). Moreover, Bussato told his readers that the engrafter had to make sure the trees and branches have good "humor . . . because if they lose too much humor, they are not good for grafting."[90]

The immensely influential book by Olivier de Serres (1539–1619), the son of a Huguenot pastor in Provence, was even more explicit. De Serres highly praised grafting. He wrote that grafting could be done in several ways and that it could serve to

> refine fruits. . . . It is universally understood that this science is the most excellent in agriculture, as that which ennobles the rest of the art of the management of the fields, and it has been not only appreciated, but almost venerated by the most important men, amazed at the contemplation of its supernatural effects (*arrestés à la contemplation de ses supernaturels effects*).

And he went on:

> it is not by chance that the science of grafting ravishes human intellect. Since what could man do which more closely resembles a miracle than to put one extremity of the branch of a tree, preserved for a long time, transported from

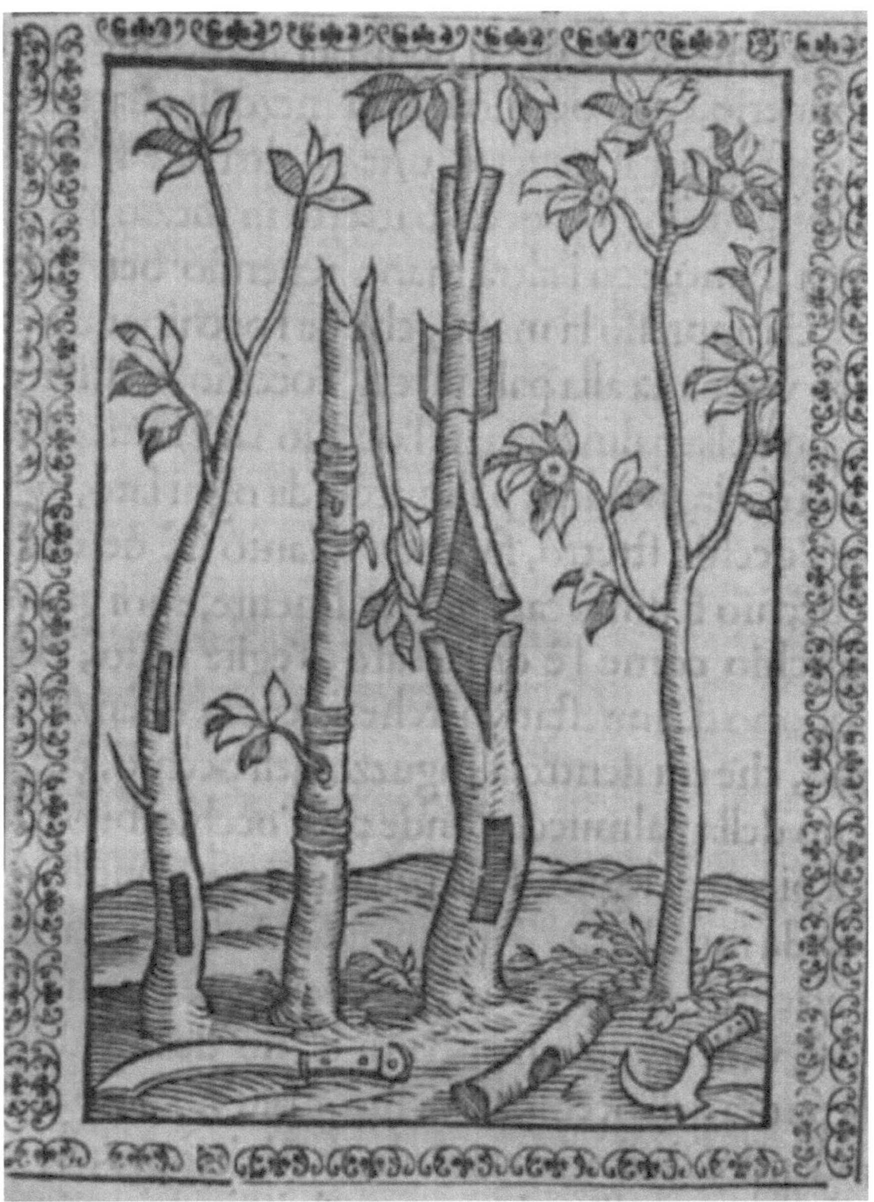

FIGURE 5.5 Marco Bussato, *Il giardino di agricoltura* (1592): grafted plants with tools.

> far away lands, on to the bark of another tree, giving it life and making it grow, and, by communication of substances, even making it to fructify?[91]

Grafting allowed men to change the natural makeup of fruits, speeding up the blooming of some, delaying that of others – in other words, grafting let the artificial take over the natural.

Tommaso Garzoni's opinion on the "professors of secrets" can serve as an introduction to the genre of which Giovanni Battista della Porta represented the learned side and Leonardo Fioravanti the more "popular" one. Garzoni wrote that the "finder of secrets" had to follow three rules: "he must make experiments concerning different things, but things that in the end serve one single goal"; he must know the six things that can be useful to people: generation, "preparation – like grafting (*la preparazione, come nell'inserto*)" – putrefaction, separation, purgation, manual operations "by means of which things are adapted, cleaned up, and joined (*con le quali s'adattano, si poliscono e si congiongono le cose*)." Finally, they had to know how to provide medicine of the body or the soul, ornament, or gain, or cunning, and so forth.[92]

Leonardo Fioravanti – certainly not a socially and professionally appealing precedent for Tagliacozzi – repeatedly insisted on the parallel between surgery and agriculture. This parallel was not entirely reducible to the traditional pairing of medicine and agriculture as perfective arts. Fioravanti did not mention agriculture in his description of the procedure of the Vianeo brothers, but in his 1570 *Cirugia*, where the reference took on a rather marked naturalistic, antiestablishment, and antitechnology meaning. Fioravanti praised agriculture as "the first of the arts which have been cultivated by Man, without which the world would not survive."[93] But the analogy was made in connection with the treatment of wounds: "He who wants to be a good surgeon must be learned and expert in agriculture, because in the treatment of wounds one must imitate agriculture, and one must be a servant of nature."[94] For example:

> when a farmer finds in his field some plant which is broken by wind, rain, etc., right away he puts it back in its place, he ties it, it bandages it, and he fortifies it with a wooden stick; once he has done all that, he lets nature act, and if the surgeons of our time could be farmers, then we could really call them the ministers of nature. But many of them could be more appropriately called destroyers of nature . . . and where the poor patient has a wound they cut his body some more, and while they should imitate farmers and simply join the edges together, they open the wound and fill it with stoup, threads, etc . . . that which is contrary to what farmers do and to the order of nature itself.[95]

This implied that treating wounds was easier than it appeared and than learned surgeons made it appear.

The same analogy between agriculture and surgery, this time based on chronological precedence, was repeated Fioravanti's *Secreti*: "Surgery is a manual art through which surgeons dress wounds and treat ulcers and aposteme. And it was discovered by shepherds and experimenters of natural things." Fioravanti then proceeded to write down a list of crafts that surgeons must know, with agriculture in the first place, most necessary "in order to understand the natural things that are necessary in surgery."[96] One very interesting passage is to be found in Book five, devoted to agricultural secrets. Among these many "farming secrets," Fioravanti discussed grafting trees and claimed to have observed and performed a new technique, less invasive and demanding for the tree, based on grafting bark (*corteccia*), not wood (*legno*).

> Therefore, while doing the anatomy of agriculture in order to understand the natural things that concern philosophy, I have found new methods to graft plants more easily and without so greatly tormenting them, unlike what all farmers do today. . . . The secret of grafting and making one plant produce different fruits lies only within its surface bark, and not in its wood. It is enough to graft the plant in its surface bark . . . and with this kind of secret one can make a tree producing different sorts of fruits, in so wonderful a way that it will appear miraculous and somehow impossible.[97]

From the point of view of a history of reading, this passage is very interesting. It must be noticed how Fioravanti tried to minimize the trees' pain and torment, as if trees were surgical patients. Most importantly, we may recall Tagliacozzi's insistence on grafting only skin and not flesh, which seems to be a precise parallel to the professor of secrets' insistence on *corteccia* over *legno*. As far as I know, at that time information on the surgical procedure as performed by the Vianeo brothers in Tropea had circulated all over Europe, but no specific reference to grafting was current. We know from Ozcho, the Polish student of Aranzi, that the Bolognese anatomist was teaching reconstructive surgery in Bologna in the 1560s, but the Polish physician made no specific reference to grafting. Ambroise Paré made such a reference, but only to oppose the analogy between plants and humans. Paré argued that there was a difference between surgery and agriculture because grafting portions of the body would need additional nourishment:

> The nose, or parts of it, can be completely cut off, and in this case the parts can never be joined together again . . . the reason is that for joining and consolidating the parts of such a nose, it needs to be nourished, and to receive life and sensation from the major members, contrary to what happens to the grafts that are attached to the trees. Therefore, those who lose their noses need to have someone make an artificial one for them, be it of silver, or made with paper and glued pieces of cloth, of the same figure and color as the natural nose.[98]

In this remarkable passage, Paré broke down the analogy between plants and humans that was so popular among scholars and argued – albeit in a rather elliptical fashion – that plants were different from humans because the juices running through their bodies did not need to be directly connected to major organs, while in humans they had to communicate with the liver and the heart.[99]

Della Porta mused on grafting both in the *Magia naturalis* and in several other works. For Della Porta, natural magic was based on observation of the operations of nature and an imitation of them, a definition that resonated with that of many who wrote on grafting.

> It appears to us that Magic is nothing else than a kind of contemplation of nature. The reason is that by examining the motions and trasmutations of the heavens, the stars, the elements, as well as of the animals, plants, minerals, their births and deaths, in this way one can discover the hidden secrets which our science uncovers from the face of nature.[100]

Della Porta talked about grafting as one of those "marvelous operations" that appeared to be "contrary to the course of nature" but that could be repeated through precise rules.[101] Della Porta was very fond of describing grafting as the coitus of plants, exploiting to its limits the metaphor of grafting as a technique. Even though he always made reference to learning from creative nature, Della Porta's emphasis was not just on how to perfect nature (better taste, color, growing plants and fruit out of season, making bigger fruits, etc.) but also on how to create new fruits. The art versus nature divide was clearly put into question.[102]

Della Porta also insisted on the fact that natural magic, in the form of grafting, only imitated and perfected nature, but he operated within the framework of a mutual imitation of art and nature in the name of creative forces. "But first we are going to describe the monstrous transmutations of plants, because agriculture has so many of these noble and pleasant experiments . . . [and] plants easily change their nature into another nature." Some plants wanted to be cultivated; others hated it and wanted to remain wild.

> If you will like to let something grow through a seed that which usually grows through a branch, or through the root, or that which grows through grafting . . . you will see that they will bear strange fruits, and you will see that these are fruits grown outside of their own nature.[103]

For Della Porta, nature worked through hidden procedures, and the magician-farmer had to discover them. In this way, he would bring about the hidden and marvelous potentialities of nature, and he would improve by "forcing and trying nature."[104] Improvement gave way to new natural entities, to ontological novelty.

In Della Porta's hands and mind, grafting became a gate toward a consideration of the unbound transformative and challenging possibilities of agriculture. An example is given by the cultivation of melons, one of the most desired and dangerous fruits of the early modern period.

> In the same way it will happen with watermelons, that is if in the summertime, when the seed is fresh, you will put their seed, the melon's seed, into the blood of a healthy man, the red blood of a mature man, as the more the warmer the blood the stronger it becomes; change it frequently, so that it does not rot, because it must be preserved in good state, and let it stay there for a week, then take the seed as you pull it out of the blood, and plant it in a fertile and well-fertilized hole in the ground.[105]

The interaction between humans and plants was made through the human blood that nourished the seed of melons (Figure 5.6).

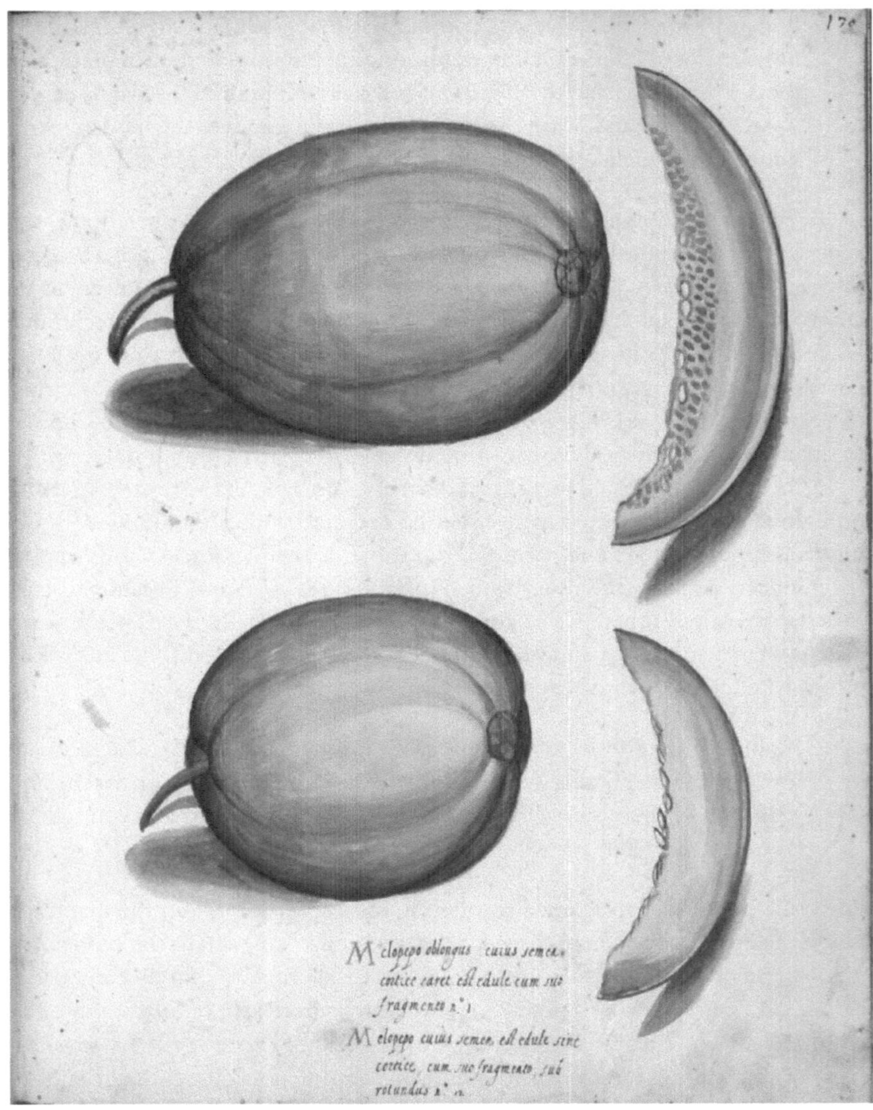

FIGURE 5.6 Ulisse Aldrovandi, *Melon* (late sixteenth century). BUB, Fondo Aldrovandi, Ms. 124, Tavole, vol. III, c. 170.

Source: © Alma Mater Studiorum Università di Bologna – Biblioteca Universitaria di Bologna.

The case of melons needs further exploration. Melon was a special fruit for sixteenth-century aristocratic families, easy to produce in southern European regions and object of complex artificial procedures in the north. The cultivation of melon represented one of the first examples of "forced horticulture" in early modern history, based on fertilization and artificial heating of the soil. For example, De Serres explained that in cold climates people let melons grow in the muck, "with no fear that the decomposition causes bad taste in the fruit."[106] At the same time, melons were considered a very dangerous foodstuff by many physicians, including most notably Girolamo Cardano.[107] A quite precise reference to the fascination for artificiality of melon cultivation and the worry for the dangers of decomposition comes from a Bolognese decree on public health in times of plague, showing how widespread these feelings about the cultivation of melons were. This July 29, 1580, decree specifically dealt with the cultivation of melons in times of "suspicion." The language employed by the officials of the Legate is worth noting:

> We understand that some people, and maybe more than a few farmers of this lands of Bologna, pushed by greed alone and thirst for money, cannot wait for the benefice of the weather and of nature, and for this reason they dare taking down unripe melons from the plants, placing them into wooden or clay jars, or directly into the earth, and then burying them; they do this because they want them to ripe faster with the biggest damage and danger for the universal health of the whole city . . . [the city government, in agreement with the Assunti di Sanità] prohibit and explicitly commands that in the future none of these farmers dare [to do these things] . . . under the punishment of 50 golden scudi, 3 blows, and if they are women 50 strokes of whip in public in the square.[108]

The danger of artificially enhancing or treating nature is echoed in a passage from Tommaso Campanella's famous utopia *La città del Sole*, composed in the early years of the seventeenth century, where it ran across agriculture and cosmetics. After having said that agriculture – and agricultural knowledge – plays a fundamental role in the utopian society, Campanella specified that the city of the Sun's farmers "make little use of manure, claiming that it causes seeds to rot and shortens the life of plants, just as women who owe their beauty to cosmetics rather than to exercise bear sickly children."[109]

There is a more direct link between grafting plants and surgery in sixteenth-century culture. Della Porta's *Natural Magic* also contained a striking passage linking agriculture and surgery, plants and humans, through a reflection on grafting. While discussing how to make the two parts of plants adhere to each other, Della Porta wrote:

> The first usefulness is that just like human flesh (*quemadmodum humanae carnis*), when wounded, can be restored by anointing it with some mixtures, in the same way the bark of the wounded plants heals more quickly when you apply this mixture." The parts had to be attached together and tied tightly, with no air passing in between them, so that their "native juice" did not dry out. The farmer was encouraged to be active and "industrious": he had to "learn to resemble nature.[110]

This is a very important passage, for the grafting technique was clearly believed to work as a bridge between humans and plants and the analogy between plants and humans was not just made in metaphoric, anatomical, or symbolic-cosmological terms but was grounded in a practical, technical, and operative level.

Della Porta's *Phytognomonica* was first published in 1588, and we can be reasonably sure that Tagliacozzi knew the book, which is a map of all the analogies – physiological, superficial, structural – existing between humans, animals, and plants. In that book, the Neapolitan natural magician never made any reference to the operative principles that one could put into practice by observing and imitating the operations of plants. There was no surgery in Della Porta's book on plants. But in the same years, 1580s, Andrea Cesalpino (1519–1603), professor of *materia medica* and botany at Pisa and pupil of Luca Ghini (1490–1556), the founder of the botanical garden in the same studio, was writing about the analogies of the pathways of blood in humans and of sap in plants in his *De plantis* (1583). In this work he identified a network of small vegetal veins that greatly contributed to the specification of the morphological analogy between plants and animals.[111] The second edition of *Magia naturalis* was published in Naples, in Latin, in 1589. It is entirely possible that Della Porta had read the letter Tagliacozzi sent to Gerolamo Mercuriale in 1586 and the latter published in the second edition of his *De decoratione*.[112] In that letter Tagliacozzi first described the procedure in terms of *inistio*, grafting.

In sixteenth-century literature on gardens, farming, agronomy, natural history, and country lifestyle (not to mention alchemy), both in Latin and in the vernacular, a slow erosion of the clear-cut distinction between art and nature was set in motion. This erosion was mediated by the reference to grafting. Either pushing to the limits the Aristotelian distinction or directly challenging it, new ideas on the ontological status of artificial entities emerged. At the same time, a few empirically minded writers made reference to agriculture as a model for surgery in a way that, albeit differently, challenged the image of learned Galenic surgery but offered inviting points of reflection for developing ideas on human grafting. The reference to grafting plants and trees allowed Tagliacozzi to insist on the technical necessity to use only the skin of the arm and not the flesh, thus replying to critics of the procedure who had written before him. Against this background, one can understand Tagliacozzi's difficulties in trying to frame his procedure in terms of the traditional natural-artificial opposition.

Reconstructive surgery and the ontology of nature

This vast and far-reaching culture of grafting sheds some light on the uncertainties and the problems that emerged from Tagliacozzi's *chirurgia curtorum*. Such difficulties concerned, on the one hand, the relationship between art and nature and, on the other hand, a shifting conception of the natural order.

At the beginning of *De curtorum*, Tagliacozzi tried to describe reconstructive surgery as included in the traditional classification of medical specialties.

He insisted on this issue in several passages of the book. The learned surgeon recalled the Hippocratic idea according to which medicine consisted in "addition and subtraction." The art of "restoring mutilations abundantly proves this assertion."[113] On the one hand, it eliminated the abundant or at least that which could be missing without damaging the body; on the other hand, through adding, it reconstructed the parts. This was a rather simplified and schematic version of a procedure that was much more complex than a simple treatment of a wound and that implied a management of time completely unknown in surgery, which was supposed to deal with urgent or present conditions. Tagliacozzi's procedure was actually based on acting on a disfigurement or a mutilation months or even years after the incident had happened, by reopening wounds (on the mutilated parts), and creating new ones (on the flesh of the upper arm). This kind of reconstructive procedure based on skin grafting was, if not completely alien, at least very different from standard descriptions of surgical techniques.

Medieval and early modern surgery textbooks generally described three "intentions" (*intentiones*) defining surgery. Bruno of Longobucco wrote in the thirteenth century that surgery "does three things: it joins separate things; it separates things that have been joined against nature; it eliminates the superfluous."[114] Dalla Croce echoed this passage three centuries later when he explained that the proper surgical "intentions" were cutting or dividing the continuity of a part (incisions of apostemes, dilatation of fistulae, etc.); joining the separated parts and preserving them in their renovated unity (wounds, fractures, etc.); and removing all superfluous parts (a sixth finger, removing flesh in excess as in polyps, etc.).[115] In this threefold partition of surgical operations there is no place for *curtorum chirurgia*. Ambroise Paré went further and broadened the array of surgical intentions, describing five of them: "removing the superfluous; putting in its place that which was lost; separating the continuous; joining the separated; adapting and helping that which is missing, by nature or by accident." Examples of this last category were "procedures such as adding an ear, an eye, a nose, one or more teeth, substituting a platinum tongue . . . a hand, an arm, a leg . . ."[116] Even when the French surgeon seemed to be making epistemological room for reconstructive surgery, he had prosthetics rather than human grafting in mind. Even when the conceptual possibility of correcting disfigurements was contemplated, this possibility did not offer a robust epistemological warranty for skin grafting.

The most important difficulties emerged when Tagliacozzi faced all the philosophical dimensions of the comparison with agriculture and horticulture. Tagliacozzi underlined that, despite the similarities, human grafting and plant grafting were also deeply different endeavors. The farmer's only preoccupation was to make plants take root. But in human surgery, once the parts were joined together, the surgeon had to model them, to shape their figure through "the ingenuity of the artist (*ex artificis industria*)."[117] This was the main goal and the specific task of grafting human body parts: "eventually the grafted parts take on the form and beauty of the parts that they replace. Although the rest of the precepts of our art can be attributed to Nature, and although the ideas borrowed from agriculture are commonplace enough, there is one aspect of our practice that is unique and remarkable. The perfection of the procedure, as performed by a careful, dexterous diligent and benevolent practitioner of the art is such that surpasses by far the learning, generosity, and ingenuity of Nature herself (*naturam ispam doctam, ingeniosam, liberalem, artifex prudens, solers, & benignus non leviter superat*)."[118] Tagliacozzi defended himself; human grafting did not really create new things in the world; it did not alter the ontological makeup of the world.

At the same time, Tagliacozzi had to admit that he was dealing with a practice that went beyond nature. In fact, reconstructive surgeons not only used nature as a resource, but they also needed to master a specific component of "human ingenuity" that complemented the principles of heat, nourishment, and the self-healing power of nature. Surgeons had to be skilled enough to shape distinctly human forms that nature alone would not be able to reshape. Tagliacozzi tried to place restoration surgery within the framework of medicine as the servant of nature, but a certain ambiguity was ineliminable. Was this improving upon nature, creating new parts of the body, or just helping nature out? The surgeon not only perfected nature but also imitated natural shapes, like in sculpture, using the human body as its material.

The same question emerged from the technical prescriptions, discussed in the second volume. Once again, Tagliacozzi tried to frame the procedure in terms of the Aristotelian-Galenic definition of medicine as a perfective art but failed. After having recalled that the surgeon's work, unlike the gardener's, did not end when the grafts took root, Tagliacozzi wrote that the surgical art had to

> make improvements on nature (*natura superari*). . . . It is therefore more fitting that our art, being Nature's most trustworthy handmaid, serve as her midwife and offer welcome help. Once it has been cut away from the upper arm, the formless mass of skin must be reshaped in the image of the missing part, and the nose or lip must be modeled in such a way that it restores glory and honor to the face (*decorum suus, & gravitas*). If one considers the condition of the material [the graft] it will be clear that Nature alone cannot accomplish this, because her laws decree that the material be pure, carefully wrought, and able to fulfill its special functions while being assigned to individual parts neither prodigally nor stingily.[119]

Later, Tagliacozzi contradicted the notion of medicine as servant of nature. The chapter devoted to how surgeons could shape the skin in order to "represent" the nostrils introduced the topic of art challenging nature or the competition between art and nature.

> Now, for the first time there was a way for our art to find access to places previously open only to Nature, to enter the same arena, and to compete with her, on equal footing, for the palm of glory.[120]

This was not an easy game, because after all nature provided the principles for joining the parts together, as well as the model surgeons strove to imitate. Art, on the other hand, tried to represent the nostrils with artificial procedures and to ensure the health and safety of the reshaped parts.

> Although Nature and our art have similar intentions and use equal zeal in accomplishing their special missions, our art takes the place of Nature by providing nourishment and perfectly emulating maternal actions. In fact, it reverses the usual order by reproducing what Nature has already wrought, creating a fruit, so to speak, that is quite similar to its antecedent.[121]

A sort of "new nature" came out of art, commented Tagliacozzi, possibly referring to the debates on grafting and the "third nature." And he made clear that it was a matter of restoring not just function but beauty as well. Just like nature, which gave beauty as an ornament to the function and usefulness of the organs, this art shaped the parts so that they could regain their original utility and beauty.[122]

Art did not achieve the same perfection and majesty of nature, but it got close. Indeed, there was a constant oscillation between the product of the surgeon-artist who made new human shapes surpassing nature in her self-healing power and the ontological subordination of art to nature as the source of all shapes, usefulness, and beauty of human bodies. In several passages Tagliacozzi talked about art forcing and subjugating nature, with a proto-experimental jargon. This art "almost subjugates nature (*quasi naturam sub iugum mittit*)," he wrote; the fact was that as soon as they created the graft, "surgeons have already overstepped the bounds of Nature (*quasi egressus naturae limites*), and the flap will slowly perish" without subtle artificial care.[123] In other passages, on the contrary, Tagliacozzi made clear that nature was superior to art. While discussing the limits of reconstructive surgery, he said that "the limits of our art demonstrate the unparalleled majesty of Nature, which is by far superior to any artifice."[124]

As in all artwork, to perfectly imitate nature was impossible. Surgeons had to realize that, as it happened to other arts, they had to pick up a model, a norm of human and animal beauty and perfection. Even the most skilled painters and sculptors could not perfectly imitate nature, so one could not ask to do so to a surgical method, which was constrained by all sorts of material obstacles. And a restored face was indeed different under many aspects from a natural face, Tagliacozzi admitted, in the "color, softness, sensitivity, size, and hirsuteness, as well as in the magnitude of the nostrils." Skin from the arm was always whiter; the restored nostrils were always softer and more pale. Sensitivity of the restored nostrils was also very different: with time it became more acute than the original. "Animal virtue" was propagated to the whole body through the nerves according to a threefold aim: transmitting "motion (*vix motrix*)," the "capacity for sensation (*virtus sentiendi*)," and the faculty of perceiving pain and injuries. Now, after a first phase of complete lack of sensitivity, this latter one increased, due to the fact that the skin coming from the arm was more sensitive and that the new nose had more vital spirits flowing in it. Moreover, the skin of the new nostrils tended to shrink with time. Hair could grow on the restored nose. Finally, the holes of the nostrils were generally narrower than normal.[125]

Tagliacozzi even attempted to establish a division of labor between human and nature's work. While discussing which was the noblest part of his surgery, whether the union of the parts or the shaping of the new skin in the form of a new nose, he wrote that

> the first is the work of Nature, the second is the product of human ingenuity. . . . I admit that Nature unites the graft with the nose, but the harmony, seemliness, and grace of this union is due to the physician alone. . . . If we entrust such important work to Nature, it cannot but become well known but she often produces unsightly and unstable scars.[126]

Reconstructive surgery dealt with the distinction between the natural and the artificial under three respects. The first was the moral problem of natural appearances: reconstructive surgery should respect the natural traits of the face and it should not deceive the eye with artificial means. The second was grafting: surgeons should not create completely artificial beings; they should not alter the ontological order of nature (however, in practice they became part of the slow process of the erosion of the distinction itself). The third was artistry: surgeons used natural principles but added human ingenuity to shape human forms by imitating nature. It is never clear in Tagliacozzi if art is to be considered superior to nature or vice versa.

This confusion was a sign of the times. For example, Tagliacozzi struggled with the idea of forcing natural limits. When surgeons shaped the nostrils, nature was forced, but it could not be forced for long, so it was crucial to act in a timely fashion with the graft. For a limited time-span, surgeons effectively went outside of nature's boundaries. It was clear that Tagliacozzi's human grafting did not fit the traditional distinction between art and nature, because it involved not only an imitation of nature, not only aiding and supporting nature, but also a human activity of reshaping that went beyond the self-healing power of nature. Galen and Aristotle thought that art could not alter the inner constitution of natural matter, because it lacked the formative power to reshape nature internally and to create something entirely new. *Cosmetics altered* superficial appearances. Medicine helped nature display its self-healing power. Curtorum chirurgia not only helped nature but overcame the borders of the distinction and reshaped the structure of nature to the point of creating new natural forms.

The passivity or activity of the work of the artist was one of the most debated issues of Renaissance art theory. For example, in the fifteenth century Leon Battista Alberti (1404–1472) claimed that art was not just a passive imitation of nature but "an imitation of the rules of nature, choosing that which appears most beautiful in the order of the cosmos."[127] Sixteenth-century theories of mannerism, with their emphasis on the fact that art and nature merged into one another, were even closer to Tagliacozzi's remarks.[128] Art theorists who devoted part of their reflections to the genre of the grotesque such as Anton Francesco Doni (1513–1574), Pirro Ligorio, and Giovanni Paolo Lomazzo (1538–1592) insisted on the "assimilation of the artist to nature" in that they both created new objects in the world.[129] Tagliacozzi seemed to join art theorists in embracing an oscillating and shaky ontology: in his work there was an "excess" of art in that nature alone could agglutinate the parts but not reshape them. In a way, perfective and mimetic arts were combined together. This could also mean that the surgically grafted nose could be considered a natural-artificial hybrid, while at the same time it was fully natural in moral terms because it stood in opposition to a cosmetically modified nose. In other words, Tagliacozzi believed that Aristotle was right and that only nature had an internal principle of motion. However, the Bolognese surgeon claimed that his reconstructive procedure went beyond nature in that it restored not just the essence of the part but its appearance, its aesthetic form. It still was a matter of restoring, and not of producing, but with an excess, a surplus of human artistry that – against the learned surgeon's intention – challenged the art versus nature divide.

Facial reconstructive surgery was both part of medicine as a science of natural bodies and a mechanical art, in that it artificially constrained nature, and in particular the nature of the human body. And that which was really troubling in the comparison with grafting was the uncertain status of its outcome: was there a new face, just like there were new fruits and flowers?

Historical narratives based on the domination of Galenic humoralism on the perception of the human body through the late seventeenth century – as well as the parallel narrative centered on its sudden collapse in favor of mechanism – should be questioned. An empiric and a charlatan like Fioravanti was able to compare the "machine" of the human body to a furnace as early as the middle of the sixteenth century, before Renée Descartes (1596–1650) described the circulation of blood by comparing the heart to an oven in the *Discourse de la methode* (1637).[130] Descartes himself recalled that William Harvey's (1578–1657) description of blood passage through the "little doors" of the veins – built on an analogy between animals and plants drawn by his master in Padua Fabrici d'Acquapendente – was confirmed by "the ordinary experience of surgeons who, by gently tying up the arm above the spot where they cut the vein, let blood more copiously than if they had not tied it."[131]

In Tagliacozzi's surgical practice one can see two concepts of nature at work. On the one hand, nature personified as a creative, generous, virtuous, insuperable artist. On the other hand, nature as a set of law-like impersonal processes that helped the reconstruction procedure, offering the principles that had to be channeled through human ingenuity. It was this second concept of nature that Tagliacozzi thought the surgeon surpassed in perfection, while the original natural creation remained divine and unattainable. This "Scientific Revolution" trademark concept of nature as a set of impersonal laws co-existed side by side with a conception of creative, divine nature, which is usually labeled as "pre-modern." Ultimately, the conceptualization of reconstructive surgery had to do with changing ontologies and changing ways of knowing the order of nature. All these epistemological and ontological changes were grounded in very specific social needs, in manual techniques of performing surgical procedures, and in the fascination of hybrids, playfulness, and marvels of art and nature.

Notes

1 On Tagliacozzi's teaching, see Miguel Angel Soto-Miranda, Andrés Romero-Y-Huesca, Alberto Goné-Fernández, and Jaime Soto-González, "Tagliacozzi: no sólo cirujano plástico," *Gaceta médica de México* 142, 5 (2006): 423–429.

2 Despite the innovations of title pages, the structure of anatomical dissections remained divided into three different roles throughout the whole sixteenth century: see Andrea Carlino, *Books of the Body*, pp. 85–92.

3 *Imago Universitatis*, vol. 1, p. 411: "ob eandem singulari industria et solertia peritissime administratam benignitate et diligentia maxima pulcherrime demonstratam."

4 See Ireneo Affò, *Memorie degli scrittori e letterati parmigiani* (Parma: dalla Stamperia reale, 1789–1797), vol. 5, pp. 19–20; Carlo Trombara, *Memorie e documenti sulla cattedra di anatomia umana normale dell'Università di Parma* (Parma: Tipografia parmense, 1958), pp. 8–10; Grendler, *The Universities*, table 4.6; Roberto Lasagni, ed., *Dizionario Biografico dei Parmigiani* (Parma: PPS, 1999), vol. 4, pp. 505–506.

5 Ranuccio Pico, *Appendice de' vari soggetti Parmigiani* (Parma: appresso Mario Vigna, 1642), pp. 202–205.

6 My reference to "ontology" is anachronistic, as it is not an actors' category. With this term I intend to underline the relevance grafting had in the eyes of sixteenth-century people for the actual constitution of the world, as it was believed to bring about new entities.

7 I borrow the expression from Lorraine Daston and Katharine Park, "Introduction: The Age of the New," in Lorraine Daston and Katharine Park, eds. *The Cambridge History of Science, Volume 3: Early Modern Science* (Cambridge: Cambridge University Press, 2006), pp. 1–17.

8 Steven Shapin, *The Scientific Revolution* (Chicago: The University of Chicago Press, 1998), p. 1.

9 Aristotle, *Physics* II.1.193b, 8–9. Intellectual historian A.J. Close, in a classic paper, has described at least eight meanings of the distinction between art and nature in the Renaissance. Many of them played a role in Tagliacozzi's self-styled epistemological and ontological conception of his procedure. I follow his account. See A.J. Close, "Commonplace Theories of Art and Nature in Classical Antiquity and in the Renaissance," *Journal of the History of Ideas* 30, 4 (1969): 467–486.

10 Aristotle, *Physics* II.8.199a, 15–17.

11 William R. Newman, *Promethean Ambitions: Alchemy and the Quest to Perfect Nature* (Chicago: University of Chicago Press, 2004), p. 16.

12 Close, "Commonplace Theories," p. 469. In Book IV of *Meteorology*, Aristotle claimed that artisans could imitate natural processes in the process of creating artifacts, thus creating natural products that are perfective of nature at the same time; see Newman, *Promethean Ambitions*, pp. 17–19; Craig Martin, *Renaissance Meteorology: Pomponazzi to Descartes* (Baltimore: Johns Hopkins University Press, 2011), pp. 1–20.

13 Galen, *On the Natural Faculties*, tr. Arthur John Brock (London: Heinemann, 1947), p. 129; quoted by Newman, *Promethean Ambitions*, p. 19.

14 To this classical discussion, medieval scholastic theology and natural philosophy added the theme of the impossibility of transmutating species and of the independence of

substantial forms from the human artifex. See Newman, *Promethean Ambitions*, pp. 49–52; Elly R. Truitt, *Medieval Robots: Mechanism, Magic, Nature, and Art* (Philadelphia: University of Pennsylvania Press, 2015), pp. 40–68.

15 Close, "Commonplace Thories," p. 477.

16 Ibid., pp. 478–480.

17 See, for example, Paolo Rossi, *I filosofi e le macchine 1400–1700* (Milan: Feltrinelli, 1962).

18 Newman, *Promethean Ambitions*, pp. 20–24.

19 Ibid., pp. 30–33. A notable case in which surgeons and barber-surgeons were involved, and whose outcome questioned the borders between natural and artificial, was that of castrati, popular in Italy by the late sixteenth century. For an account of castrati's voice as a hybrid of art and nature, see Bonnie Gordon, "It's Not about the Cut: The Castrato's Instrumentalized Song," *New Literary History* 46, 4 (2015): 647–667.

20 See, respectively: Paula Findlen, *Possessing Nature: Museums, Collecting, and Scientific Culture in Early Modern Italy* (Berkeley: University of California Press, 1996); Bernard W. Ogilvie, *The Science of Describing: Natural History in Renaissance Europe* (Chicago: The University of Chicago Press, 2006); Mary Baine Campbell, *Wonder & Science: Imagining Worlds in Early Modern Europe* (Ithaca: Cornell University Press, 2004); Harold J. Cook, *Matters of Exchange: Commerce, Medicine, and Science in the Dutch Golden Age* (New Haven: Yale University Press, 2008); Lorraine Daston and Katharine Park, *Wonders and the Order of Nature, 1150–1750* (New York: Zone Books, 1997); Harold J. Cook, "The History of Medicine and the Scientific Revolution," *Isis* 102, 1 (2011): 102–108; Pamela Smith, *The Body of the Artisan: Art and Experience in the Scientific Revolution* (Chicago: The University of Chicago Press, 2004).

21 Daston and Park, *Wonders*, pp. 215–253.

22 Paula Findlen, "Jokes of Nature and Jokes of Knowledge: The Playfulness of Scientific Discourse in Early Modern Europe," *Renaissance Quarterly* 43, 2 (1990): 292–331, p. 293.

23 Bacon, "Descriptio globi intellectualis," in James Spedding, Robert Leslie Ellis, and Doglas Henon Heath, eds. *The Works of Francis Bacon*, 15 vols. (Boston: Houghton, Mifflin, and Company, 1857), vol 5, pp. 503–560.

24 Paolo Rossi, *Francesco Bacone. Dalla magia alla scienza* (Rome: Laterza, 1957), pp. 54–62.

25 Daston and Park, *Wonders*, pp. 291–292.

26 Newman, *Promethean Ambitions*, p. 261. These historiographical discussions are fascinating. I believe that Newman is right in seeing an echo of Aristotle in Bacon, but that the collapse of the ontological distinction is more radical than what he believes. Craig Martin has described the impact of critiques of Aristotelianism on early modern natural philosophy and the sciences as paradoxically stemming from religious motivations. In his account, early modern natural philosophers were pushed to develop alternative forms of scientific methods by the fact that Aristotelian philosophy could be interpreted as impious. See Craig Martin, *Subverting Aristotle: Religion, History, and Philosophy in Early Modern Science* (Baltimore: Johns Hopkins University Press, 2014), pp. 1–10.

27 Tagliacozzi, *De curtorum*, p. 54 (1:39). Translation is slightly modified.

28 Ibid., p. 59 (1:42).

29 Ibid.

30 Pliny, *Natural History*, 10 vols., tr. H. Rackham (Cambridge: Harvard University Press, 1938–1963), vol. 5, p. 71 (XVII.24). On the sixteenth-century fortunes of Pliny, see Charles G. Nauert, "Humanists, Scientists, and Pliny: Changing Approaches to a Classical Author," *The American Historical Review* 84 (1979): 72–85.

31 Lucretius, *De rerum natura*, tr. W.H.D. Rouse (Cambridge: Harvard University Press, 1943), pp. 484–485 (V.1361–1378). On the importance of Lucretius in the Renaissance, see Alison Brown, *The Return of Lucretius to Renaissance Florence* (Cambridge: Harvard University Press, 2010); Ada Palmer, *Reading Lucretius in the Renaissance*

(Cambridge: Harvard University Press, 2014). On grafting as a bridge between art and nature in Roman culture, see Marco Beretta, *La rivoluzione culturale di Lucrezio. Filosofia e scienza nell'antica Roma* (Rome: Carocci, 2015), pp. 212–213.

32 See Antonio Saltini, *Storia delle scienze agrarie. Venticinque secoli di pensiero agronomico*, 4 vols. (Bologna: Edagricole, 1984), vol. 1, pp. 47–57. Living in the fisrt century CE, contemporary of Seneca and Pliny the Elder, Columella was native of Southern Spain, and he spent most of his life in the surroundings of Rome as an agricultural entrepreneur, owning several farms. His *De re rustica* was printed for the first time in 1472 by Nicolas Jenson in Venice in a collection of agricultural texts, and then again in 1482. The first Venetian critical edition of by Aldus Manutius dates to 1514, and a second to 1533, while the first vernacular translation was printed, once again in Venice, in 1544, translated by the Modenese humanist Pietro Lauro.

33 Columella, *On Agriculture*, 3 vols., tr. Harrison Boyd Ashe (Cambridge: Harvard University Press, 1941–1955), vol. 1, pp. 3–5.

34 Columella had said that up to his times, farmers had given men three methods of grafting. (1) The tree, which has been cut and cleft, receives the scion, which has been cut in turn; (2) the cut tree takes in grafts between the bark and the hard wood; (3) the tree receives actual buds with some bark attached into a part that has been stripped of the bark. The first two had to be practiced in the spring; the last was called "emplastration" or "inoculation" (*emplastratio* or *inoculatio*) and was to be implemented in the summer. Columella mentioned a fourth method that he had "discovered," concerning vines and based on either a "split" technique – putting a scion with its shaped extremity into a split made in the main tree – or a "drill" technique – putting a pointed scion into a hole made on the main tree with a drill; see Ibid., vol. 2, pp. 101–103.

35 Ibid., vol. 2, pp. 103–107.

36 Ibid., pp. 106–109. I have modified the translation: the Loeb translators' version reads "daub the joints of the wound," introducing an analogy between plants and humans which the Latin text lacks.

37 Tagliacozzi, *De curtorum*, p. 61 (1:45).

38 Ibid., p. 63 (1:46).

39 Ibid., pp. 74–75 (1:57–58).

40 Ibid., p. 62 (1:45).

41 Ibid., pp. 111–114 (1: 90–92).

42 Dalla Croce, *Cirugia universale*, fol. 56v-57r: "Quando poi è totalmente amputata, & portata via un particella del naso, & tanto più la cartilaginosa, bisogno è perdere della sua sanità ogni speranza, essenda essangue, & parte spermatica, la quale nè cresce, nè si cònglutina, quando è rimossa. Tutte le parti, diceva Galeno, che sono generate dal sangue, quando mancano, non è impossibile, che rinaschino, ma quelle, che nascono dal seme, è quasi impossibile, la sua regenerazione . . . non sono degni d'esser uditi coloro, chef anno professione di regenerare uno naso totalmente perduto: conciosia, che non si trova artificio di natura, nè meno dono di artifice, che goda di così ampio privilegio, che possi un naso intieramente separato dalla faccia nè unire, nè rigenerare. per questo non vi essorto, trovando un naso ferito, & mezzo morto, riseccarlo in tutto, & gettarlo via, imperoche ne ho veduti di simili ristaurati, agglutinati, & guariti." On this important Venetian surgeon, see Berardo Di Matteo, Vittorio Tarabella, Giuseppe Filardo, Anna Viganò, Patrizia Tomba, and Maurilio Marcacci, "The Renaissance and the Universal Surgeon: Giovanni Andrea Della Croce, a Master of Traumatology," *International Orthopaedics* 37, 12 (2013): 2523–2528. On the spermatic and sanguinary members in Galenic physiology, see Karine van't Land, "Sperm and Blood, Form and Food: Late Medieval Medical Notions of Male and Female in the Embryology of *Membra*," in Manfred Horstmanshoff, Helen King, and Claus Zittel, eds. *Blood, Sweat, and Tears: The Changing Concepts of Physiology from Antiquity into Early Modern Europe* (Leiden: Brill, 2012), pp. 363–392.

43 Cortesi, *Miscellaneorum*, p. 82.

44 Tagliacozzi, *De curtorum*, pp. 66–67 (1:49).
45 Ibid., p. 62 (1:45).
46 Marcel Mazoyer and Laurence Roudart, *A History of World Agriculture: From the Neolithic to the Current Crisis* (London: Earthscan, 2006), pp. 313–353; Mauro Ambrosoli, *The Wild and the Sown: Botany and Agriculture in Western Europe, 1350–1850* (Cambridge: Cambridge University Press, 1997), pp. 1–11; Mauro Ambrosoli, "Cultivation and Diffusion of Species Diversity in Northern Italy: Peasant Gardeners of the Renaissance and After," in Michael Cronan and W. John Kress, eds. *Botanical Progress, Horticultural Innovation and Cultural Change* (Washington, DC: Dumbarton Oaks Research Library and Collection, 2007), pp. 177–198; A.G. Morton, *History of Botanical Science* (London: Academic Press, 1981), pp. 115–164; and the invaluable Antonio Saltini, *Storia delle scienze agrarie*, especially vol. 1, pp. 285–298 and vol. 1, pp. 469–482. On gardens and knowledge, see Richard Palmer, "Medical Botany in Northern Italy in the Renaissance," *Journal of the Royal Society of Medicine* 78 (1985): 149–157; Cristina Bellorini, *The World of Plants in Renaissance Tuscany: Medicine and Botany* (Farnham: Ashgate, 2016), pp. 1–14.
47 Ambrosoli, *The Wild and the Sown*, p. 13.
48 See Ruggiero Romano, *Tra due crisi: l'Italia del Rinascimento* (Turin: Einaudi, 1971), pp. 51–68; Donati, *L'idea di nobiltà*, pp. 56–57; Adriano Prosperi, *Dalla peste nera alla guerra dei trent'anni* (Turin: Einaudi, 2000), pp. 170–174; Gregory Hanlon, "In Praise of Refeudalization: Princes and Feudataries in North-Central Italy from the Sixteenth to the Eighteenth Century," in Nicholas A. Eckstein and Nicholas Terpstra, eds. *Sociability and Its Discontents: Civil Society, Social Capital, and Their Alternatives in Late Medieval and Early Modern Europe* (Turnhout: Brepols, 2009), pp. 213–225.
49 Quoted by Donati, *L'idea di nobiltà*, pp. 160–161.
50 Ambrosoli, *The Wild and the Sown*, p. 103; Bellorini, *The World of Plants*, pp. 40–51 on the Medici Grand Dukes' passion for garden design in the second half of the sixteenth century (including explicit references to grafting trees, p. 43).
51 Ambrosoli, "Cultivation and Diffusion." On the typology or Renaissance gardens, see Raffaella Fabiani Giannetto, "Types of Gardens," in Elizabeth Hyde, ed. *A Cultural History of Gardens in the Renaissance* (London: Bloomsbury, 2013), pp. 43–72. On the different social characters gathering around villas and fields, see Elide Casali, "Catechesi di villa tra *oeconomica* e *res rustica*," in Luisa Avelini, Roberto Finzi, and Leonardo Quaquarelli, eds. *Testi agronomici d'area emiliana e Rinascimento europeo* (Bologna: CLUEB, 2007), pp. 7–34.
52 Luke Morgan, *The Monster in the Garden: The Grotesque and the Gigantic in Renaissance Landscape Design* (Philadelphia: University of Pennsylvania Press, 2016), pp. 1–16. See Alexander Samson, "Locus Amoenus: Gardens and Horticulture in the Renaissance," *Renaissance Studies* 25, 1 (2011): 1–23; Claudia Lazzaro, *The Italian Renaissance Garden: From the Conventions of Planting, Design, and Ornament to the Grand Gardens of Sixteenth-Century Central Italy* (New Haven: Yale University Press, 1990), pp. 8–19, 26–27; on grafting and alchemy, see Newman, *Promethean Ambitions*, pp. 65–66. On the ancient Aristotelian tradition of including plants and animals within the same kingdom of living beings, see Morton, *History of Botanical Science*, pp. 27–43.
53 Andrew Cunningham, "The Culture of Gardens," in Nicholas Jardine, Emma Spary, and Jim A. Secord, eds. *Cultures of Natural History* (Cambridge: Cambridge University Press, 1996), pp. 38–56, especially pp. 47–52.
54 Lazzaro, *The Italian Renaissance Garden*, pp. 2–11; Eugenio Battisti, "*Natura artificiosa* to *Natura artificialis*," in David C. Coffin, ed. *The Italian Garden* (Washington, DC: Dumbarton Oaks, 1972), pp. 63–80; Philippe Morel, *Les Grotesques. Les figures de l'imaginaire dans la peinture Italienne de la fin de la Renaissance* (Paris: Flammarion, 1997), pp. 139–204, has insisted in a very convincing way on the relationships between the visual language of the grotesque and hybrids between animals, plants, and humans and, on the one hand, the juxtaposition of naturalia and artificialia typical of the

late-sixteenth-century culture of collection and, on the other, the innovations of medicine and natural history.

55 John Dixon Hunt, *Garden and Grove: The Italian Renaissance Garden in the English Imagination, 1600–1750* (Philadelphia: University of Pennsylvania Press, 1996), p. xiii.

56 Aristotle, *On plants* (*De plantis*), 818a, 15–20, in *Minor Works*, pp. 160–161. Aristotle considered animals and plants as part of one and same kingdom of living beings: on his and Theophrastus' works on plants, see Morton, *History of Botanical Science*, pp. 27–43.

57 Spanish natural philosopher Oliva Sabuco used the metaphor in the late sixteenth century to claim for the preminence of the brain on the liver and to advance a new theory of how food became blood in the human body. This use of the metaphor of the inverted tree has important iatrochemical ramifications; see Gianna Pomata, "Introduction," in Oliva Sabuco de Nantes Barrera, *The True Medicine*, ed. and tr. Gianna Pomata (Toronto: Center for Reformation and Renaissance Studies, 2010), pp. 42–48.

58 Torquato Tasso, *Il mondo creato*, III, 1278–1285: "Ma quel che maraviglia in vero apporta/è che ritrovi in lor, se ben riguardo,/I diversi accidenti, e i vari essempi/Di gioventude e di vecchiezza umana/Perché le piante ancor novelle e verdi/Han polita la scorza e quasi estesa/Ma s'advien che per molti anni invecchi,/S'empie di rughe, ed increspata inaspra." Quoted by Piero Camporesi, *Le officine dei sensi* (Milan: Garzanti, 2009), p. 26.

59 Camporesi, *Le officine*, pp. 26–27.

60 Ibid., p. 42.

61 Marie-Christine Pouchelle, *Corps et chirurgie à l'apogée du Moyen Age: savoir et imaginaire du corps chez Henri de Mondeville, chirurgien de Philippe le Bel* (Paris: Flammarion, 1983), pp. 277–284.

62 Ulisse Aldrovandi, *Monstrorum Historia* (Bologna: Bernia, 1642); on this topic, see Enrico Baldini, "Prodigi, simulacri e mostri nell'eredità botanica di Ulisse Aldrovandi," in Giuseppe Olmi, Luca Tongiorgi Tomasi, and Attilio Zanca, eds. *Natura-cultura: L'interpretazione del mondo fisico nei testi e nelle immagini* (Florence: Olschki, 2000), pp. 215–243.

63 Giovanni Battista Della Porta, *Phytognomonica* (Naples: apud Horatium Salvianum, 1588), pp. 10–12: "virium plantarum investigandi methodus, ex partibus, & vitae, quae insunt signis fixis, & mobilibus."

64 Ulisse Aldrovandi, *Dendrologiae naturalis scilicet arborum historiae libri duo* (Bologna: ex typographia Ferroniana, 1667), pp. 3–5: "Plantae igitur omnes, maximeque Arbores similaribus non solum, sed compositis constant evidentissime partibus, quas ratio demonstrative suadet, convincitque *autopsia* . . . unde aliquam in Arboribus partem Caput, & Cerebrum appellamus, aliam Pedes, & sic Brachia, Digitos, Ungues, Capillos, Aures, & Oculos saepe saepius adnotamus; quae omnia faciunt totius ad Arboris perfectionem, vegetatiuumque nobilissimum complementum . . . sic Plantae omnes, & Arbores Dermata, & Epidermata, cutaneas scilicet, atque cuticulares partes, veluti fascias totius conservatrices habent vitae, ubi naturales omnes facultates vigent, & propriis mediantibus organis exercentur, variis quae illae praerogativis tum specificis, tum individualibus insigniuntur." Like almost all of the works by Aldrovandi, this one was composed in the late sixteenth century and published posthumously. On Renaissance readings of classical botanical works, see Karen Meier Reeds, "Renaissance Humanism and Botany," *Annals of Science* 33, 6 (1976): 519–542.

65 Aldrovandi, *Dendrologia*, pp. 5–6.

66 Ibid., p. 60.

67 Tomaso Tomai, *Idea del giardino del mondo* (Venezia: appresso Domenico Imberti, 1611), p. 46. This book was first published in 1582 and by the end of the sixteenth century was reprinted 7 times.

68 On the history of grafting, see Ken Mudge, Jules Janick, Steven Scofield, and Eliezer E. Goldschmidt, "History of Grafting," *Horticultural Reviews* 35 (2009): 437–493, p. 439; Gianmaria Venturi, *Trattato degli innesti* (Reggio: G. Davolio, 1816), pp. 426–474. Incidental notes on the relevance of grafting for the history of early modern science can

be found in Daston and Park, *Wonders*, pp. 262–265; Lorraine Daston, "The Nature of Nature in Early Modern Europe," *Configurations* 6, 2 (1998): 149–172; Kjell Lundquist, "Reconstruction of the Planting in Uraniborg, Tycho Brahe's Renaissance Garden on the Island of Ven," *Garden History* 32, 2 (2004): 152–166.

69 Saltini, *Storia delle scienze agrarie*, vol. 1, pp. 285–298; Douglas Fairchild Ruggles, *Gardens, Landscapes, & Vision in the Palaces of Islamic Spain* (University Park: The Pennsylvania State University Press, 2006), pp. 15–32; George Sarton, *Introduction to the History of Science*, 3 vols. (Washington: The Carnegie Institute, 1927–1948), vol. 2.1, p. 425. I have already shown that by the time of Lucretius and Pliny the Elder grafting was already a topic for naturalists. Greek sources indicate that grafting was practiced by the fifth century BCE. The Hippocratic text *On the Nature of Child* is the first Greek reference to grafting, where it was described as a common technique. There emerged the notion of a "specific fluid" responsible for the success of grafting, which remained in currency throughout the early modern period. Theophrastus in the fourth century BCE reiterated the Hippocratic view about grafting as a propagation in another tree. Then came the Roman writers of husbandry: the first one was Cato's, *De agri cultura, which* described grafting in the second century BCE. Jewish tradition presents important traces of the technique as well. In several Talmudic parables, grafting is compared to marriage. In the third century CE the Talmudic school of Shmuel compared grafting to breeding, and in general grafting became a matter of debate in Jewish religious culture down to the sixteenth century, when grafting medicinal citrus on lemon was prohibited. The first reliable evidence of practices of grafting in China dates to the first century BCE. The great synthesis of Arabic agronomy, written in twelfth-century Seville, the *Book on the art of the farmer (Kitāb al-filāḥa)* by Ibn al-'Awwam (d. late twelfth century), also described classical grafting techniques and represented the peak of an intense flourishing of the botanical sciences in medieval al-Andalus. Grafting was practiced throughout the Middle Ages, and a thirteenth-century text by Albertus Magnus, titled *De vegetabilibus*, described it as an important agricultural technique. See Mudge et al., "History of Grafting."

70 Indeed, alchemy and medicine had a long history of shared techniques of manipulating natural matters and conceptions of the human world; see the essays in Chiara Crisciani and Agostino Paravicini Bagliani, eds., *Alchimia e medicina nel Medioevo* (Florence: SISMEL/Edizioni del Galluzzo, 2003). On the history of plant symbolism before the early modern period, see Agostino Paravicini Bagliani, ed., *Le monde vegetal: Médecine, botanique, symbolique* (Florence: Sismel/Edizioni del Galluzzo, 2009).

71 Quoted by Newman, *Promethean Ambitions*, p. 64.

72 Ibid., pp. 112–113.

73 Vannoccio Biringuccio, *De la pirotechnia* [1540] (Milan: Polifilo, 1977), fol. 8r.

74 Ibid., fol. 123r-v.

75 Bartolomeo Taegio, *La villa* (Milan: dalla stampa di Francesco Moscheni, 1559), p. 157: "Et io vi dico che se bramate vedere nelle zucche marine, o cedri (se n'havete) novi, & strani volti, debbiate far fabbricare un vaso di cristallo di quella forma, che più vi piace, e poi chiuderle dentro quando sono nella loro più acerba età, onde vedrete a poco a poco la zucca crescendo farsi simile al vaso, & reuscir l'effetto ch'io vi dico."

76 Ibid., pp. 157–158: "sopra di questo pero e di quel vermiglio moro si possono innestar gli aranzi, l'agrezza de quali volendola voi addolcire fa di mestieri, che foriate mezzo il tronco da basso, dando in questa maniera luogo al tristo humore fin tanto, che i pomi si veggano ben formati, poi bisogna con loto fermar la piaga loro; onde ne vedrete effetto meraviglioso."

77 Ibid., p. 55: "chiaramente si vede come la natura cede alla industria, & per longo uso muta costume."

78 Ibid., p. 58: "quivi sono senza fine gl'ingeniosi innesti, che con si gran meraviglia al mondo mostrano, quanto sia l'industria d'un accorto giardiniero *che incorporando l'arte con la natura fa, che d'amendue ne riesce una terza natura*, la qual causa, che i frutti sieno quivi più saporiti, che altrove."

79 On "third nature" in early modern European horticulture and botany, see Thomas Beck, "Gardens as a 'Third Nature': The Ancient Roots of a Renaissance Idea," *Studies in the History of Gardens & Designed Landscapes* 22, 4 (2002): 327–334.

80 Pietro Andre Mattioli, *Commentarii inex libros Pedacii Dioscorides Anarzabei de materia medica* (Venice: apud Vincentium Valgrisium, 1554), vol. 1, p. 8.

81 Rembert Dodoens, *Histories of Plants* (Antwerp, 1578), pp. 154 and 213; quoted by Daston and Park, *Wonders*, p. 262.

82 Aldrovandi, *Dendrologia*, p. 344.

83 Francis Bacon, "The New Atlantis," in *The Works*, vol. 5, p. 401. The Royal Society of London notoriously took up some of Bacon's ideas on learning from craftsmen and improving their techniques, including gardening and grafting: see Michael Hunter, *Science and Society in Restoration England* (Cambridge: Cambridge University Press, 1981), pp. 92–94; Kathleen H. Ochs, "The Royal Society of London's History of Trades Programme: An Early Episode in Applied Science," *Notes and Records of the Royal Society of London* 39, 2 (1985): 129–158.

84 Vincenzo Viviani, *Vita di Galileo* [1667] (Rome: Salerno, 2001), pp. 72–73: "Egli stesso di propria mano le [viti] potava e legava nelli orti delle sue ville, con osservazione, diligenza et industria più che ordinaria; et in ogni tempo si dilettò grandemente dell'agricoltura, che gli serviva insieme di passatempo e di occasione di filosofare intorno al nutrirsi e al vegetar delle piante, sopra la virtù prolifica de' semi, e sopra l'altre ammirabili operazioni del divino artefice."

85 Agostino Gallo, *Le vinti giornate dell'agricoltura* (Venice: Appresso Camillo Borgominerio, 1578), p. 2: "il veder da una semenza uscir tanto numero di grani; da una sottil verga, grossissimi alberi; & da un tenero innesto, saporiti frutti."

86 Ibid., p. 102: "produrrà frutti più grossi, più saporiti, e di maggior licore, che non farà quell'altro."

87 Ibid., p. 106: "VIN. Veramente che l'arte dell'incalmar'è una delle più belle cose, che siano nell'Agricoltura, poiche tramutano gli arbori selvatichi ne i domestichi, gli sterili ne i fruttiferi, gli insipidi ne i delicati, i tardi ne i temporiti, & e i temporiti ne i tardi. Oltra che non tanto si tremuta una specie nell'altra, e s'acomodano piu frutti diversi sopra d'un arbore, ma anco si tarsportan le sorti forastiere a noi, e le nostre ne i paesi alieni. GIO. BAT. Chi potrebbe mai esplicare le utilità, le commodità, & i gran contenti che si prendono nell'incalmare, & nel racogliere i primi frutti con le medime mani, che gli hann'incalmati, nutriti, & allevati? Che se dovessi dire quanto fu sempre celebrata questa cosi gloriosa arte da' Principi, da' Duchi, & da' primi Signori del mondo, non so quand'io potessi finire."

88 Marco Bussato, *Giardino di agricoltura . . . nel quale con bellissimo ordine si tratta tutto quello, che s'appartiene a sapere a un perfetto Giardiniero* (Venice: appresso Giovanni Fiorina, 1592). Very little is known of Bussato. He published a fortunate *Giardino di agricoltura*, a relatively brief manual almost entirely devoted to grafting techniques. The book went through three further editions (1593, 1599, 1612) and had been published in Ravenna with less material in 1578 with the title *Prattica historiata dell'inestare gli arbori*. See Giuseppe Olmi, "L'agronomia illustrata. Osservazioni sull'iconografia dei trattati agronomici della prima età mdoerna," in *Testi agronomici*, pp. 89–126, especially pp. 101–103.

89 Bussato, *Giardino*, "Ai lettori," pages not numbered: "all'incontro poca fatica basta a coltivar gli arbori: i quali poi bene e giudiciosamente coltivati quanta vaghezza, quanta gratia, quanto piacere arrecano alla vista dell'uomo?"

90 Ibid., fol. 16r-v: "humore . . . perché perdendo l'humore, elle non sarian bone da innestare."

91 Olivier de Serres, *Le Théatre d'Agriculture et de mesnages des champs* [1600] (Arles: Thesaurus Actes-Sud, 2001), p. 981.

92 Garzoni, *La piazza*, vol. 1, p. 325: "che isperimenti molte cose fra lor diverse a un tratto, ma tutte tendenti ad un fine . . ."

93 Fioravanti, *La cirugia*, fol. 1v: "che fu la prima arte che al mondo si facesse, senza della quale il mondo malamente si potrebbe sostentare."

94 Ibid., fol. 8v: "chi vuol esser buon cirugico, & intender bene la cirugia, bisogna essere esparto agricoltore, percioche nella cura delle ferrite, bisogna imitare la agricoltura, & esser ministro della natura." More on Fioravanti's naturalistic approach in chapter 4.

95 Ibid., fol. 8v-9r: "quando lo agricoltore truova nel suo campo alcuna sorte di piante, che sia rotta o scavezzata, dal vento o dalla pioggia, subito la rimette al suo luoco, la liga, la infascia, e la fortifica con un legno, & fatto tutto questo, lascia poi operare alla natura. ma se i cirugici del nostro tempo, fossero agricoltori, si potriano dire ministri della natura. ma molti si potrieno chiamare distruggitori della natura . . . & dove il poveretto ha una ferrite, gli ne danno un'altra, & dove a imitatione dell'agricoltore doverieno unire le parti separate, & strenger la ferita, loro la aprono, & dentro vi mettono stoppa, fila, & taste . . . il che è tutto in contrario dello agricoltore, & contra l'ordine di natura."

96 Fioravanti, *Del compendio dei secreti*, fol. 38r: "La cirugia è un'arte manuale, con la quale i cirugici curono ferrite, ulcere, & aposteme. Et questa fu trovata da Pastori, & esperimentatori delle cose naturali . . . per havere cognition delle cose naturali, che nella Cirugia si convengono."

97 Ibid., fol. 148r-v: "Ma imperò facendo la Notomia dell'Agricoltura per venire in cognition delle cose naturali della filosofia, ho trovato altri nuovi modi da insitire le piante con maggior facilità, & senza dare un così gran tormento come oggidì fanno tutti gli Agricoltori . . . Il secreto adunque dell'insitire & far produrre altre sorte di frutti ad una pianta è solamente nella scorza e non nel legno . . . & con questo secreto si potrà far produrre ad un arbore diverse sorte di frutti, che parerà cosa miracolosa, & che habbia dell'impossibile."

98 Paré, *Oeuvres*, vol. 2, p. 605.

99 Ibid., pp. 605–606.

100 Della Porta, *Magia naturalis*, p. 2: "Nobis vero non nisi universae Naturae contemplationem esse videtur. Ex coelorum enim motus consideratione, stellarum, elementorum eorumque transmutationibus, sic animalium, plantarum, mineralium, eorumque ortus, & interitus occulta vestigantur arcana, ut tota scientia ex Naturae vultu dependere videatur, ut latius videbimus." In the Renaissance tradition of natural magic, the magician was often compared not only to the physician, but to the farmer too: see Paola Zambelli, *White Magic, Black Magic in the European Renaissance: Ficino, Pico, Della Porta to Trithemius, Agrippa, and Bruno* (Leiden: Brill, 2007), pp. 24–26. For a synthetic but excellent overview on Della Porta's epistemology and practical endeavors, see Eamon, *Science and the Secrets*, pp. 194–233, and the relative bibliography; Gabriella Belloni, "Conoscenza magica e ricerca scientifica in Giambattista Della Porta," in Giambattista Della Porta, ed. *Criptologia* (Rome: Centro Internazionale di Studi Umanistici, 1982), pp. 45–101; and the old but extraordinarily relevant and up-to-date Luisa Muraro, *Giambattista Della Porta mago e scienziato* (Milan: Feltrinelli, 1978), especially pp. 21–58.

101 Della Porta, *Magia naturalis*, p. 84.

102 Della Porta also authored a 12-volume book on agriculture: see Francesco Tateo, "Arte e scienza della 'villa' in Giambattista Della Porta," in Milena Montanile, ed. *L'edizione nazionale del teatro e l'opera di G. B. Della Porta: atti del Convegno, Salerno, 23 maggio 2002* (Pisa: Istituti editoriali e poligrafici internazionali, 2004), pp. 9–17.

103 Della Porta, *De i miracoli et miracolisi effetti dalla natura prodotti* (Venice: appresso Ludovico Avanzi, 1560), fol. 31r-v: "Ma prima insegnamo le mostruose trasmutationi delle piante, percioché l'agricoltura ha di molti nobili esperiementi, & dilettevoli . . . con facilità le piante si mutano in una natura aliena . . . Ma se tu vorrai far nascere per via di seme, quello che nasce per via di ramo, o di radice, o quello che per innesto . . . darà frutti stravaganti, & vedrai che sono venuti frutti fuori della natura sua." This book is the vernacular version of the first edition of Della Porta's, *Magiae naturalis.*

104 Ibid., fol. 32v.

105 Ibid., fol. 34v-35r: "Et similmente l'istesso de' cocomeri avverrà, se il seme suo, overo de' meloni, lo metterai la state, quando il seme è fresco, dentro del sangue dell'huomo sano, che sia huomo maturo, & sia di color rosso, percioché è più caldo il suo sangue, e più gagliardo: muttalo spesso, che non si marcisca, che bisogna che si conservi buono

senza marcire, lassavelo stare per una settimana, poi piglia il seme così come lo cavi del sangue, e farai le buche in terra che sia fertile, & bene spolverizzata."

106 Saltini, *Storia delle scienze agrarie*, vol. 1, p. 454.

107 Siraisi, *The Clock and the Mirror*, p. 74. On the complexity of the social perception of melons in the Renaissance, see Allen J. Grieco, "The Social Politics of Pre-Linnaean Botanical Classification," *I Tatti Studies* 4 (1991): 131–149, especially pp. 141–146.

108 ASB, Sanità, *Bandi Bolognesi sopra la peste*, n. 1: "Intendendosi, che alcuni, e forse non pochi Hortolani di questa Guardia, & Territorio di Bologna spinti da mera avaritia, & avidità del guadagno non potendo aspettare il beneficio del tempo, & della natura, ardiscono dispicare dalle lor Piante li Meloni acerbi, sotterrandoli, & ponendoli in vasi di legno, o di terra, o nell'istesso terreno, o Locco, per più tosto violentemente maturarli in gravissimo danno, & periculo della Sanità universale di tutta la Città . . . [il Senato in accordo con gli Assonti di sanità] prohibisce, & espressamente ordina, & comanda, che per l'avenire non sia alcuno di detti Hortolani, o qual si voglia lara persona di si sia conditione, ardsichi [fare queste cose] . . . sotto pena di cinuqanta Scudi d'oro, & de tre tratti di corda, & se saranno Donne, di cinquanta Staffilate da darsi pubblicamente in Piazza."

109 Tommaso Campanella, *The City of the Sun: A Poetical Dialogue*, tr. and ed. Daniel J. Donno (Berkeley: University of California Press, 1981), pp. 83–85.

110 Della Porta, *Magia naturalis*, pp. 47–48.

111 Andrea Cesalpino, *De plantis libri XVI* (Florence: apud Georgium Marescottum, 1583), pp. 1–30, with particular reference to grafting on pp. 6–8.

112 Girolamo Mercuriale, *De decoratione* (1587 edition), pp. 115–120. An English translation of the letter can be read in Teach-Gnudi and Webster, *The Life and Times*, pp. 136–139.

113 Tagliacozzi, *De curtorum*, p. 1 (1:1).

114 Bruno da Longobucco, "Chirurgia magna," in *Ars Chirurgica* (Venice: apud Iuntas, 1546), fol. 103r. On Galenic surgery, see Luis H. Toledo-Pereyra, "Galen's Contribution to Surgery," *Journal of the History of Medicine and Allied Sciences* 28, 4 (1973): 357–375.

115 Dalla Croce, *Cirugia universale*, fol. 5r.

116 Paré, *Oeuvres*, vol. 1, p. 27.

117 Tagliacozzi, *De curtorum*, p. 62 (1:46).

118 Ibid. Translation modified.

119 Ibid., p. 119 (2:3).

120 Ibid., p. 195 (2:73): "Qua de causa factum est ut inconcussis in hoc usque aevi naturae foribus, ad cuius penetralia accedere impossibile fuerat, haec una aditus primum perrumpere, eadem in arenam provocare, & de gloria decertare cum illa non erubuerit."

121 Ibid.

122 Ibid., pp. 195–196 (2:74).

123 Ibid., p. 160 (2:41).

124 Ibid., p. 109 (1:88).

125 Ibid., pp. 110–111 (1:89).

126 Ibid., p. 169 (2:49–50).

127 See Castelli, *L'estetica*, p. 89 (Leon Battista Alberti, *De pictura* II, 42).

128 See Morel, *Les grotesuqes*, p. 312.

129 Ibid., pp. 85–110, quotation on p. 89.

130 Fioravanti, *Cirugia*, pp. 22r and 156r.

131 Renée Descartes, "Discours de la méthode," in Charles Adam and Paul Tannery, eds. *Oeuvres de Descartes* (Paris: Cerf, 1897–1913), vol. 5, p. 51.

6

SURGERY AND THE MORAL ECONOMY OF PAIN

Surgeons had to cut and prepare a skin flap on the upper region of the arm, make it adhere to the defective nose by keeping the two parts bound together for about three weeks, sever the flap from the arm, shape the new parts of the nose, and finally make sure that the outcome lasted by using special molds. Tagliacozzi commented:

> We all know that extreme pain not only causes prostration but also interrupts the normal functions of the body. I have yet to see this happen during my operation. But if by some chance a patient were to faint, I would attribute it not to the violence of the procedure but rather to the patient's abject soul. This type of effeminate and weak man (*molles, & effoeminatos*) is terrified at the prospect of suffering pain, and the only virile thing about him is the appearance. The cowardly man should not participate in this procedure.[1]

Tagliacozzi both denied that his procedure was extremely painful and argued that only morally defective men – men who were not masculine enough – were not able to endure it. This is just one example of the gendering and moralization of pain and pain endurance that are characteristic of Tagliacozzi's book and reflect his attitude to his patients. This chapter investigates whether this attitude toward patients in pain was something common in sixteenth-century surgical literature or whether it was specific of reconstructive surgery.

Pain in history

I will consider pain not primarily as the object of medico-theoretical definitions but rather as something inherent to surgical operations and, as such, as a tool for mediation in the surgeon-patient relationship, as it can be read between the lines of texts written by surgeons.[2] To employ an anachronistic concept, my focus is on cultures of "pain management" rather than on theoretical thinking on pain. I consider pain as part of a social negotiation involving both the senses and social status.

Historiography on pain forms a relatively new and expanding body of literature.[3] It has been argued that in Renaissance Europe medicine and surgery were neither the exclusive nor the most important places where reflection on painfulness was produced.[4] This remark contains some truth. Nevertheless, the history of surgical management of pain can tell us something about the history of pain in general. It must also be noticed that Renaissance medicine and surgery were much broader and culturally richer endeavors than their modern "scientific," laboratory-based, and neuro-biologically driven counterparts. Renaissance medicine and surgery were concerned with many "non-medical" affairs. One must not make the mistake of projecting back the coherence of a present-day discipline to past practices.

The history of pain – and in general the history of the body – in pre-modern contexts does not belong to the history of medicine by its own right.[5] Nonetheless, surgical pain can be treated as a historical object independent and different from medicine in its present state, as part of a history of experience. In the early modern pre-anesthesia period, techniques for easing pain were generally not meant to suppress pain as such, as in modern times. Rather, such techniques and medicaments aimed at suppressing pain as a symptom and as something that would endanger patients.[6] Twentieth-century French surgeon René Leriche wrote about a "living pain" experienced outside of the laboratory and impossible to be reduced to a universal code of neural impulses.[7] This living pain is the only kind of pain sixteenth-century women and men were experiencing, in and outside surgery.

The present chapter follows the methodological approach adopted by recent scholarship on the history of pain, particularly by Esther Cohen, Joanna Bourke, and Javier Moscoso.[8] These historians all suggested that pain must be treated as a historically determined social event or a complex experience that takes place among people in specific political, linguistic, gendered, and epistemic contexts. Joanna Bourke espouses Ludwig Wittgenstein's approach to pain as a language game and argues that such an approach can be extremely fruitful for historians. According to her view, the essence of pain is not the point, because pain is always grasped when it performs social functions. In other words, pain always refers to ways of feeling and not to the incommunicable, subjective content of feeling. Speaking and expressing pain are ways of describing a social and cultural experience.[9] In a similar way, Javier Moscoso treated the history of pain as part of a "historical epistemology of experience" that makes use of the methods of, but is not the same thing as, history of science, on the one hand, and history of emotions, on the other. According to him, the history of pain is rather a history of the ways in which pain has been made intelligible and representable.[10]

The official 1979 definition by the International Association for the Study of Pain – "an unpleasant sensory and emotional experience associated with actual or potential tissue damage, or described in terms of such damage" – allows for considerable conceptual flexibility and avoids a rigid distinction between "physical" or "bodily" pain and "mental" or "psychological" pain.[11] I will try to avoid this distinction too. I will ask how, why, and in what contexts the distinction itself could be articulated, built, and enforced.

Tagliacozzi made surgical pain (an intense "bodily" pain) a matter of social honor and masculine identity (the matter of what moderns would call "psychological" pain) in unprecedented ways, playing with early modern conceptions of surgical pain that included both fear of expected pain and reaction to inflicted pain. I will highlight Tagliacozzi's strategies in replying to accusations of performing a much too painful procedure. Then I will take a look at some ways of treating pain caused by surgical treatment in the second half of the sixteenth century, trying to focus on the following question – why was Tagliacozzi's attitude toward patients in pain so different?

Tagliacozzi's view

Surgical technology that would eventually be re-purposed by Tagliacozzi was already in place by the sixteenth century, like metallic cannulas to be inserted in the nostrils and rounded forceps to operate on the interior parts of the nose with swiftness and finesse. But in general, among the most learned and famous surgeons of the sixteenth century, skepticism about reconstructive surgery was the norm.

As we have seen, Ambroise Paré was skeptical about the case of the "cadet de Saint-Thoan." In a very interesting passage, Paré seemed to imply that it was ethically disturbing and epistemologically ambiguous to wound the patient in his healthy parts, inflicting patients a great pain, given that the outcome would be ugly to see anyway. It was one thing to cut near the wound to treat it directly, or to cut in order to extract a bladder stone, and quite another to wound a healthy arm once the wound to repair was already distant in the past and for the sake of a dubious outcome. The second example is Gabriele Falloppio's sentence in *De decoratione*: "I would rather have my nose cut off than to suffer through such torments."[12]

Tagliacozzi needed to defend and justify his procedure. First of all, he distanced himself from the Southern Italian empirical practitioners who performed the operation "casually and not rationally."[13] He then went on to claim that, contrary to what some illustrious physicians were writing, only a portion of the superficial skin of the arm should be used for the graft, thus avoiding the much more painful asportation of flesh and muscles.[14] And he added a step-by-step review of his procedure, showing that the pain was inevitable but bearable. Most interestingly, he embarked on a revision of past and present surgical literature up to his times, with the purpose of showing that facial surgery was much less painful and demanding than many other operations advocated for by glorified authors such as Celsus, Paul of Aegina (c. 625–690), Albucasis (Ibn al-Abbas Al-Zahrawi,

936–1013), and even Galen.[15] Tagliacozzi described all sorts of eye, hernia, and stone treatments, notoriously the most painful ones, and paused to criticize such medically insignificant and purely aesthetic operations as the reconstruction of the prepuce and the reduction of exaggeratedly big male breasts.

> Good Lord! What kind of practices are these? The ancient physicians had no fear of subjecting their patients to the most savage torment and obvious peril. And why? For a minuscule gain in dignity in a part that no one should even see [the prepuce], and whose absence is not even remotely life threatening![16]

Compared to these cases, Tagliacozzi argued, the pain patients suffer during his surgery was minimal.

This contemptuous reference to a purely aesthetic procedure is particularly interesting. Tagliacozzi was referring to the Byzantine surgeon Paul of Aegina, who discussed "male breasts resembling the female." In most cases, Paul argued, puberty brought about a certain swelling up of the female as well as the male breasts, but as time passed by the situation normalized. There were cases, however, in which

> having acquired a beginning they go increasing, owing to the formation of fat below. Wherefore, as this deformity has the reproach of effeminacy, it is proper to operate upon it. Having, therefore, made a lunated incision below the breast, and dissected away the skin, we unite the parts by sutures.[17]

This procedure was also described by Albucasis, Haly Abbas (Alī ibn ʿAbbās al-Majūsī, d. 982–994), and Rhazes, thus indicating an Arabo-Byzantine agreement on the necessity to treat such a condition.[18] But for Tagliacozzi this was only a cruel, worthless procedure. This implies a shift in the history of cultural sensibility to pain: for Tagliacozzi, the balance between the painfulness of the procedure and the desired outcome did not make the procedure itself worth the attempt.

From Tagliacozzi's passage, another shared feature of late Renaissance learned surgery emerges: a sense of the historicity of techniques and of the progresses of human sympathy – coupled with a certain anti-Arabic attitude typical of some humanist physicians.[19] This is confirmed by one of the most important Italian physicians and anatomists of the time, Girolamo Fabrici D'Acquapendente. In his *Observationes chirurgicae* (1617) Acquapendente showed similar historical sensibility in reviewing past operations. Acquapendente wrote that some operations were "so cruel, and horrible" that it was not by chance that they were not practiced anymore: "If they are in use today, only Barbarians and Turks practice such things as making a hole in the forefront and inserting a feather for aesthetic reasons, or wounding themselves as a sign of love."[20] In such cases, inflicting pain was not connected to saving lives but to useless aesthetic procedures and "barbarian" rituals. Only "inferior" civilizations from the past and from foreign lands could tolerate such painful procedures. "We do recall these surgical operations, which are cruel and cause horror and pain; even if they are described by Celsus, he does that more to report others' opinions than to state his own."[21] 'Excruciating" (*atroce*) and "cruel" were the words used by the Padua professor to describe eye surgery.

> Up to our times we can read about such excruciating and painful operations, to the head and other parts, which I believe are not practiced, because patients prefer to suffer from the illness of their eyes for their whole life than to subject themselves to these cruel procedures. But in our lands physicians are more modest and merciful.[22]

For a delicate procedure such as that of removing cataracts (*suffusione*), Fabrici suggested "to abstain from surgery, whenever possible." He also claimed to have seen some specialized eye surgeons performing the procedure with a needle, sometimes successfully, sometimes blinding their patients, and more often operating empirically rather than according to a rule. He himself tried such operation two or three times,

> 'then I stopped performing it, because patients would hate me, and also because in such operations one has to look with painstaking attention and for a long time into the patient's eyes, and I felt that I was damaging my own sight, so that while I was restoring a patient's sight I was losing mine at the same time,' and finally because the risk of damaging the eyes was too high.[23]

The learned surgeon showed that both for the sake of the patient and for the sake of his reputation and physical integrity he had to refrain from performing too painful procedures. Pain represented a practical obstacle for both patients and surgeons. Moreover, empiric practitioners were exposed as those who inflicted pain on patients due to their lack of proper medical education.

Besides correcting technical errors, reviewing past painful surgery, and appealing to "real men," Tagliacozzi employed a fourth strategy: a broad moralization of the pain felt in surgery, casting it as one instance of the adverse and painful circumstances of life. Uncharacteristically, it looks like our author began to address not his fellow physicians and learned surgeons but patients directly. Tagliacozzi mixed up the fashionable Stoic moral philosophy, the example of the Christian martyrs remaining impassible in torture, and chivalric ethics of bravely facing pain and danger. The teaching of Stoic ethics showed that a moral man knew that pain was not a real evil, because his willpower could make him endure it. According to this view, pain depended – at least in part – on the state of mind of the sufferer.[24] Michel de Montaigne, in a famous description of his experience with bladder stones, more subtly explained that there could be pleasure associated with bearing pain.

> There is pleasure in hearing people say about you: There indeed is strength, there indeed is fortitude! They see you sweat in agony, turn pale, turn red, tremble, vomit your very blood, suffer strange contractions and convulsions, sometimes shed great tears from your eyes, discharge thick, black, and frightful urine, or have it stopped up by some sharp rough stone that cruelly pricks and flays the neck of your penis; meanwhile keeping up conversation with your company with a normal countenance; jesting in the intervals with your servants, holding up your end in a sustained discussion, making excuses for your pain and minimizing your suffering. Do you remember those men of past times who sought out troubles with such great hunger, to keep their virtue in breath and in practice?[25]

Tagliacozzi echoed these ideas:

> Because there is nothing the physician can do, the patient must simply endure the pain. Is there anyone so cowardly and pathetic that he cannot accept an immutable and universal fact of life, and expects, even in misfortune, that everything will be pleasant and agreeable, and cannot bear the thought of suffering in any circumstance?[26]

And he went on by saying that the projected outcome, namely the restoration of the dignity of the human face, was more than enough to elicit bravery.[27] But there was more: "anyone who cannot withstand three or four days of the mildest discomfort is obviously of ignoble and dishonorable origin."[28] Tagliacozzi appealed to his patients' pride and prompted them not to act like a lower kind of men. Finally, a few examples of ancient martyrs should have humbled patients in front of the much bigger torments holy men and women faced with an impassible demeanor. But examples of martyrdom were also meant to uplift the patients' spirit: "Who can object to my procedure, which offers wonderful recompense in exchange from minor suffering?"[29]

Torture was actually an analogical trope running under the surface of sixteenth-century surgery. This illustration taken from the Venetian surgeon Giovanni Andrea Dalla Croce's European best-seller *Chirurgiae universalis opus absolutum* (1573) may serve as an example. The image shows a Christian soldier heroically enduring the work of battlefield surgeons, who are extracting an arrow from his chest (Figure 6.1). The visual analogy with the catalogue of illustrated martyrdom contained in a 1591 work by the Oratorian Brother Antonio Gallonio (1556–1605) is striking. Specifically, the expression of impassibility is very similar (Figure 6.2).[30] It is also interesting to notice that Della Croce had a parallel illustration of what looked like a Turkish soldier, beardless and agonizing in pain with eloquent gestures and contortions of the body (Figure 6.3). While the Christian knight was represented as impassible like a martyr, the Turk was represented as not being capable of enduring pain with dignity.[31]

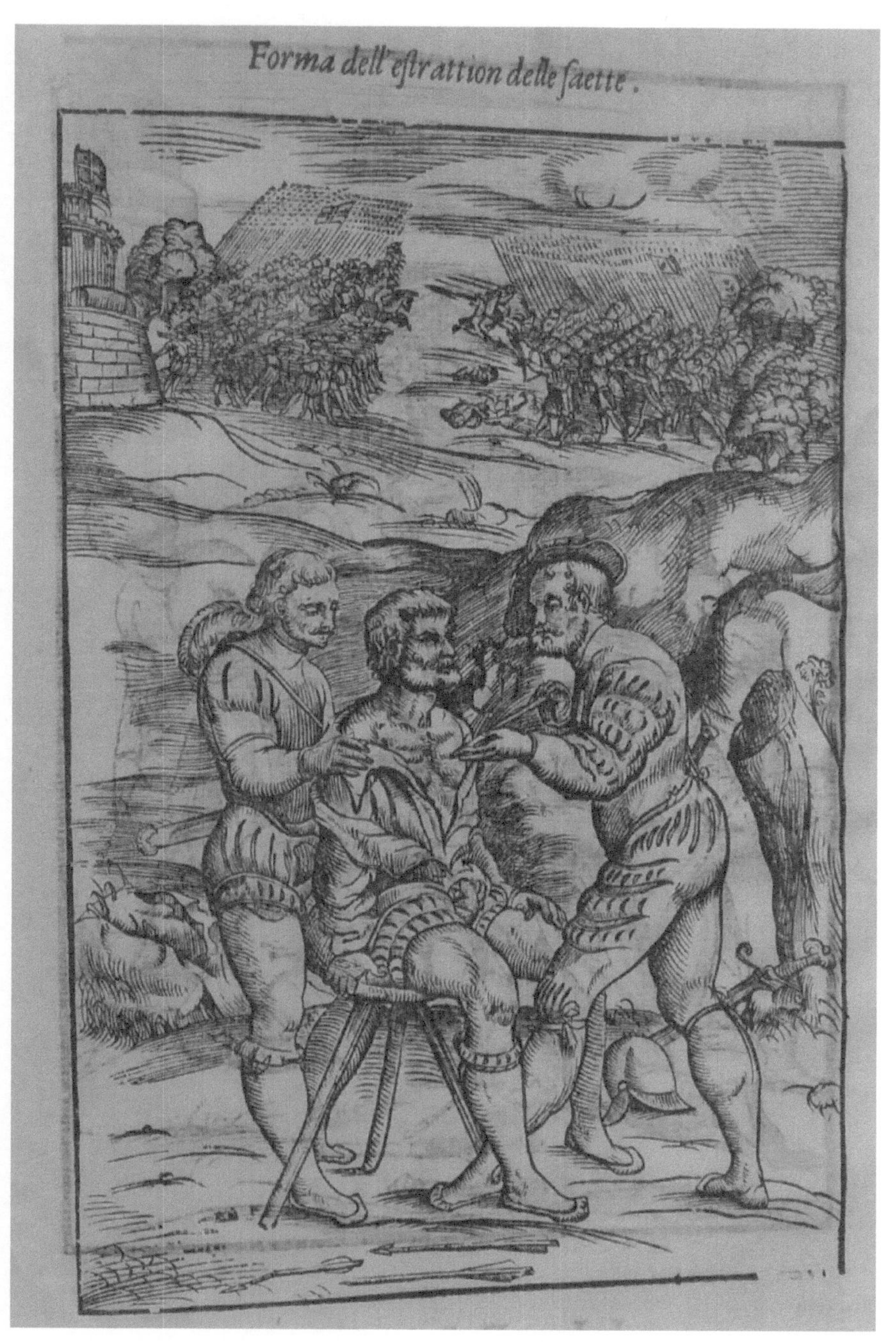

FIGURE 6.1 Giovanni Andrea dalla Croce, *Cirugia Universale e Perfetta* (1583): Christian knight.

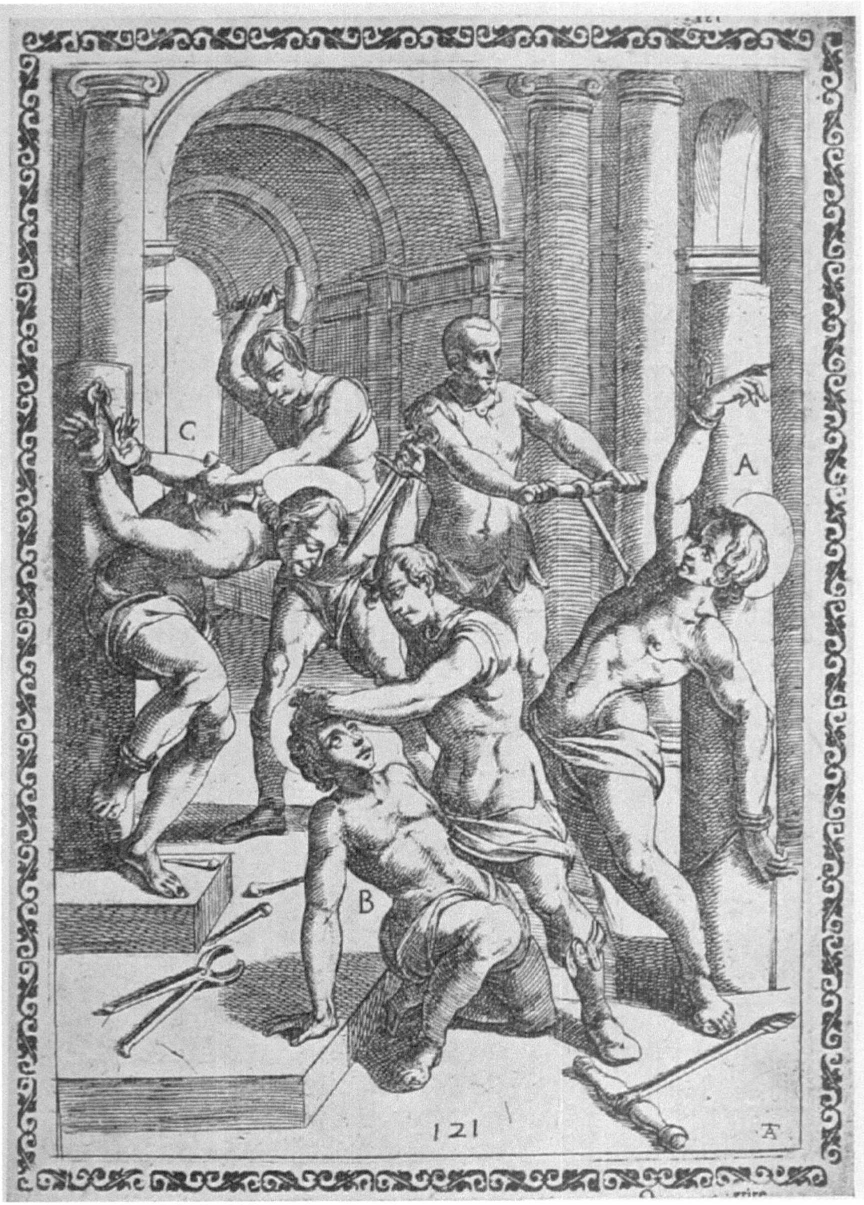

FIGURE 6.2 Antonio Gallonio, *Trattato degli instrumenti di martirio e delle varie maniere di martoriare* (1591): scenes of torture.

It would not be correct, however, to say that Tagliacozzi had only an aggressive and moralizing attitude toward his patients. He also showed a certain will to minimize pain. First of all, the Bolognese surgeon recognized pain as a fundamental site of difference between humans and plants. Human grafting was

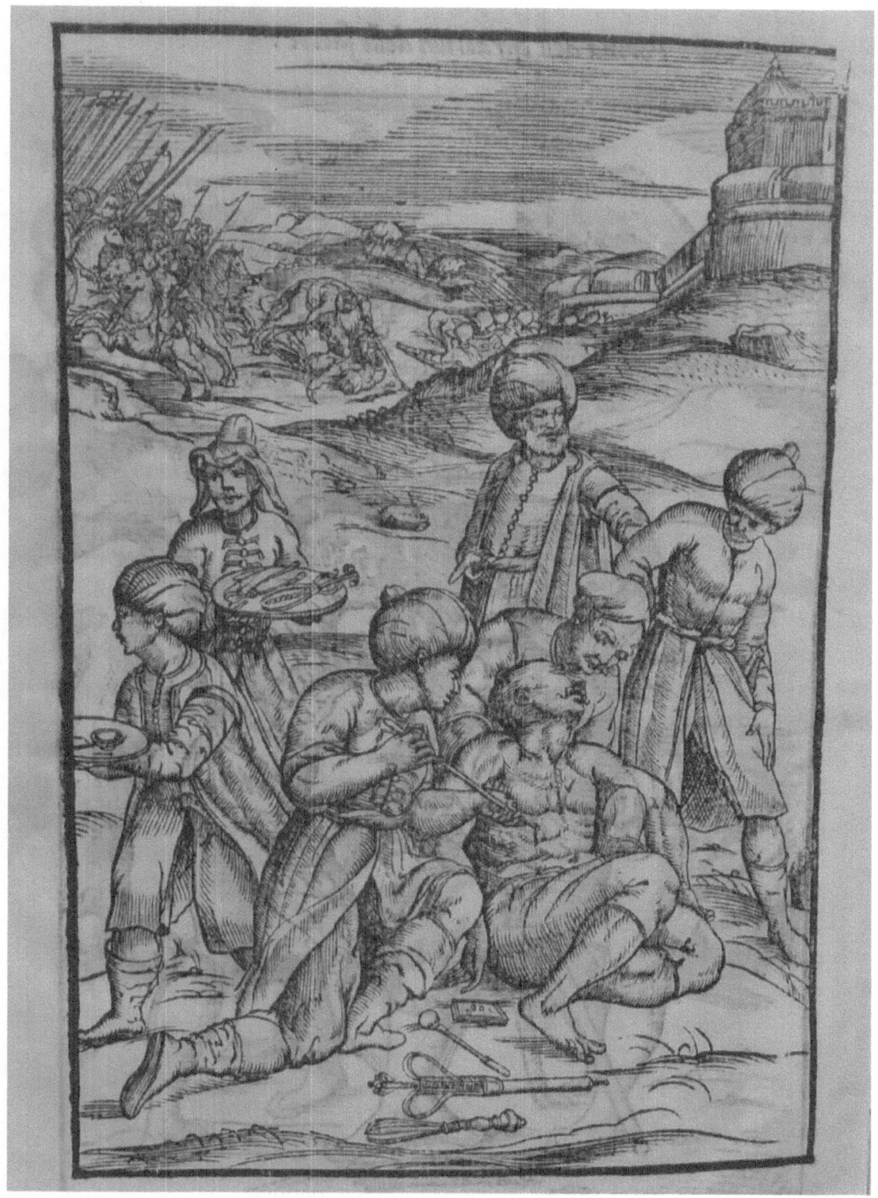

FIGURE 6.3 Giovanni Andrea dalla Croce, *Cirugia Universale e Perfetta* (1583): a "Turk."

different from plant grafting in that plants did not experience any feeling of pain.[32] The need for more time and the many more difficulties to overcome in human grafting did "not make our art less noble." On the contrary, "the worthiness of an act is proportional to the thought and attention required to perform it," and usually what took longer had also more *dignitas*.[33] The emphatic beginning of Book II of *De curtorum* underlined this same proud attitude. Enough with beauty and theory, wrote Tagliacozzi,

> now is the time for us to sharpen our knives and prepare our needles, razors, and cautery irons, for the skin must be cut and parts must be wrenched or removed. These actions are inevitably accompanied by pain, damage, and serious symptoms. . . . I wish to render drowsy minds alert to make the surgeon's hand readier to undertake this mission.[34]

Tagliacozzi chose a rather masculine epic and military tone to emphasize the manual work of the surgeon and the fact that pain was something inevitable that the surgeon had to be ready, and equipped, to manage. The graduate surgeon wished to show that he was not only learned but a surgeon too: he was perfectly capable of combining erudition with the specific physical and moral skills required for an activity that involved inflicting pain on other human beings.

Tagliacozzi claimed that the most acute pain was caused by the artificial position of the arm that had to be fixated to the face for three weeks. The procedure was gradual and took time, so it "must be accomplished with the least possible amount of inconvenience (*incommode*) to the patient."[35] But "if we consider how much the arm, when it is raised to the face, deviates from a middle posture (which is painless), the answer to our question will be evident."[36] However, once the procedure ended, this part – the internal part of the upper arm – was particularly safe because there were no nerves, no arterial channels, or no blood vessels. As a counterexample, Tagliacozzi showed how ridiculous it would have been to take the skin from the leg and attach the leg to the face, thus causing "unbearable pain."[37]

In any case, children and old men could not bear the procedure: "Not every single age is suitable for this operation: its success in old age and childhood is by no means assured." Old age brought about a lessening of the vital heat and an increased desiccation. Childhood, on the other hand, "possess great heat and purity of humor," two favorable conditions, but

> their [of children] continuous movement and exquisite sensitivity to pain are serious impediments (*ob motus impetus & sensuum vivacitatem*). A child would find it unbearable to be immobile; moreover, the pain of the incisions and sutures, although short-lived, is severe. Constancy and fortitude can overcome pain, but children lack these attributes.[38]

The perfect pain-bearer was a young man capable of focusing on healing, of standing still for a long period of time, and strong enough to endure all this without screaming and kicking.

Pain behavior was codified in a series of bodily structures and gestures in the late sixteenth century. These bodily schemes of pain behavior can be grasped by looking at art theory. One of the most famous art treatises of the century, Giovanni Paolo Lomazzo's *Trattato dell'arte de la pittura, scoltura, et architectura* (1584), detailed how to represent pain. According to Lomazzo, pain induced the body to make painful movements, according to the kind of torment it made people suffer through. For example, Prometheus tied to the rock with the vulture eating up his liver "pulled back his belly and his ribs, for the acute pain he held his thigh . . . he stretched his nerves down to the tip of his toes, showing pain in the rest of the body too, by reclining his eyelids, closing his lips, and uncovering his teeth."[39] Pain was also made visible through the contortions of the body and the eyes, as it could be seen in the Laocoon statue. Lomazzo said that in those who are prey to pain, one sees

> pulling back of body parts, abandoning of arms, wrapping of the eyelids, twisting, closing up the eyes, tightening and opening mouths, trembling, screams, agitations, inflammations, fears, sweats, howls . . . fainting, crying, loosing of the self, opening up the arms, despairing, closing up the hands, and other similar gestures.[40]

Tagliacozzi's ideal male, self-controlled, upper-class patient was someone who was able to control all this.

Pain played a role in the discussion on whether it was advisable to take the skin graft from a donor or not.

> Some have argued that one motive for taking the graft from another person lies in sparing the patient as much pain as possible. I will now enumerate all the painful aspects of the procedure so the reader can make an informed decision about the best source of the graft.[41]

Tagliacozzi believed that this would be possible in principle but impossible in practice. In fact, two persons – the patient and the donor – could not be forced to be attached to each other for three weeks. However, what followed was indeed a catalogue of painful procedures. Lifting and preparing the skin flap was not possible "without causing violent wrenching and severe pain." Surgeons "must excise the skin with a knife, pierce it with needles, and suture it; he must force the arm into unnatural position and immobilize it." The arm that suffered the cut was temporarily weakened and impaired. Finally, "the flow of irritating humors (*excrementa*) causes the arm to swell and ulcerate," thus causing further pain.[42]

Tagliacozzi did not abstain from quoting the Galenic surgical mantra (*De methodo medendi* 14.13), according to which in surgical operations one had to take into account "the swiftness with which the treatment can be completed, its freedom from pain, and its safety." The surgeon then showed that it was rare to find all these three conditions united in one kind of surgery and that, despite this rarity, his procedure actually complied with the Galenic prescriptions. Contradicting himself, the Bolognese physician argued that the stage of taking up the skin flap was

> so swift that some patients do not notice it until the act is accomplished. The surgeon uses a very small blade to cut the skin, which is held with a forceps. The incision can be completed very quickly, often before the senses perceive it.[43]

But "the grafting of the skin to the base of the nose cannot, however, be carried out without pain. After all, parts that are endowed with acute sensitivity must be excoriated, incised, and pierced with needles."[44] In any case, the pain of this phase was still lesser than the one caused by other operations.

Tagliacozzi always accompanied his description of painful procedures with the claim that such pain was far from unbearable, thus implicitly reinforcing the appeal to men to show their masculine strength of body and soul. While in Tagliacozzi's book there is a certain respect for the patients' suffering, and a sense of the historical progress of surgery based on its ability to minimize pain, he also vigorously appealed to his patients' sense of upper-class masculinity and moral values in order to invite them to bear pain for the sake of the highest goal: the restoration of their face.

Surgical pain

Respect and concern for the patients' pain were common in sixteenth-century surgery books. Galen and Avicenna (Ibn Sinā, c. 980–1037) had provided standard definitions and physiological models of pain, individuating its causes in humoral imbalance and in a "dissolution of continuity" of the soft or hard parts of the body.[45] As showed by the Neapolitan Aristotelian philosopher Simone Porzio (1496–1554), professor of philosophy in Pisa in the 1540s and physician at the Medici court, there was a certain consensus about what pain was and what caused it. Porzio recalled that there were three basic conditions for a human being to feel pain: the body had to able to receive impressions and to feel sensations; a sudden and violent mutation had to happen; and, finally, a change "against nature" had to take place, contrary to pleasurable feelings of the body.[46]

The five medieval "rational surgeons" all dealt with the painfulness of surgical operations, agreeing upon the precept that one of the most basic duties of surgeons was to minimize patients' pain.[47] The treatment of wounds, fractures, and ulcers, as well as more complex operations like the extraction of bladder stones and the elimination of cataracts, were all accompanied by in-passing remarks on easing pain, cheering patients up with artful conversation, and preventing patients from moving, so as not to put their lives in danger. It is true that surgical pain never became the object of explicit focus, but the concern for it, albeit indirectly expressed, was there and formed something like a tradition for Renaissance and early modern surgeons.

The manual for examining aspiring university-trained surgeons found in the papers of the College of Physicians of Bologna, written by the Roman surgeon Mariano Santo (1488–1577), summarized contemporary conceptions of pain. What is pain? – it asked in the pedagogical format of question and answer.

> Pain is a thing contrary to sensibility, or contrary to the quality of a body part. Or I will say that pain is that which happens through sensibility by

> a dissolution of continuity or an alteration of the substance, affecting one particular sense or the common sense.

What are the causes of pain? "Pain is caused either by a dissolution of continuity or by a sudden alteration." How can a dissolution of continuity happen? "By incision, corrosion, tumefaction, or fracture." How an alteration can happen? "Because of heat, cold, dryness, humidity, or a mixture of them." Finally, spasms, "illnesses of the nerves that dilates or breaks them," could be caused by repletion or evacuation. Spasms could be of two kinds: "proportionate" or "not proportionate" to the material, namely caused by some kind of noxious humoral impediment from which the nerves tried to get away to expel it. Among the causes of this second kind of spasm "there is pain."[48]

Pain in surgery was considered to be a liability from a purely technical-medical point of view. Physicians and surgeons believed it was accompanied by dangerous inflammation and that it attracted bad humors to the damaged parts of the body. Moreover, it was a symptom of the patients' weak state and inability to undergo treatment. In a few particularly serious cases, pain could be the cause of death too. Dalla Coce wrote:

> When pain is powerful it attracts to the wounded part other materials and causes inflammation, and there is not a more powerful cause of the filtering of evil humors than pain; fever can cause a strong pain too, when it produces a sudden change in natural operations. . . . When pain is cruel, it weakens the vital virtue, corrupts digestion, hinders sleep, and sometimes causes death: for all these reasons it is commonly said that pain is an evil accident, and one must take care of it with great solicitude and before attending to other things.[49]

More specifically, from sixteenth-century literature on surgery emerges a peculiar use of the term "virtue" (*virtus*) to indicate the patients' physical and physiological state, their strength and acceptable temperament. This use of the term can be found in Avicenna already, and it became more frequent in the Renaissance. Avicenna, while explaining the procedures of bloodletting (which among other things he thought could be used as painkiller), discussed "syncope," or fainting, during phlebotomy. Syncope was rare – he said – unless a great amount of blood was lost. The cases in which the patient was more likely to faint were fevers, apoplexy, inflammatory swellings, and severe pain. The physician had to make sure "the strength [*virtus*] of the patient was adequate" before attempting a demanding treatment.[50] Guy de Chauliac defined syncope as

> a sudden and acute decrease of virtue which usually follows excessive evacuation and pain, and which you will know by weak pulse, paleness, and slow and difficult mobility (especially of the eyelids and the extremities, as it would be impossible for them [patients] to move about), and cold sweat.[51]

Dalla Croce recommended that the first thing surgeons had to take into account before starting such a demanding procedure as trephination of the skull had to be

> the patient's virtue, that is the one which governs every other operation, and that can be weakened by cruel and unbearable accidents, by the great quantity of blood lost by the patient, or by the size of the fracture itself.[52]

Commenting upon the treatment of inguinal hernias, Paré described a long and painful treatment with a cannula to be inserted into the penis and pushed inside an incision made in the peritoneum. He then remarked: "However, this operation cannot be performed unless the patient's virtues are strong enough to bear it, and also unless you have made a favorable prognostic to his friends and relatives before touching him."[53]

In the physiological models dominating in the sixteenth century, surgical pain weakened the patients' strength and could generate powerful responses, ranging from kicking and screaming to fainting. Typically, one or two strong male assistants were required for particularly painful procedures. Descriptions of the assistants' role were ubiquitous in surgical literature. Paré, when giving instruction on how to extract kidney stones, one of the most painful pre-anesthesia surgical procedures, offered precise instruction about how surgeons could make use of their assistants. In this case, there were four of them.

> You must place the patient on a table – he wrote – the kidneys on a pillow, a folded cloth under the buttocks; he must be half-reclining, his tights folded, heels almost touching the buttocks: you must tie his feet at the height of his ankles with a resistant bandage three fingers wide, which must pass behind his neck two or three times; from there, his hands will be tied against his knees, as you see in this figure. Having placed and tied the patient this way, you need four strong men who are neither afraid nor shy: two of them have to keep the patients' arms, and the other two will block his knee and feet, so firmly that he will not be able to move his legs or his buttocks, but he will remain immobile.[54]

Pain is never mentioned by the author in this passage, but patients can almost be heard screaming and seen moving around, trying to free themselves from the assistants' hold.

Tagliacozzi gave a long description of the role of assistants in rather similar terms. At least two assistants were needed for reconstructing noses, "who are not only agile and dexterous with booth their hands and bodies, but also extremely vigilant and obedient." They had to prepare a comfortable bed over which the patient would be placed. The room had to be "well illuminated" for the purpose of outlining the skin flap. The bed had to be in the middle of the room, far from the wall, because the surgeon and his assistants had to be able to go around it. The patient had to lie in bed, with one of the assistants holding his arm, which had to be kept perfectly still. Making the patient sit on a chair would ensure better illumination, but that would be the only advantage; moreover, "when he sees the scalpel approaching he will resist because of the anticipated pain and will pull his arm back no matter how tightly he is restrained."[55] After the incision, patients had to lie down and rest for several hours in order for their excited humors to calm down. The surgeon had to handle forceps and knives with a sharp edge, placed on a special plate in order to be easily grabbed. "The patient must not be allowed to see these instruments, so the surgeon should cover them with a cloth or some other item."[56] In the scene of complex surgical procedures, pain – anticipated pain, fear of pain, and the actual painfulness of the cuts – was always the silent major character: no one talked about it, but it governed the whole ritual.

Surgery books also included recipes, classifications of painkillers, and remedies to ease operatory pain but much more often postoperative pain and collateral pain. From the times of Avicenna, things changed very little. The Persian physician explained that pain relief was based on the use of contraries. According to him, "pain is relieved either by modifying complexional balance, or by eliminating the material which causes it, or by stupefying by destroying the power of sensation in the part."[57] Some medicinals could have a relaxation effect, such as dill, linseed, melilot, chamomile, celery seed, bitter almond, especially when mixed up with the gum of prunes, starch, lead carbonate, saffron, marsh mallow, cardamom, cabbage, turnip, and various kinds of oils. The most powerful of the stupefacients was opium, to be used with great caution, said Avicenna. Phlebotomy, cupping, poultices, and so forth were also listed as remedies to ease pain. Avicenna also mentioned a series of psychological remedies as well: patients could be encouraged to "walk about gently," listen to "pleasant songs," because in general to be "occupied with something that cheers you up removes the severity of pain."[58]

Sixteenth-century health-care culture was not indifferent at all to pain, as surgery textbooks and collections of recipes attest. Giovanni Battista della Porta listed in his *Magia Naturalis* a series of sleep-inducing plants and recipes explaining that such remedies "are in high esteem among physicians, because with them they can soothe many pains." These were mandrake, already described by Dioscorides, poppy seeds, and a special essence gained by mixing together poppy, opium, mandrake, and hemlock juice into a device described as a "little lead basket" that had to be placed under the nose of the patient or the sufferer.[59] Surgeon Tarduccio Salvi da Macerata devoted several chapters of his vernacular surgery book to painkillers. Standard ingredients were "seasoned olive oil, almond oil, egg yolk; milk, fatty butter, chicken fat, rabbit fat, duck fat, and similar things."[60] Other resources were the

> stupefacients, which have a nature cold and dry in the fourth degree, and are used to induce sleep when pain becomes extreme; because when a great pain has neither been eased by removing its cause nor by the anodyne medicaments, then we are forced to use stupefacients.

There were strict conditions for this use: the patient had to have his "able virtue (*valida*)" in the whole body as well as in the affected part, he had to be purged, and the medicaments had to be of very modest quantity. Ingredients for the common stupefacient were poppy seeds and leaves, "the condensed juice of poppy, which is called opium," mandragora (both roots and leaves), hemlock, and so forth.[61] Standard remedies in the sixteenth century included oil of roses, egg's white, several other kinds of oils, lettuce, cabbage, turpentine (pine distilled raisin), and warm baths. Dalla Croce systematized the whole matter of painkillers. They could be of three kinds: anodyne medicaments (the abovementioned oils and local agents and ointments); medicaments that acted on the cause of pain and changed the altered balance of humors (pharmacy and diet); medicaments that made the hurting part dull or insensitive. If the cause of pain was occult, or hidden, Della Croce suggested phlebotomy. As all medieval and Renaissance surgeons did, he finally warned that "narcotic medicaments" – mostly compounds with opium – had to be used only in extreme cases of absolute necessity, because they could prove to be lethal.[62]

Pain treatment was directed mostly at post-operatory states and not at the actual surgical procedure. Physician Elideo Padoani's collection of cases, published in Frankfurt in 1607 but compiled in the mid-sixteenth century, included a telling example. Padoani narrated that he extracted one arrow from the hand of a patient and then prescribed a series of recipes and a plaster to help his patient cope with the pain, but no mention is made of techniques to ease the pain during the procedure itself.[63]

Licensed empirics provide another way to understand how widespread was the culture of pain relief, and how important it was for patients, well beyond official medical written culture. I mention here only one letter, written in 1613 by a professional actor to the College of Bologna, a Joseppho Scarpetta, perhaps a mountebank performing in the piazzas. Scarpetta was petitioning to obtain an official license to sell

> an oil called Balm by him, which has been given to him by a learned man in Paris, which is a wonderfully excellent remedy for all kind of pains, and which has been administered to several people, who were all freed from pain. . . . Therefore, he wishes to obtaining a licence from your Most Illustrious Lords, as you have given to others; and asks that no one but him and his heirs can administer this balm.

As the letter made clear, this was not an isolated case, and Joseppho had prepared and sold his balm for a long time. He even attached a "certification of a cure (*fede di guarigone*)" prepared by one of his patients.[64]

Cognitive innovation

Besides the historicizing attitude described earlier, I have identified three other models according to which surgical pain was dealt with by surgeons and acted as a mediator in the doctor-patient relationship which are specific of the sixteenth century: a cognitive use of pain; pain as seen by barber-surgeons; and pain as a subject for professors of secrets and empiric surgeons.

The Bolognese physician and professor of surgery Bartolomeo Maggi (1477–1552) exemplifies what can be called "a cognitive use of pain" as a marker of innovation. In his 1552 book on gunshot wounds, Maggi corrected the widespread view according to which harquebus balls were poisoned or heated, thus burning the flesh. In doing so, he advanced two claims. First, the pain felt by patients came from the bruises and lacerations caused by the bullet, not by its inherent heat. Maggi came to this conclusion by making use of his patients' accounts, gathered on the battlefield.

> I did not hear from any of the many wounded soldiers in the siege of Mirandola [a city nearby Modena where he was serving as military surgeon] any complains about suffering burning or a feeling of heat when injured by harquebus, but rather they all said that they were feeling a sense of heaviness, like that coming from a severe bruise.[65]

Maggi went on replying to an anticipated objection: critics might counter that – following Hippocrates' aphorism that of two pains, only the stronger is perceived – the stronger pain caused by the bruise silenced the less acute pain caused by the burning. Maggi replied that since the two pains were felt in the same place, the burning sensation should have been perceived before the second one kicked in: but this was not the case.[66]

Second, Maggi combined his patients' narratives with an experiment. He explained that if you fired a bullet with a harquebus to a highly inflammable substance hanging from a tree (like straw or wool), this substance would not be set on fire, as it should have according to the Aristotelian theory of heat. Moreover, there were no signs of burning on the clothes and armor of the people who were shot.[67]

Ambroise Paré's famous 1575 discourse on gunshot wounds narrated the events of his first experience with these injuries when he was serving as a war surgeon in Piedmont in 1536.[68] Paré recalled that up to that time he had only read about such wounds in Giovanni Da Vigo's (c. 1450–1517) book, which taught that there was poison in the cuts, due to the poisonous nature of gunpowder. Da Vigo recommended cauterizing such wounds with oil of elder and theriac. Paré noticed that other surgeons did the same with boiling oil, causing "extreme pain to patients." One day he found himself short of oil on the battlefield, and he simply put oil of roses, eggs, and turpentine on the wound. Greatly fearing that the patient would die poisoned, the morning after Paré rushed to his bedside and, to his great surprise, he found the patient "feeling very little pain, with neither inflammation nor tumor." After having repeated the procedure on several other patients with the same successful outcome, he concluded: "From that moment I decided not to burn anymore those poor men injured by shots of harquebus in such a cruel way."[69] In Paré's case, inflicting less pain to patients was both a sign and an outcome of progress and technical innovation.

Sixteenth-century surgery books are filled with similar examples of how minimizing pain accompanied technological innovation. Famous French empiric surgeon Pierre Franco (1505–1578) described a method of his invention for extracting bladder stones. Surgeons had to make an incision close to the peritoneum and insert a silver cannula into the penis to push the stone toward the bladder and the open cut. Franco then suggested the use of a *gorgeret*, a hollow and pointed tube. Surgeons would insert the extraction forceps through the cut into the *gorgeret*; the forceps then would grab the stone, which had to be extracted "with the greatest dexterity." The extraction forceps and the hollow tube were new inventions. Franco proudly described their action as much less painful, as it had the effect of keeping the incision small-sized.[70]

Another similar meaning of pain in surgical procedures can be inferred from the passages concerning a sort of modulated use of pain. Pain could be a guide for the progress of certain procedures. Military surgeon Girolamo Crasso, when treating the setting of the bones broken by firearms, described a procedure involving the help of two "assistants" holding the patient. He considered surgical pain as a guide for the success of the operation:

> Once you are done lightly bandaging the sick part, it is necessary to make sure that the part keeps still until the bone is consolidated and repaired; and if the patient feels pain, you will know for sure that the bone is not well repaired yet, or that some pointed fragment causes an alteration. The sign of the bone being repaired is the absence of pain.[71]

Pain could be a sort of plastic matter to mold and use for cognitive purposes concerning the outcome of the whole procedure.

In his Latin book on "tumors," the learned Giulio Cesare Aranzi devoted four chapters (on polyps, ozenae, warts, and herpes) to tumors affecting the nose. In the chapter on nose polyps Aranzi claimed that, historically, more pain than relief had come from surgeons and physicians. In fact, the internal parts of the nose were very sensitive and likely to feel pain when invasive remedies such as red-hot cauteries were employed. Paul of Aegina had suggested the use of scalpels when it came down to manual operations, but scalpels "easily injury the healthy parts, and most seriously so, if the patient moves." Aranzi boasted the invention of a special instrument for nose polyps: "for this reason, as a long practice has taught me, I have invented an oblong forceps, which erases the majority of the polyps with very light pain."[72] Interestingly enough, Fabrici d'Acquapendente too claimed to have invented a new instrument for treating nose polyps. This was supposed to be one single instrument that did all the procedures (cutting, extracting, cleaning the remnants, and cicatrizing) on the polyp in one single step, "with no pain, quickly, and safely: and with positive outcome, while, on the contrary, the tools described by the ancients make the operation slow, painful, dangerous, and only sometimes successful."[73]

Less pain, more effectiveness: innovation was measured against the minimization of surgical pain.

The view of the barber-surgeon

Pietro Paolo Magni's vernacular manual of phlebotomy (1584) provides an example of the barber-surgeons' view on pain. Magni's book showed a great deal of attention to minimizing pain in cutting veins and to reassuring frightened patients – much more so than his learned Latin-writing counterparts. Contrary to medieval writers on bloodletting, Magni addressed the issue of its inherent painfulness (Figure 6.4).[74] The barber-surgeon treated Roman cardinals and noblemen, and thus, writing from a much lower social standing than his patients', he was very respectful and eager to put into practice the Galenic prescription of performing painless, swift, and safe procedures. For example, when evaluating the tools of the trade – lancets – and making suggestions to the apprentice barber-surgeons, he argued that the lancets had to be "very well sharpened, so that they do not inflict too much pain on patients."[75] Bandages had to be soft "so that they do not cause pain." Barber-surgeons always needed to have some oil at hand to anoint the veins: "oil has the property of being a lenitive . . . barbers should dip in it a piece of cloth and then they should put it on the cut, so that they will not let the patient feel pain at all."[76]

In a chapter devoted to instructions on how to cut the veins of "frightened and pusillanimous" men, Magni told the story of a man who was supposed to be the epitome of virility but fainted only at hearing the word "bloodletting."[77] Another case involving a soldier had more explicit implications.

> [In 1558] I was called to bleed an ensign-bearer at the *hosteria del sole al paradiso* . . . and while I was tying the band around his arm, he was taken by the strongest syncope [he fainted] I had told him many times to lie down on the bed, but he had replied me that he was a soldier, that he was not afraid of harquebus shots, so bloodletting was nothing for him. But to cut it short: he was taken by this syncope and suddenly fell down, making awful grimaces with the eyes and the mouth, and water, wine, or vinegar in his wrists were not nearly enough to calm him . . . [he then stood for a while quite still, as if dead]. There were in attendance two nephews of him, who were knights, and at this sight they threatened me saying: you killed our uncle, we will bring you to court; but in that moment God decided to wake up the ensign-bearer.[78]

Magni noted that

> even if some people claim that only pusillanimous men can be taken by such syncope, in my opinion they are wrong: I have seen several strong men (*valenti uomini*) be taken by a syncope during bloodletting, and the same thing I have seen happening to men much experienced in war affairs and who overcome many tests in their lives.[79]

Fear and painfulness of surgical operations were not moral issues but physical ones.

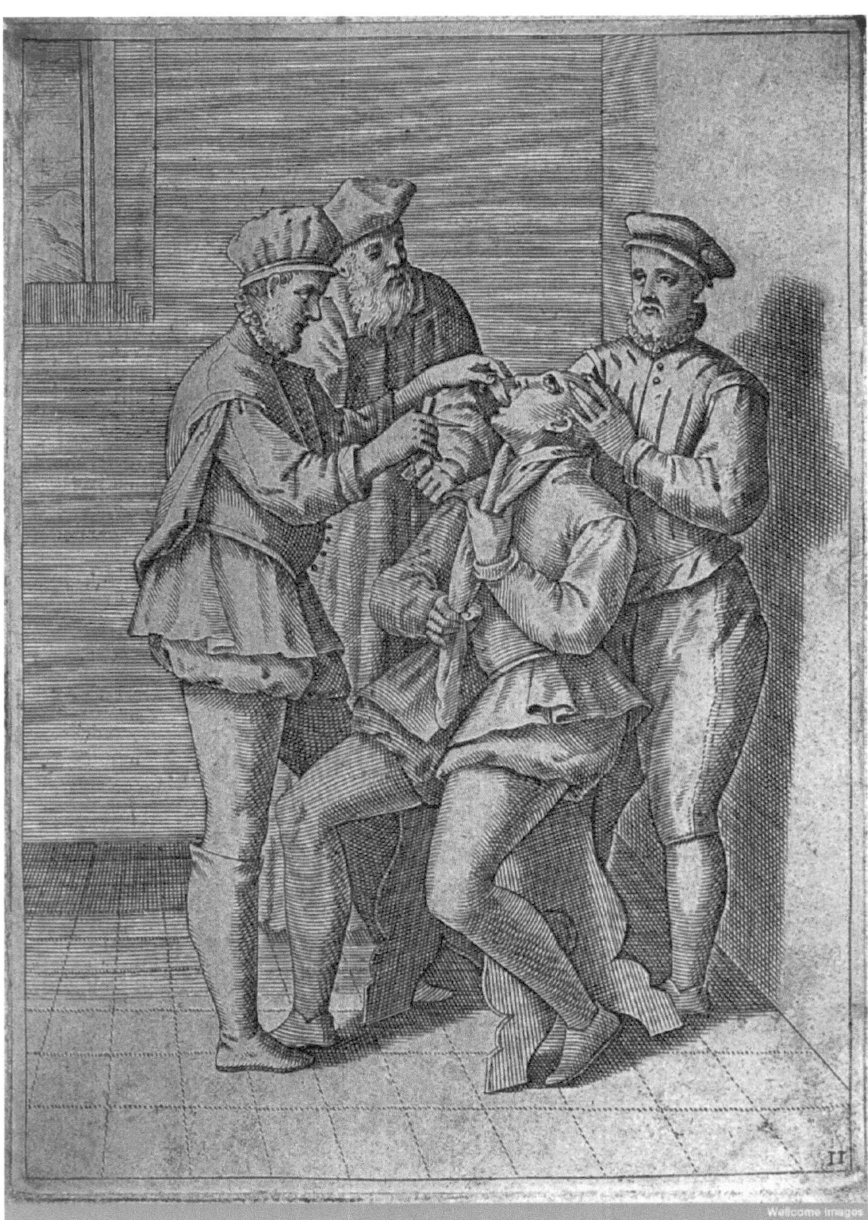

FIGURE 6.4 Pietro Paolo Magni, *Discorsi intorno al sanguinar i corpi humani* (1584): phlebotomy.

Source: Courtesy of the Wellcome Collection

In other cases, Magni suggested that the barber-surgeon simply tricked his patients whenever he realized that they were too afraid and risking fainting. He told the case of a patient who was angry because a few barbers had tried to bleed him with no success, because he did not want them to use the lancet. Magni recounted that "in a very friendly manner" he told the patient that he had no intention to use the lancet, but he only wanted to check his arm. In order for the patient to believe him, he gave him his case containing the lancets and said: "you see? I don't have any intention to bleed you, and without these tools I couldn't, even if I wanted to." At this point, the patient relaxed and showed the barber-surgeon his arm, and the operator, who had a small lancet hidden in his robe, all of a sudden made the incision without the patient having the time to notice it.[80]

Ambroise Paré described similar tricks; for example is a case of cauterization of a "phlegmon" (a hardened swelling) with a red-hot iron (1572).

> There are patients who are so afraid of having their phlegmon opened that they run away at the mere sight of it, and they greatly fear the pain: they will kick and move, hiding the part in question, and the incision cannot be made in the necessarily precise way.[81]

To this, Paré's reaction was to fool the patients. He claimed that the surgeon had to trick the patient by covering the point of the lancet, hiding the lancet with a poultice, and then suddenly making the incision without leaving the patient any time to react. "Another way of fooling the patient is this: let the Surgeon wear a ring, on which he must have placed a little lancet, suitable to make the incision of the aposteme."[82] Just like Paré, barber-surgeons did not judge patients; they simply reassured them and tried to figure out methods for minimizing pain, strengthening their physical forces, and occasionally overcoming their fear with a few tricks.

Barber-surgeons' books usually present another striking tendency: a sort of naturalism.[83] They generally considered the human body as part of a cosmological conception of nature, in touch with other life forms. Human bodies were endowed with an innate power of self-healing that practitioners had simply to support through bloodletting and the purgation of the flow of bad humors traveling in the blood. For example, Salvi's definition of phlebotomy reads as follows: "a universal evacuation of the whole body, and of all humors, made through the cutting of a vein: indeed, it evacuates blood, choler, phlegm, and melancholy from all the veins of the human body." Moreover, it was a method of evacuation and purgation that was safer than oral remedies, because it was entirely in the physician's hands to draw bad blood and to let good blood stay – while with oral drugs "we do not have the same grasp on humors."[84]

And here is how Salvi represented the origins of phlebotomy – in much the same way that ancient naturalists like Pliny and Lucretius had narrated the discovery of grafting (Figure 6.5).

> Naturalists say that the inventor of phlebotomy was the hippo, an animal that lives on the Nile river, as big as a Frisian horse, of both earthly and aquatic nature; when it feels heavy for the excessive quantity of blood in its body, it goes into a reed bed or a similar place and under the push of a

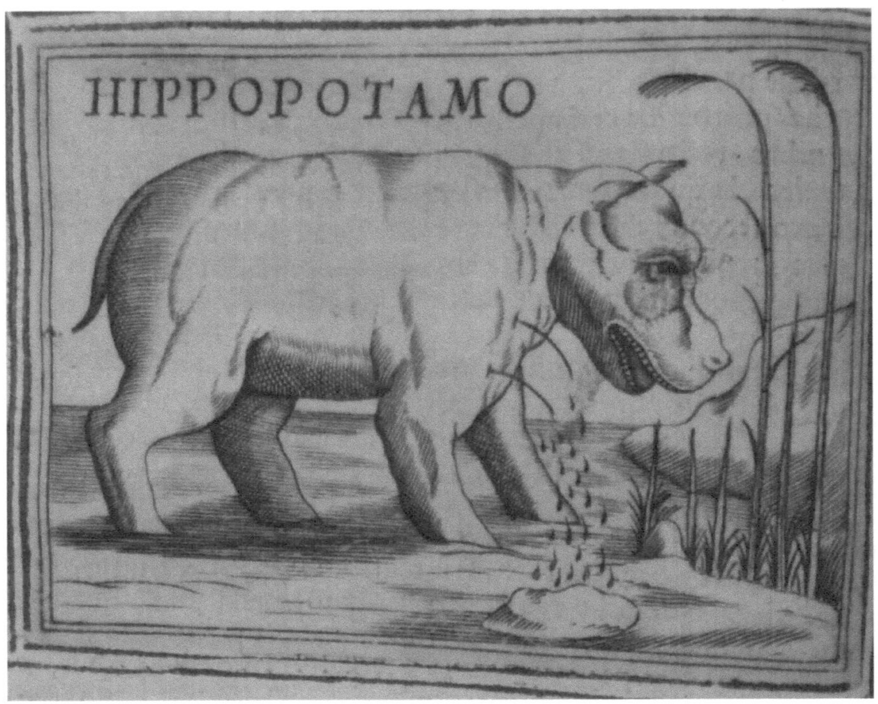

FIGURE 6.5 Tarduccio Salvi da Macerata, *Il ministro del medico* (1613): a hippopotamus inventing phlebotomy.

> natural instinct he cuts its veins and lets blood out until it feels better; then the hippo finds out some mud and patches up its wounds.[85]

There was no doubt: the author of phlebotomy was nature "which operates through the expulsive virtue." In the second place, it was the barber-surgeon operating with the proper tools as an assistant to nature.

> To those who deny that such operation is made by nature, this can be proved through the senses with an experience (*sensatamente con l'esperienza*): if you open the vein of a dead body, it is impossible to draw the blood, because in a dead body there is no expulsive virtue.[86]

Malfi's *Il barbiere* shows how the care of barber-surgeons for managing pain, anxiety, and fear became a true art and the focus of close attention at the beginning of the seventeenth century. Malfi engaged in a detailed anatomical description of nerves and muscles, which the barber-surgeon had to learn to recognize from the very start, unless he wanted to cripple his patients. It seems like patients were aware that barber-surgeons could commit such dreadful errors:

> [S]ometimes we see a patient who fears and trembles, even if he is someone who in other circumstances would be so brave to face a thousand swords and spears; but when he needs to face such an accident [that might happen during phlebotomy] he is terrified. Therefore, sometimes these patients expose themselves to the risk of being perpetually impaired.[87]

In this passage an otherwise brave patient is terrified by the idea of being impaired during bloodletting, and there is no moral judgment whatsoever directed at him, only understanding.

Letting blood was a difficult and dangerous operation. The main senses involved were sight and touch. Through them, the barber had to figure out what was the individual complexion of his patients and in a way to visualize the body as it would appear "under the skin,"[88] said Malfi. The barber-surgeon even compared bloodletting with sharp razors and lancets to sculpture in that both arts did not allow for errors: if the artisan made one mistake he could not correct it, in marble as well as in humans.[89] Therefore, barber-surgeons needed to gain perfect knowledge of the dangers they had to face.

> Properly speaking, and only under the respect of the materiality of the body, opening up the veins is contrary to nature, because it divides and separates that which nature has joined. And this is signaled by the fact that all men abhor and try to escape it: both for the above mentioned reason, and because it causes pain, since it is a dissolution of continuity, which always causes pain.

If someone would claim not to have felt pain during bloodletting, he could not be trusted, because that was impossible and could only be a false impression caused by a light hand, the numbness of sensation, or "the power of distraction given by the patient's imagination which blocks the painful sensation."[90]

Syncope was discussed at length as well. According to Malfi, there were four reasons for the syncope (fainting) or "appearance of death (*sembianza della Morte*)": the loss of too many spirits, pain, abundance of choleric humors, and fear. With respect to fear, Malfi stated that

> fear is a very frequent cause in pusillanimous patients, who believe bloodletting is a terrible thing. . . . In such cases, one has to behave in the following way: he must change the patient's fear by knowing his pusillanimity, because it only comes from the patient's imagination. Therefore, one has to address the patient's imagination with all that can serve to divert it, such as persuading him that bloodletting is an easy procedure and that the phlebotomist is skilled and experienced; besides, one must let the patient believe that some kind of occult property of an herb or a stone can strengthen his heart and block all fears . . . but the main faculty is the imaginative, which can alter everything and turn a man upside down.[91]

Malfi insisted on the power of the mind, of inducing the right thought and on distracting the patients' attention away from pain through a thoughtful and skilled manipulation of their imagination.

> The remedy for pain will be this: if you see that the person is very delicate, and soft (*molto delicata, e molle*), you can anticipate some troubles, and thus you must adapt your ingenuity in order to be light-handed, and cut as little as possible. And if by any chance to the insistent pain follows fainting, you must all at once comfort the patient with good smells, and ease the pain with water, oil, and warm wine, at the same time making frictions, and cleaning up the offended part.[92]

As far as the "resolution of the spirits" is concerned,

> one must let the man lay down and put some spirituous wine in his mouth, or soak some bread in wine, and even more so if the patient has a fever; one must soak the bread in water of roses and then in the wine. . . . I praise the good wine above all, as it is approved by the Salernitan school and Arnaldo [of Vilanova] the commentator. . . . I do comfort patients with these things and then I make the incision on the vein, an incision which must be small and narrow. I am not even talking about spraying water on the face, smelling vinegar and odorous essences, making ligatures at the extremities, pulling hair and ears, since everyone knows about them.[93]

Barber-surgeons had to become experts of the human mind, all for the sake of managing fear and pain.

The view of the professor of secrets

Leonardo Fioravanti, empiric surgeon and "professor of secrets," was highly skeptical about learned surgery. He often exalted natural remedies learned from the wisdom of nature herself as opposed to the complex, painful, and technologically advanced procedures of graduate surgeons. In his 1570 *Cirugia*, Fioravanti bitterly criticized the trephination of the skull, used as a treatment for fractures, by describing it as too "artificial." He wrote that he could not understand which reasons physicians could adduce to justify their treatment of skull fractures, which consisted in cutting and dilating the bones of the head. "But I mostly marvel – he added – at how the wounded patients let themselves be tortured without any plausible reason."[94] Patients should rebel against the pain graduate surgeons uselessly inflicted on them. Fioravanti was arguing for a treatment of the wounds of the skull that was based on ointments and application of external remedies – of his invention and sold by him, of course. Elsewhere, he pushed his arguments so far as to criticize one of the sacred tenets of sixteenth-century learned medicine: the key value of anatomy for surgeons.

> Instead of learning so much anatomy, we would do better by learning agriculture, to treat surgical conditions more easily and in a simpler manner, without tormenting the patient. . . . I am astonished by the fact that all the Princes of the world let their subjects earn such an art, which is so noxious to human bodies. But I am much more astonished at the men of the world, who, when they are wounded or suffer some kind of injury, let themselves be treated by those who always want to use anatomy, as if nature would have no power to heal . . . because for patients it is much better to have the right remedies than to let their wound be observed in detail: for this reason, the former [the caring surgeon] comforts and the latter [the anatomically-skilled learned surgeon] tortures; the former heals, the latter kills.[95]

Nature is a self-healing process that the surgeon's art must second, while learned surgery inflicts unnecessary pain by focusing on solid organs.

Men's pain, women's pain

Although not all sixteenth-century surgery books mentioned the idea, it was generally understood that different bodies felt pain differently. Dalla Croce remarked that surgeons had to be quick and minimize pain in treating and bandaging wounds "and much more so when their patient is noble and delicate."[96] In another passage, while the Venetian surgeon was discussing the conditions that needed to be observed in order to evaluate the possibility of an operation on the skull, he listed as the sixth of these circumstances "age, sex, and way of life of the patient." And he went on:

> children's bones are less resistant than those of older and more robust men; women's bones, or those of the timid, are less resistant than those of the valorous men; less resistant are the bones of a delicate body who is used to live among comforts of all sorts than those of the sailor, the peasant, the soldier, or another man used to live under the sun."[97]

Clearly, there was the idea that noble bodies and bodies of women, children, and people who did not work were more sensitive and delicate than the bodies of those who worked with their hands and of those who were hardened by the training and practice of the military arts.

The gender division between men and women operating in Tagliacozzi's book referred much more to the conceptual oppositions analyzed in Chapters 3 and 4 (natural versus artificial, medicine versus cosmetics) than to gendered norms of expression of pain or to different ways of moralizing male and female pain. In a patriarchal society in which issues of inheritance were crucial, male medical writers writing on women were much less interested in the ways they behaved when in pain than in questions revolving around the physiology of birth and the functions of the organs of generation. Overall, in Renaissance surgical literature – and despite the fact that Seneca had thought that the experience of childbirth predisposed women to a greater tolerance of pain –[98] there is little to be found on how men and women perceived pain. It was widely understood that the inferior quality of women's complexion, leaning toward the cold and moist, could make them more sensitive to painful sensations.[99] However, there were exceptions.[100]

Let us take as an example the 1567 book on honor by the Sicilian humanist lawyer, trained at Bologna, Girolamo Camerata da Randazzo.[101] Camerata summarized all the reasons why men were considered superior to women in medical, theological, and moral terms.[102]

But Camerata had a much more nuanced view on this matter. He said that one could discuss it in two ways: according to what there is or according to what there could be. There was no doubt that men were better than women "if we refer to the present state of affairs (*parlando dello stato presente*)." Not that there were not excellent women, but they were rare.[103] However, with respect to "possibility (*quello che potria essere*)," we could not be certain. Camerata thus invited readers to take a look at male and female complexions, because "the body is an instrument of the soul; therefore when the body has a good complexion and is well organized, the soul operates more or less perfectly."[104] Camerata believed the complexions of man and woman were part of the human species, the "most perfect" one. Qualities had degrees, and saying that women were cold and moist was not an absolute but a relative assessment, compared to men's complexion. This meant that in a way women were closer to the mean temperament – the Golden Mean – than men: "and therefore we could conclude that women have a better complexion than men."[105]

With respect to enduring physical pain and effort though, Camerata had to agree that man's body "because of its dryness is more apt to tolerate hardness and stronger, and because of its greater heat is braver and more audacious . . . ready to take action, and better for the most active endeavours."[106] In this respect, man was superior to woman, because he was more apt to military affairs, to commerce, and to those intellectual pursuits that were finalized to actions. On the other hand, women were "more stable, more honest, more healthy, and with a longer lifespan." Women were not as inclined as men to active practices but they could still engage in them and were able to learn all the intellectual disciplines:

> [O]n the contrary, they are superior to men in learning the letters and busy themselves in contemplative things; because if all our cognitions come from the senses, since they are closer to the perfectly temperate complexion, they have a better tempered sense; therefore, their intellect too is more perfect.[107]

To sum it up: women were better in letters and contemplative sciences; men were better at war, commerce, and practical sciences.

Despite such exceptions – partial exceptions, because even Camerata had to admit that men were more apt than women to endure physical distress – it is clear that in the surgical literature women were considered less capable of enduring pain and were not even expected to do so. On this point, a binary behavioral division emerged.[108]

The tradition of barber-surgeons' manuals was once again the most explicit on the topic of gendered endurance to pain. Pietro Paolo Magni claimed that it could happen that bloodletting procedures failed because the veins on the feet were too difficult to find or because "the assistant who holds the foot lets it go when he hears the cries and screams of the patient, who being most of the times a woman, is naturally timid and weak (*timida e frullosa*)."[109] Here Magni was much harsher than with his male patients:

> I have to say that [in such cases of weak female patients] I do not wonder at the poor work of the barber, but at the ignorance and foolishness (*balordaggine*) of the patient: and I would say that they deserved to be crippled, but the barber must be punished too.[110]

In the middle of the seventeenth century, famous Neapolitan barber-surgeon Cinthio D'Amato wrote that if the patient was a woman, "you would do better to take care of her lower parts, given that the uterus is the main cause of a syncope which she might suffer: for this reason it will be a very good remedy to fumigate her nose with stinky and dirty things." This was a remnant of ancient practices based on the conception of the mobile uterus.

> It will be wise neither to talk about blood or bloodletting in their presence, nor to let them see the blood, because they are so pusillanimous that these discourses would induce terror in the patient, and from terror comes the syncope.[111]

So, women were pusillanimous. It was implicit that men who behaved like women were pusillanimous too, but that was never stated, and D'Amato spoke clearly of moral defect and cowardice only when he talked about female patients. The Milanese learned surgeon Gabriele Ferrara (1543–1627) suggested in his 1596 collection of secrets and medicaments not to let women and children be around male patients when performing surgery. In fact, their expressions, cries, and gestures of fear and horror could discourage the patient and compromise the outcome of the surgical procedure.[112]

Esther Cohen has shown that some Renaissance physicians believed that female pain par excellence, labor pain, had its own code of expression. While the *Trotula* collection was silent on the matter, all medieval and Renaissance midwifery textbooks had recipes for hastening birth and easing postpartum pain. However, they did not address childbirth pain as such. In any case, male surgeons writing on women's health and birth process were not indifferent at all to labor pain. As François Rousset (1535–1590), the physician of the Duchy of Savoy, wrote in his *Traitté nouveau de l'hysterotomotokie* (1581):

> I have been led to do this [to write a book on the matter of childbirth] by the pitiful sight of the agonies, helplessness, prayers, and pitiful looks of those poor creatures who are so tortured, and cry murder, as they appeal only to us, begging with clasped hands for such help as we may be able to give them. For it is in this more than in any other calamity that the greatest women suffer everything.[113]

It seems that the reason was neither masculine callousness to feminine pain nor some reminder of Eve's burden but rather that uterine contraction and pain were considered one and the same thing, and therefore easing childbirth pain would compromise the whole process – at least those were the ideas of the fifteenth-century eminent physician Michele Savonarola (1385–1468). While the subject of labor pains was avoided by medical texts, other sources examined by Cohen suggest precise reasons to prescribe a specific pain behavior. In 1490 Saragoza, the childbirth of the noblewoman Isabel de la Cavalleria was recorded in minute detail by a notary and several witnesses for inheritance reasons. In this case, pain was often mentioned and had a crucial function: that of testifying that the childbirth was not a fraud and was actually taking place. These lay persons considered pain as the inevitable and involuntary mark of childbirth. Indeed, the idea that crying and screaming in labor were a required part of the delivery can be evinced by a sixteenth-century case of a German woman reported for "not having acted during her labor as she should." The norm, Cohen argues, was crying out. Women who did not follow the script were suspected of misbehavior or of faking the delivery, and, in any case, they would not receive all the sympathy they wanted.[114]

The 1563 vernacular manual on women's illnesses by Giovanni Marinello (d. 1585) implies that women *must* cry out their pain in childbirth: "So we require that women, feeling the most acute pain, do cry: because this behavior brings great relief to such pain."[115] However, it is hard to find a shared norm on the subject of childbirth pain. This norm, if it ever was a norm, was not universally accepted. Some texts suggested that women restrain themselves. French physician Jean Liebaut (1535–1596) wrote in his popular gynecological and obstetrical vernacular book, first published in 1582, that a good midwife "will tell her [the laboring woman] to hold her breath, and to restrain herself as far as possible, and instead of shouting to block her nose and close her mouth."[116] Likewise, Scipione Mercurio in 1596 explained that different women suffer through childbirth pain in different ways and mentioned the capacity to hold breath for a long period of time among the conditions for a less painful delivery.[117] Childbirth pain could make an impression in the lay male observer as well. I have found a trace of that left in the diary (*libro dei ricordi*) of the patrician Gozzadini family of Bologna. One Camillo Gozzadini narrated how he came to name one of his male children Giovanni Battista. In October 1584 his wife Lodovica gave birth to a boy "whom I have named Gio. Battista, both to honor my father who had this name, and because when she [my wife] was tormented by such serious pain I have been won over by compassion and piety in seeing her in such trouble and even risking her life."[118] In this period, doctors, surgeons, and natural philosophers also took up stories of "primitive" women in the New World, Africa, or the Near East who, unaccustomed to the luxury of the European lifestyle and fortified by their natural way of living, could give birth almost with no pain.[119]

Helen King, taking up a suggestion by Nicole Loraux, noted that, in the Greek language, the work *ponos* meant a kind of pain "that cannot be treated because it was seen as a necessary part of the process." She underlined that there is an analogy linking together labor in childbirth and pain at war to defend the state – an analogy that reverberated through the early modern period.[120] Screaming for pain was more than acceptable as a female behavior and therefore the opposite of a male behavior, especially if the men in question were upper-class heirs of the chivalric tradition.[121] The field of reactions to pain – not pain itself – was the arena of the construction of gender norms.

The role of pain management

In his analysis of early modern medical practice in England, Andrew Wear has described three functions of surgical pain. Pain was a matter of negotiation between surgeons and patients; a diagnostic sign; and a practical concern to be integrated in the surgeons' work.[122] Despite the institutional differences between London, Bologna, Paris, and so forth, I have identified these very same features in a variety of books by Italian and French practitioners of the body, no matter their social and professional rank. Michael McVaugh has emphasized how in the fourteenth century Guy de Chauliac devoted a constant attention to minimizing pain. He also persuasively argued that in extremely dangerous and difficult operations, like hernia treatment, patients did not necessarily look for a permanent cure but rather for a "minimization of their fear and pain" and "increasing control over the kind of operation – and of agony – that they would have to endure."[123]

Indeed, the rate of success of past surgical operations must be evaluated as historically and socially determined, rather than against modern standards. Sixteenth-century surgery writers – in both Latin and vernacular, both university-trained and self-taught – had great respect for patients' pain and were deeply concerned by the inherent painfulness of surgical procedures. Some of them associated pain control with epistemic and technological innovation; some others considered it a tool with which to attack competing professional categories; others believed that minimizing pain was a sign of professional status. Inflicting too much pain was not simply the mark of the empiric as it was in late medieval Latin surgery literature. Being skilled in pain management was a shared value among the different kinds of practitioners of the body. Indeed, the empiric surgeon could accuse the learned surgeon of being cruel and inhuman, of inflicting torture-like treatment to patients for the sake of knowledge and prestige. In turn, the graduate Latin-writing surgeon could accuse the empiric surgeon of treating wounds, fractures, and ulcers blindly, thus greatly damaging and hurting patients.[124]

It is true that pain never became the object of explicit focus, being confined to in-passing remarks and marginal sub-paragraphs, at best implicitly present and indirectly readable between the lines of descriptions of surgical operations.[125] But all surgery books I have examined agreed in considering painfulness, and emotional reactions to perceived and expected pain, both as something to take care of and as a result of weakened bodies and unbalanced temperaments, much more than of faulty moral character or questionable masculine identity. Moreover, in the Galenic tradition pain was never a purely corporeal matter, as separate from what we would call "psychological" reactions and sensations. Besides being a phenomenon of the body and of the soul, or the imagination, elements like patients' social status, political opportunity, and the practitioner's professional reputation must be taken into account in order to paint an accurate picture of pain management in sixteenth-century surgery.

In Tagliacozzi's monograph, pain as a matter of negotiation between patient and surgeon took a quite unique turn. This is not because *De curtorum* involved extra-medical factors but because it played with social and political factors in a different way. From the point of view of pain management, Tagliacozzi's approach to surgery appears to be an exception that requires explanation.

Moral economy

Surgery writers of the sixteenth century used to justify pain as an element in a delicate balance that had as a possible outcome death or the impossibility to carry on a normal life. The general moral economy of pain between surgeons and patients implied a justification of severe pain only insofar as it was the only way to prevent death or of removing the causes that made living a normal life impossible. Ambroise Paré explained very clearly the terms of the metaphorical – and often real – contract between surgeons and patients in the introduction to his complete works (1575).

> To tell the truth – he wrote – surgical procedures cannot be performed without causing pain: indeed, how would it be possible to cut an arm, or a leg, or to make incisions on the neck of the bladder and put there several instruments without inflicting pain? In the same way, treating a luxation, when you have to push and pull a part that is already in pain; opening apostemes, cutting a tendon or a nerve which is already half-broken, suturing the flesh to join the edges of a wound, applying burning irons . . . and other procedures that cannot be accomplished without causing great and often extreme pain. However, without the surgeon's help, people would

> die miserably. Is performing such operations enough to call surgeons cruel and inhuman, and to despise them?[126]

Durante Scacchi (1540–1620), the first author who in 1596 put on paper the century-long and well-respected empirical art of the *norcini*, also commented upon the pain-death balance while discussing the Hippocratic ban on cutting for bladder stones.[127] Scacchi suggested that patients had to be encouraged to bear pain with bravery and strength. A priest had then to administer the sacrament of confession, and finally their relatives had to be informed of the extreme danger of such an operation, "which is never certain, and often brings about death." But if the stones were left in the bladder, he went on, one day they would close all the passages and the patient would die anyway. Therefore, "even if Hippocrates said that he would have never cut for the stone, it would be impious to leave patient with no help. Anything must be tried for the patient's sake."[128] In other words, when the patient faced death or constant and ultimately unbearable pain, any procedure that offered even a small chance of success could legitimately be tried, despite the pain and danger involved. The patient's voice begging for a remedy entered Scacchi's picture and justified the painfulness of the treatment:

> The necessity of such a procedure is shown by the fact that people who suffer from stones often envy the dead, and say that they wish to die soon rather than live with such atrocious pain; for this reason the operator who successfully removes the stone can get much glory. Therefore, moved by their sense of charity and by the patients' great suffering, these operators always invoke the help of God, and carefully assess the age and strength of patients, the time of the year, the brightness of the day, the right place.[129]

The balance between bearing pain and living a relatively normal life is a more or less explicit and constant theme in the history of pre-modern surgery. For example, a story told by the eleventh-century scholar al-Biruni about the great physician and surgeon Rhazes, well known in medieval and Renaissance Europe, went like this. Rhazes was becoming blind because of a growing cataract, and the best oculist of the times offered to treat him. After he had heard the description of the procedure, the great surgeon replied:

> I acknowledge that you are the most learned of oculists. You know, however, that this operation is not without pain, which the soul loathes, and long-drawn-out discomfort which men find wearying. But perhaps [my] life may be cut short and the time of death may be near; and in that case it is repugnant to someone like myself at the end of his days to choose pain and discomfort over repose. So depart, with thanks for what you intended to do.[130]

Surgical patients shared with martyrs, anatomical models, and soldiers the fact that they could reveal some kind of truth by paying the price of being subject to violence needed to have their pain, fear, and endurance placed within meaningful contexts.[131] Pain must have a meaning in order to be tolerable.[132] The balance between death-impairment on the one hand and pain on the other had the function of legitimizing painful surgical procedures.

Against this background, the concept of "moral economy" advanced by E.P. Thompson becomes more than a metaphor.[133] Gianna Pomata used this conceptual tool to show how the College of Medicine and the Protomedicato in Bologna were integral parts of the system of power of the old regime and of its mechanisms of legitimization based on "a set of reciprocal expectations between aristocracy and the common people."[134] The Protomedicato was in charge of establishing and enforcing a "moral economy of medicine" – or, better, of health – in that its role was to ensure a fair price and steady supply of medicaments and treatment for the people. For such institutions, health was a gift to the people, not a citizen's right. Collegiate physicians were with lower-class patients in a relation similar to that of the powerful aristocrat with the client: a vertical relation of dependence based on benevolence, Christian charity, and concession of a favor.[135]

Gaspare Tagliacozzi was part of the College of Physicians of Bologna, the most elite medical institution of the city, but he had come a long way. The encounter between surgeons and patients was mediated by violence: noblemen's violence and the violence of surgical procedures. This question of violence is linked to that of the relationships between men of different social rank. The flourishing of duel and of treatises on duel in the sixteenth century has been used as a counterargument to Elias' thesis of the civilizing process and the decrease of violence in the early modern period. Jean-Claude Chesnais has divided violence into two subcategories: "interpersonal," including criminal violence and deviancy, both lethal and nonlethal; and "collective," including crimes against the state, state measures against the individual, and war.[136] Stuart Carroll has welcomed the distinction and claimed it has eliminated the difference between war and violence, one supposedly rational and the other irrational. Many historians have also opposed Elias' *longue-durée* view and embraced a more historically specific approach to violence; others have emphasized the perspectival character of violence, which is dependent upon the kind of society it takes place in.[137] Historians like Carroll and Dewald have criticized Elias' theory on the birth of the modern self-restrained self, according to which violence became less and less tolerated in the early modern period, as the state claimed its monopoly. Elias believed that knights channeled their competitive drives into the court and that self-constraint became the center of the new ethos, while Carroll and Dewald registered an increase of violence in the same period and emphasized the existence of networks of negotiation and compromise between centralizing states and the noble classes that ultimately benefited both. In other words, violence must be treated not like the expression of a meta-historical, primitive, basic human impulse but as part of systems of human relationships governed by rules within historically determined contexts.

Noblemen were violent before and after Tagliacozzi, and surgery was a learned discipline in Italy before and after that time as well. So, what happened in the late sixteenth century? Several phenomena came together in this period. On the one hand, it was a sort of paradoxical and short-lived golden age of noble culture. On the other hand, social mobility for learned surgeons like Aranzi, Tagliacozzi, and Cortesi, the chance they had to improve their wealth and status, thanks to their studies and patients, was a short-lived phenomenon, as seventeenth-century proofs of citizenship for admittance to the College of Medicine of Bologna show. In that century, these proofs obsessively focus on checking that candidates and their relatives did not work as "*mechanici*."[138]

It was in this precarious social and political scene that a book under many respects exceptional like *De curtorum* could come into being. In a period in which the Papal state tried to centralize power and established its new bureaucratic authority at the cost of fighting against aristocratic privileges and codes of honor, Tagliacozzi had to face a delicate situation. He had "made it" thanks to state structures, but his best chance to really become wealthy and famous came from violent, unruly, dueling noblemen. This was a common feature of sixteenth-century urban life and government. Surgeons and physicians served as military doctors, advisors for public health in times of plague, public lecturers, and hospital officials. At the same time, they knew that they needed to build a good reputation among the noble class if they wanted both wealth and social prestige.

The moral economy of pain took a peculiar shape in facial reconstructive surgery precisely in the sense of preserving a legitimizing balance: that between the ultimate goal of the operation and the pain that had to be tolerated. In the facial reconstruction operation, patients were not in immediate danger and could decide whether to undergo the procedure or not.[139] This moral economy cut across all modern distinctions between the private and the public – private feelings and public expressions. Subjecting themselves to painful "private" procedures to have their appearance restored could become for sixteenth-century upper-class men a display of braveness and "public" honor. In turn, this balance included the sub-balance of three factors. (1) The ethical values of noble, ruling-class, male patients, and the mechanics of social distinction that marked them as a certain type of men. (2) The relationship between cosmetics, associated with women and condemned by Tagliacozzi in many passages of the book, and the restoration of men's face, namely their identity and social honor. (3) The key importance of not looking like a monster and not bringing about horrified reactions for men involved in constant social gatherings and in taking political decisions. In a way, Tagliacozzi's work looks like an attempt to bend the usual moral economy of pain of sixteenth-century surgery and to create a different "emotional community" or system of feelings among surgeons and patients.[140]

Tagliacozzi often emphasized the socially mutilating nature of disfigurements related to missing noses: "But no one will deny that there is nothing more disgusting (*foediore*) than the sight of the nasal cavities gaping open and allowing the onlooker to see the unwelcome spectacle of mucus dripping forth."[141] It is significant that Tagliacozzi in another passage justified pain in surgery taking into account the moral economy of the social and political system he lived in, a system in which punishment, war, and even torture were necessary.

> The State – he wrote – demands that evil or arrogant citizens be punished with the sword, the whip, the rope, banishment, and other tortures in order to preserve its dignity and safety. Likewise, in wartime, a soldier must endure hunger, thirst, heat, cold, and lack of sleep, and must value the well-being of his country more than his own life. Just as no great or memorable deed can be accomplished without danger or inconvenience, so no disease can be cured without the potential for harm or danger. Those who use a painful treatment to cure a cruel disease should be praised, not condemned, so long as they accomplish this end with the least possible pain for the patient, for it is indeed impossible to cause no pain at all.[142]

Facial surgery was an element in a moral economy of pain within a moral economy of medicine, within a moral economy of power. As noted by Joanna Bourke, pain performs ideological functions, and the content of pain, what counts as "being-in-pain," is a political matter of "legitimation, inclusion, exclusion."[143] Bravely bearing pain was a behavior functioning as one important element in the construction of masculinity in the sixteenth century. However, such element became part of surgical culture only under specific circumstances in late Renaissance Bologna. The kind of man Tagliacozzi had in mind was neither the "mechanical man," an artisan working with his hands to make a living, nor that of the soft and too much refined, effeminate, and "slavish" courtier. The world of reconstructive surgery patients was a male world of differentiated forms of masculinity, populated by upper-class men competing for honor, for whom saving face literally meant saving their public appearance.

The man from the artisanal class who promised to restore their sense of selfhood needed to boost his authority by appealing to upper-class values of traditional masculinity. At the same time, he was confident that his role as public officer would grant him a sufficiently high moral standing facing noblemen, who were not always willing to be integrated into the political order. The decisive push for a physician to write an entire monograph on the surgical reconstruction of noses can be found at the local level, and it involves – combined with the fact that surgery was esteemed enough for a College physician to practice and to write about – a complex politics of masculinity, a specific social context in which the upper class' rituals fell under both admiration and suspicion, and a moral economy of pain which by far exceeded the boundaries of medicine.

As we have seen, both sixteenth-century surgery and late twentieth-century pain studies do not make a sharp distinction between moral and physical pain. Of course, this is much more a contingency than a repetition, as contemporary biomedicine has very little to do with humoral theory. However, both traditions are different from a mechanistic conception of human beings, which has come to be firmly associated with the Scientific Revolution of the seventeenth century. This mechanistic physiology that supposedly explained all the workings of the body in terms of matter and motion would make psychological pain disappear, or better, it became a sort of by-product of the motions of the bodily matter, more precisely of the nervous system.

This illustration from Descartes' *Traité de l'homme*, published after his death (Figure 6.6), has often been interpreted as a manifesto for dualism and mechanism. Fire hits the nerves, nerves touch the brain, and the brain gives the order to remove the suffering leg from the fire. As we have seen, such a rigid interpretation and periodization of the history of science have been widely criticized. But if we look at the history of pain as a history of social, political, and scientific

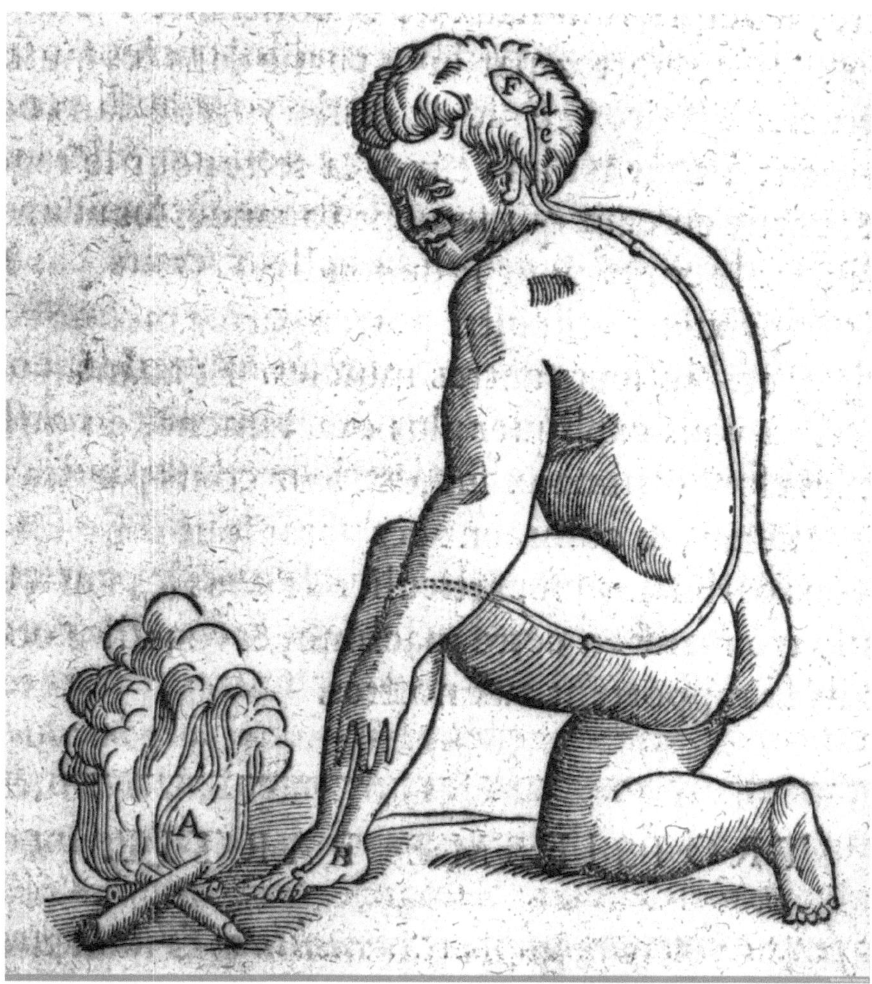

FIGURE 6.6 Descartes, *L'homme* (Paris: chez Charles Angot, 1664): pain provoked by fire.

Source: Courtesy of the Wellcome Collection

relationships – without separating them – we will come to the conclusion that there has never been a real distinction between physical and psychological pain but only historical ways in which humans have dealt with each other through the social events of inflicting, feeling, and showing pain.

Notes

1 Tagliacozzi, *De curtorum*, p. 105 (1:83–84).
2 For a similar approach applied to seventeenth- and eighteenth-century French surgery, see Lisa Silverman, *Tortured Subjects: Pain, Truth, and the Body in Early Modern France* (Chicago: The University of Chicago Press, 2001), pp. 133–151. On the history of pre-modern physiology of pain, see Daniel De Moulin, "A Historical-Phenomenological Study of Bodily Pain in Western Man," *Bulletin of the History of Medicine* 48, 4 (1974): 540–570; Moreno Rodríguez, Rosa María, and Luis García Ballester, "El dolor en la teoría y práctica médicas de Galeno," *Dynamis* 12 (1982): 3–24; Aurélien Gautherie, "Physical Pain in Celsus' *On Medicine*," *Studies in Ancient Medicine* 42 (2014): 137–154; Peregrine Horden, "Pain in Hippocratic Medicine," in Roy Porter, ed. *Religion Health & Suffering* (London: Routledge, 2013), pp. 295–315.
3 Katherine Walker, "Pain and Surgery in England, circa 1620-circa 1740," *Medical History* 59, 2 (2015): 255–274.
4 Jan Frans Van Dijkhuizen and Karl A.E. Enenkel, "Introduction," in Jan Frans van Dijkhuizen and Karl A.E. Enenkel, eds. *The Sense of Suffering: Constructions of Physical Pain in Early Modern Culture* (Leiden: Brill, 2009), pp. 1–18, quotation on p. 9.
5 Park, "Was There a Renaissance Body?," p. 325.
6 David B. Morris, *The Culture of Pain* (Berkeley: University of California Press, 1991), pp. 9–30; Esther Cohen, *The Modulated Scream: Pain in Late Medieval Culture* (Chicago: The University of Chicago Press, 2009).
7 Renée Leriche, *The Surgery of Pain*, tr. Archibald Young (London: Baillière, Tindall, & Cox, 1939), pp. 13–15.
8 Interestingly enough, with the exception of Moscoso, they are not historians of science and medicine.
9 Joanna Bourke, *The Story of Pain: From Prayer to Painkillers* (Oxford: Oxford University Press, 2014), pp. 6–9.
10 Javier Moscoso, *Pain: A Cultural History*, tr. Sarah Thomas and Paul House (New York: Palgrave Macmillan, 2012), p. 2.
11 Morris, *The Culture of Pain*, p. 16.
12 Falloppio, *De decoratione*, fol. 43v: "ego teneo, quod maximus est cruciatus, et vellem totum admittere nasum potius, quam, hunc subire laborem."
13 Tagliacozzi, *De curtorum*, p. 3 (pages in the original edition are not numbered; my translation).
14 Ibid., pp. 80–81 (1:64).
15 Ibid., p. 91 (1:72).
16 Ibid., p. 85 (1:67).
17 Paul of Aegina, *The Seven Books of Paulus Aegineta*, 3 vols., tr. Francis Adams (London: The Sydenham Society, 1844–1847), vol. 2, p. 334.
18 Ibid., p. 335.
19 Peter E. Pormann, "The Dispute Between the Philarabic and Philhellenic Physicians and the Forgotten Heritage of Arabic Medicine," in Peter E. Pormann, ed. *Islamic Medical and Scientific Tradition* (London-New York: Routledge 2010), vol. 2, pp. 283–316.
20 Girolamo Fabrizi d'Acquapendente, *L'opere chirurgiche* (Padua: appresso Giacomo Cadorino, 1671), p. 197. The first edition of Acuapendente's surgical works, published in Latin, dates 1592. As it is well known, Edgar Zilsel argued that the sense of collaboration and progress of early modern science derived from the artisans' attitude;

these humanist and learned surgeons seem to be another source for this idea. See Edgar Zilsel, "The Genesis of the Concept of Scientific Progress and Scientific Cooperation," in Edgar Zilsel, ed. *The Social Origins of Modern Science* (Dordrecht: Springer, 2003), pp. 128–168.

21 d'Acquapendente, *L'opere*, p. 197: "Memoriamo però noi queste operationi chirurgiche, le quali son crudeli, & apportano orrore, e dolore; che tuttoche proposte da Celso, egli lo fa più tosto per opinione d'altri, che per la propria."

22 Ibid., p. 198: "Sin qui si leggono appreso molti autori si atroci, e dolorose operationi, tanto nel capo, quanto altrove, le quali affermo non esser praticate, perche gl'infermi vogliono più tosto portare tutto il tempo della lor vita i mali d'occhi, che sottoporsi a queste crudeli operationi. Mà nei nostri paesi i Medici sono più modesti, e pietosi."

23 Ibid., p. 206: "le quali poi ho tralasciate, si perché questi tali mi havevano in odio, si ancora perché bisognando in coteste operationi guarder fissamente con gli occhi, lungo spatio di tempo, sentiva da questa fissatione negli occhi una offesa di rilievo, ho temuto, che mentre desiderava di giovare all'altrui occhi, perdessi i miei."

24 See Cicero, *De finibus bonorum at malorum*, tr. H. Rackham (Cambridge: Harvard University Press, 1931), pp. 246–249, 260–263 (3.8.29 and 3.12.42).

25 Michel de Montaigne, *The Complete Essays*, tr. Donald M. Frame (Stanford: Stanford University Press, 1965), pp. 836–837.

26 Tagliacozzi, *De curtorum*, p. 186 (2:65).

27 However, Tagliacozzi admits that the outcome can hardly equal the beauty of the "original" face and that problems can arise: the skin of the new nose can become more sensible, it can shrink, the holes of the nostrils are generally smaller, and sometimes hair can grow on the nose, which will need to be shaved: Ibid., pp. 109–111 (1:88–89).

28 Ibid., p. 187 (2:65): "hoc servile est, & indignum . . ."

29 Ibid., p. 188 (2:66).

30 On Antonio Gallonio's representation of martyrdom, see Jetze Touber, "Articulating Pain: Martyrology, Torture, and Execution in the Works of Antonio Gallonio (1556–1605)," in *The Sense of Suffering*, pp. 59–89. On impassibility, see Cohen, *The Modulated Scream*, 2009, pp. 227, 256.

31 An article exploring the genesis of this representation in post-Lepanto Venice is in press.

32 Tagliacozzi, *De curtorum*, pp. 159–160 (2:41).

33 Ibid., p. 160 (2:41).

34 Ibid., p. 117 (2:1).

35 Ibid., p. 64 (1:47).

36 Ibid., p. 65 (1:48).

37 Ibid., p. 66 (1:49).

38 Ibid., p. 74 (1:57).

39 Giovanni Paolo Lomazzo, *Trattato dell'arte de la pittura* (Milan: appresso paolo Gottardo Pontio, 1584), p. 166: "ritirava adietro il ventre, & il costato, & a suo danno raccoglieva la coscia . . . distendeva a basso i nervi dritti fino all'estremità delle dita, dimostrando anco dolore nel resto del corpo coll'inclinar le ciglia, stringer le labra, & discoprire i denti."

40 Ibid.: "ritiramenti di membra, abbandonar di braccia, incarnamenti di ciglia, travolgimenti, chiuder d'occhi, stringer, & aprir di bocca, tremor, gridi, agitationi, infiammationi, paure, sudori, gemiti . . . svenire, gridare, smarrirsi, piangere, aprir le braccia, disperarsi, chiuder le mani, & simili affetti." It is remarkable that Lomazzo described what we would call moral and physical pain in the same terms, and said that both forms of pain should be represented with the same palette of movements and emotions. On Lomazzo's knowledge of the human body see Barbara Tramelli, *Giovanni Paolo Lomazzo's* Trattato dell'Arte della Pittura*: Color, Perspective and Anatomy* (Leiden: Brill, 2017), pp. 174-210.

41 Tagliacozzi, *De curtorum*, p. 76 (1:60). For a survey of aeraly modern knowledge of human skin, see Craig Koslofsky, "Knowing Skin in Early Modern Europe, c. 1450–1750," *History Compass* 12, 10 (2014): 794–806.

42 Ibid. Although these are serious reasons to choose another person as a donor and the physician is free to choose, as we have seen in Chapter 4, Tagliacozzi's strong suggestion is not to do it.
43 Ibid., p. 105 (1:83).
44 Ibid.
45 "I remember often saying that the two types of pain are the sudden change of temperament and the rupture of continuity": Galen, *Of the Affected Parts*, quoted by Cohen, *The Modulated Scream*, p. 88.
46 Simone Porzio, *De dolore* (Florence: apud Laurentium Torrentinum, 1551), p. 7.
47 McVaugh, *The Rational Surgery*, pp. 106–110.
48 ASB, Studio, 234 [pages are not numbered]: "Dolor est rei contrariae sensibilitas, aut contrariae qualitatis existenti in membro. Vel dicas, quod dolor est quodam adveniens ex sensibilitate, & re contraria solutionem, aut alterationem faciente, sensum particularem vel communem affligens . . . Causa doloris aut est solutio continui, aut subita alteratio . . . Aut solvitur incisione, aut corrosione, aut tumefactione, aut fractione . . . Fit aut caliditate, aut frigiditate, aut siccitate, aut humiditate, vel horum mixtionibus." See also the summary of the causes of pain given by Porzio, *De dolore*, p. 10: "Pain is an bad, preternatural sensation caused by bad temperament, with dissolution of continuity (*Dolor est sensus asper, praeternaturalis, consertim factus a mala temperie, cum solutione continui*)."
49 Dalla Croce, *Cirugia universale*, fol. 27r.
50 Avicenna, *Canon medicinae* (Venice: industria ac sumptibus Juntarum, 1608), p. 219 (1.4.5.20).
51 Chauliac, *Inventarium*, vol. 1, p. 154: "subita et acuta concisio virtutis que consuevit sequi inmoderatas evacuaciones et dolores, quam cognosces per pulsum deficientem et per colorem pallidum et motum (precipue palpebrarum et extremorum) difficilem, et per sudorem frigidum."
52 Dalla Croce, *Cirugia universale*, fol. 25v.
53 Paré, *Oeuvres*, vol. 1, p. 411.
54 Ibid., vol. 2, pp. 478–479. On the history of lithotomy, see Owen H. Wangensteen, Sarah D. Wangensteen, and John Wiita, "Lithotomy and Lithotomists: Progress in Wound Management from Franco to Lister," *Surgery* 66, 5 (1969): 929–952.
55 Tagliacozzi, *De curtorum*, pp. 127–128 (2:10–11).
56 Ibid., p. 130 (2:13).
57 Avicenna, *Canon*, p. 233 (1.4.5.30); see also E. Aziz, B. Nathan, and J. McKeever, "Anesthetic and Analgesic Practices in Avicenna's Canon of Medicine," *The American Journal of Chinese Medicine* 28, 1 (2000): 147–151.
58 Avicenna, *Canon*, p. 234 (1.4.5.30).
59 Della Porta, *Magia naturalis*, pp. 150–151: "maximeque apud Medicos sunt existimationis, ludificando per somnum aliquorum dolores." Similar recipes for opium-based anesthetic for surgery circulated in the literature on secrets.
60 Salvi da Macerata, *Il chirurgo*, p. 155: "l'olio di oliva maturo, d'amandole dolci, di rosso d'uovo; latte, botiro, grasso di pollo, d'oca, di coniglio, e simili."
61 Ibid., pp. 155–156.
62 Dalla Croce, *Cirugia universale*, fol. 89v-90r. Medieval and Renaissance surgeons were highly skeptical of opium-based narcotics, including the almost mythical *spongia soporifera*, because they believed them to be too dangerous and difficult to dose; see McVaugh, *The Rational Surgery*, pp. 106–110; Cohen, *The Modulated Scream*, pp. 108–110; De Moulin, "A Historical-Phenomenological Study," p. 559; Walton O. Schalick, III, "To Market, to Market: The Theory and Practice of Opiates in the Middle Ages," in Marcia Meldrum, ed. *Opioids and Pain Relief: A Historical Perspective* (Seattle: IASP Press, 2003), pp. 5–20.
63 Elideo Padoani, *Processus, Curationes et Consilia in curandis particularibus morbis, quæ prosperos habuerunt eventus . . . Medicinæ Candidatis in praxi cum sequentibus communicata* (Leipzig: Nicholas Nerlicht, 1607), pp. 308–310.

64 ASB, Assunteria di Studio, 100 (pages are not numbered).
65 Bartolomeo Maggi, "De vulnerum, a bombardarum, & sclopetorum globulis illatorum, & de eorum symtpomatum curatione, & medicamenta ipsis ulceribus curandis idonea [1552]," in *De sclopettorum et tormentariorum vulnerum natura, et curatione, libri IIII* (Venice: apud Guglielmum Valgrisium, 1566), fol. 2v: "Principio nullum audivi, (licet quamplurimos in Mirandulensi obsidione perconctatus fuerim) cui a bombardicis, seu sclopetariis globulis, ictus infixus fuerit, qui in ipso ictu, caliditatem se percepisse, dixerit, sed contusionem quondam, perinde ac si trabs aliqua, vel ruina ingens, in se ictum fecisset." This book is a collection of short treatises on gunshot wounds circulating independently in the middle of the sixteenth century by Maggi, Francesco Rota, Alfonso Ferri, and Leonardo Botallo and signals the novelty of, and the growing interest for, the treatment in question. On Maggi's life and work, see Giulio Gentili, *La vita e l'opera di Bartolomeo Maggi (1516–1552)* (Bologna: Università di Bologna, 1967).
66 Maggi, *De vulnerum*, fol. 2v-3r. On the lack of incorporation of patients' pain narratives in scholastic medicine, see Fernando Salmon, "From Patient to Text? Narratives of Pain and Madness in Medical Scholasticism," in *Between Text and Patient*, pp. 373–395.
67 Maggi, *De vulnerum*, fol. 3v-5r.
68 For an introduction to the topic, see Kelly DeVries, "Military Surgical Practice and the Advent of Gunpowder Weaponry," *Canadian Bulletin of Medical History* 7, 2 (1990): 131–146.
69 Paré, *Oeuvres*, vol. 2, pp. 126–127.
70 Pierre Franco, *Chirurgie*, ed. Edouard Nicaise (Paris: Félix Alcan, 1895), pp. 99–101.
71 Crasso, *Diario empirico*, fol. 5r-v: "Finito ch'havrai di legare leggiermente il luogo offeso con qualche fascia, bisogna che non si muova, ma che stia fermo, & riposato perfino alla consolidatione, & fermezza dell'osso: Et, se il patiente, stando in questa maniera, sentisse dolore, in tal caso sarai certo, o che l'osso non sia ancora ben riposto, o che per qualche fragmento acuto proceda tale alterazione. Il segno, che l'osso sia ben riposto . . . è, che sia levato il dolore."
72 Aranzi, *De tumoribus*, p. 172.
73 Acquapendente, *L'opere*, p. 217.
74 Pedro Gil-Sotres, "Derivation and Revulsion: The Theory and Practice of Medieval Phlebotomy," in Luis García Ballester, ed. *Practical Medicine from Salerno to the Black Death* (Cambridge: Cambridge University Press, 1994), pp. 110–155. Sixteenth-century Latin short books and pamphlets on phlebotomy written by learned physicians and surgeons usually are commentaries on Galen and Avicenna's, *De sanguinis missionis* opinions, closer to scholastic discussion than to pain management manuals.
75 Magni, *Discorsi*, p. 8.
76 Ibid., p. 9.
77 Ibid., pp. 10–11. On Magni's manual multiple editions and illustrations, see Elizabeth Lincoln, "Curating the Renaissance Body (Pietro Paolo Magni's Illustrated Treatise 'Discorsi Sopra Il Modo Di Sanguinare, Attaccar Le Sanguisughe, & Le Ventose, Far Le Fregagioni Vessicatorij a Corpi Humani')," *Word & Image* 17, 1–2 (2001): 42–61.
78 Magni, *Discorsi*, p. 11.
79 Ibid., pp. 11–12.
80 Ibid., p. 13.
81 Paré, *Oeuvres*, vol. 1, pp. 333–334.
82 Ibid., p. 334.
83 Besides Magni's, the other early modern famous manuals for barber-surgeons were published by Tarduccio Salvi da Macerata in 1613, by Tiberio Malfi in 1628, and by Cinthio D'Amato in 1669. For the sake of diachronic consistency, I will discuss briefly some of the aspects of Savi's and Malfi's books.
84 Tarduccio Salvi da Macerata, *Il ministro del medico* [1613] (Rome: appresso Gio. Battista Robletti, 1650), p. 1.
85 Ibid., p. 4: "Dicono i naturali, che l'inventore della phlebotomia è stato l'Hippopotamo animale, che habita presso il fiume Nilo, di grandezza simile a qualsivoglia Cavallo di

Frisia, & è di terrestre, & acquatica natura, il quale, quando si sente aggravato dalla copia del sangue, va in un canneto o cosa simile, e per istinto di natura si ferisce la vena, e ne lassa uscir tanto sangue, fin che si senta sgravato: poi trova la belletta, o fango, & ivi si imbelletta, si stagna, e serra le ferita della vena."

86 Ibid.

87 Malfi, *Nuova prattica*, p. 76: "Che però, vedesi talvolta temere, e tremare il suggetto, ancorche per altro volentieri ne starebbe egli fra mille spade, e mille lancie, con intrepido cuore; sol che di non incorrere in uno di sì fatti accidenti, par che naturalmente dubiti, e s'atterrisca. Onde gli occorra, che per star migliore, si ponga a periglio di starne per sempre manco, e storpiato."

88 Ibid., p. 79.

89 Ibid., pp. 79–80.

90 Ibid., p. 81.

91 Ibid., pp. 136–137: "Il timore veramente è cagione frequentissima ne' pusillanimi, che apprendono per terribil cosa la sagnìa . . . Il modo poi da notarsi in simili occorrenze sarà; quanto al timore, conoscendo la persona di colui per pusillanimità mutarsi; perché dalla sola immaginatione viene il male; ella sola similmente attendasi con altra contraria a divertire, come di persuadere, che'l salasso sia cosa assai facile, e che colui, che l'essercita avveduto, esparto, e destro ne sia; & oltre a ciò dando a credere al patiente, che per virtù oculta d'herba, o di pietra, quali forza ottengono di corroborare il cuore, facil cosa sia impedire ogni timore, . . . ma la virtù è nella immaginativa, che alterna, e volge l'huomo tutto."

92 Ibid., pp. 137–138.

93 Ibid., p. 138: "facciasi stare l'huomo coricato, e mettasi in bocca un pochetto di vino spiritoso, o in questo bagnate alcune fette di pane brustolato, e quando pure l'infermo tenesse febre; intingasi prima il pane nell'acqua rosa, e poi nel vino . . . Io più di tutti do lode al buon vino, lo che approva la Scuola Salernitana, & il commentator Arnaldo . . . Con queste cose confortato il patiente facciasi l'apertura della vena, ma picciola e stretta. Io non dico qui (per rivocare li diffusi spiriti) gli spruzzamenti dell'acqua in faccia, o sia pura, o nanfa, gli odoramenti dell'aceto, e delle specie odorose, non le ligature delle parti estreme, non i tiramenti de' capelli, e dell'orecchie; perché son cose a tutti note, e usate."

94 Fioravanti, *Cirugia*, fol. 12r-12v: "ma molto più mi maraviglio, di quei, che son feriti, che si lasciano così tormentare senza alcuna ragione che sia probabile."

95 Ibid., fol. 130v-131r and 134r. On the relevance of this criticism for learned surgeons in Italy, see Cynthia Klestinec, "Renaissance Surgeons: Anatomy, Manual Skill, and the Visual Arts," in Peter Distelzweig, Peter Benjamin Goldberg, and Evan R. Ragland, eds. *Early Modern Medicine and Natural Philosophy* (Dordrecht: Springer, 2016), pp. 43–58.

96 Dalla Croce, *Cirugia universale*, fol. 11r.

97 Ibid., fol. 8v.

98 Seneca, *Epistolae*, xcv; quoted by Ian MacLean, *The Renaissance Notion of Woman: A Study in the Fortunes of Scholasticism and Medical Science in European Intellectual Life* (Cambridge: Cambridge University Press, 1985), p. 42.

99 On sexuality, gender and sexual difference in pre-modern Europe, see Danielle Jacquart and Claude Thomasset, *Sexuality and Medicine in the Middle Ages*, tr. Matthew Adamson (Princeton: Princeton University Press, 1988), pp. 67–120; Cadden, *The Meanings*, pp. 167–227; Pomata, "Menstruating Men," pp. 110–152; Katharine Park, "Cadden, Laqueur, and the 'One-Sex Body'," *Medieval Feminist Forum* 46, 1 (2010): 96–100; Monica Green, *Making Women's Medicine Masculine: The Rise of Male Authority in Pre-Modern Gynaecology* (Oxford: Oxford University Press, 2008), pp. 141–162; King, *The One-Sex Body*, pp. 49–70.

100 See MacLean, *The Renaissance Notion*, pp. 28–46; Francine Daenens, "Superiore perché inferiore: il paradosso della superiorità della donna in alcuni trattati italiani del Cinquecento," in Vanna Gentili, ed. *Trasgressione tragica e norma domestica: esemplari di*

tipologie femminili dalla letteratura europea (Rome: Edizioni di Storia e Letteratura, 1983), pp. 7–50; Ray, *Daughters of Alchemy*, pp. 73–110. On "Renaissance feminism," see Sarah G. Ross, *The Birth of Feminism: Woman as Intellect in Renaissance Italy and England* (Cambridge: Harvard University Press, 2009), pp. 1–16.

101 Camerata's life is not well known. He was active at the court of the Spanish courts of Naples and Madrid and dedicated the section on men's and women's honor to Ana Mendoza de Silva (1540–1592), princess of Eboli.

102 For the whole discussion, see Girolamo Camerata da Randazzo, *Trattato dell'honor vero et del vero dishonore* (Bologna: per Alessandro Benacci, 1567), fol. 10v-14r.

103 Ibid., fol. 14r-15r.

104 Ibid., fol. 15r-v: "il corpo è instrumento dell'anima; onde quando il corpo è ben complessionato, & organizato tanto opera l'anima più, o meno perfettamente."

105 Ibid., fol. 16v: "e perciò potremmo concludere, la Donna essere temperata rispetto all'Huomo)."

106 Ibid., fol. 17r: "per la siccità più atto alle fatiche, e più forte, & per la calidità più audace e animoso . . . presto nelle attioni, & atto molto alle cose attive."

107 Ibid., fol. 17r-v: "più stabili, più honeste, più sane, atta ad haver più lunga vita . . . anzi, esse sono superiori a gli Huomini nel poter imparare lettere, & attendere alle contemplative; percioché se ogni nostra cognitione viene dal senso, & per essere elle più vicine alla temperatura hanno ben anco senso più temperato; seguita che l'intelletto loro sia anco più perfetto." Camerata also mentioned a "Gentil Donna" in Bologna who studied not only poetry but also the philosophy of Aristotle in all its branches.

108 Surgical conditions such as bladder stones were considered to affect mostly men, and the procedure of extraction was much more complex and painful in men than in women, but this was for physiological and anatomical reasons, not moral.

109 Magni, *Discorsi*, fol. 64r.

110 Ibid.

111 Cinzio D'Amato, *Prattica nuova et utilissima. Di tutto quello, ch'al diligente Barbiero s'appartiene: cioè di cavar sangue, medicar ferrite, & balsamar corpi humani* (Venice: appresso Gio. Battista Brigna, 1669), p. 19.

112 Gabriele Ferrara, *Nova selva di cirugia* (Venice: per Bartolomeo carampello, 1596), fol. 12r-13r.

113 François Rousset, *Traitté nouveau de l'hysterotomotokie* [1581], tr. Valerie Worth-Stylianou, *Pregnancy and Childbirth in Early Modern France. Treatises by caring Physicians and Surgeons (1581–1625)* (Toronto: The Other Voice in Early Modern Europe: The Toronto Series, 2013), p. 23.

114 Cohen, *The Modulated Scream*, pp. 102–103, 131–133.

115 Giovanni Marinello, *Le medicine pertinenti alle infermità delle donne* (Venice: appresso Francesco de Franceschi, 1563), fol. 268r: "Però imponiamo, che la donna sentendosi da gravissimi dolori punta gridi: percioché è atto, che porge gran refrigerio alla sopravvenuta noia."

116 Jean Liebaut, *Trois livres appurtenant aux infirmitez et maladies des femmes* [1582], in *Pregnancy and Childbirth in Early Modern France*, p. 119.

117 Scipione Mercurio, *La commare o raccoglitrice* (Venice: appresso Gio. Battista Cion, 1596), pp. 55–56.

118 BAB, Gozzadini, Documenti 2, 1, fol. 126r: "al quale ho posto nome Gio. Battista, sì per rinovare mio Padre, che havea questo nome, come perché trovandosi lei, aggravata da estremi dolori vinto io da compassione, et pietà, in vederla stare in tanta pena, non senza pericolo della vita."

119 Liebaut, *Trois livres*, in *Pregnancy and Childbirth in Early Modern France*, p. 124, note 194; for the colonial implications of the idea that black women could give birth with no pain, see Malcomson, *Studies of Skin Color*, pp. 147–168.

120 Helen King, "The Early Anodynes: Pain in the Ancient World," in Ronald D. Mann, ed. *The History of the Management of Pain: From Early Principles to Present Practice* (Carnforth: Parthenon, 1988), pp. 51–62, especially pp. 58–59.

121 On the ethics of knights, see Mazo Karras, *From Boys to Men*, pp. 20–66; Gehl, "Military Courtesy," pp. 55–76; Vigarello, "The Upward Training," pp. 148–199.

122 Andrew Wear, *Knowledge and Practice in English Medicine, 1550–1680* (Cambridge: Cambridge University Press, 2000), pp. 241–248. Despite his alternative theory of diseases and the physiology of human bodies, Paracelsus never developed a deeper conception of pain than the one discussed in the Galenic tradition. The Swiss reformer of medicine, who used to define himself a surgeon more than a physician, avoided all knife surgery, put forward chemical remedies for all surgical conditions, was respectful of patients' pain, and tried to minimize it whenever possible. For example, he considered that the pain patients felt in dislocations came from the acidity of the liquid that broke from the damaged parts; or, prior to treating wounds, he recommended to soothe the pain with fairly standard remedies, such as chamomile and olive oil. See, respectively, Paracelsus, *Chirurgiae minoris*, p. 16 and *Chirurgia Magna*, p. 12 in *Opera omnia medico-chemico-chirurgica, vol. III: Chirurgica opera complectens* (Geneva: Jean-Antoine and Samuel De Tournes, 1658). See also Walter Pagel, *Paracelsus: An Introduction to Philosophical Medicine in the Era of the Renaissance*, 2nd ed. (New York: Karger, 1982).

123 Michael McVaugh, "Treatment of Hernia in the Later Middle Ages: Surgical Correction and Social Construction," in Roger Kenneth French, ed. *Medicine from the Black Death to the French Disease* (London: Ashgate, 1998), pp. 131–155, quotation on pp. 145–146.

124 There is only one exception in which patients were blamed in moral terms. It was the case of the application of the so-called actual cautery, namely red-hot iron tools to induce cicatrization and stop the blood flow, and "potential cautery," or the application of caustic topic remedies for the same purposes. In the sixteenth century, this distinction between forms of cauterization and the relative blaming of patients who appeared to regularly choose the "wrong" one had already become traditional. Indeed, in such cases, surgeons reported that patients did greatly favor the application of caustic remedies over red-hot iron, because they were afraid of the latter. Doctors thus blamed them for choosing the remedy that was, despite appearances, the most painful. But in this case patients were blamed because they claimed they knew better than their healers. In other words, patients were guilty not of being cowards but of not trusting the epistemic authority of surgeons – not because they were not men enough to tolerate pain. Many surgeons repeated this point for centuries. See, for example, Guy de Chauliac, *Inventarium*, vol. 1, p. 414; Paré, *Oeuvres*, vol. 2, p. 588.

125 The partial exception being the brief booklet of theoretical commentary on the authorities' ideas and definitions of pain by Simone Porzio, *De Dolore*, quoted above. I say partial exception because this is not a surgery booklet but rather a learned commentary on Galen, Aristotle, and Avicenna; it could be called a book on the philosophy of pain.

126 Paré, *Oeuvres*, vol. 1, pp. 30–31.

127 The passage is from the Hippocratic Oath and says: "I will not use the knife on sufferers from stone, but I will leave it such as are craftsmen therein;" quoted by de Moulin, *A History of Surgery*, p. 6. The *norcini* were highly specialized empiric surgeons who performed the most painful procedures such as bone-setting, treatment for hernias and stones, tooth extraction, and the cure of cataracts. They were well-respected practitioners and frequently hired as public servants and hospital surgeons from the fourteenth well into the eighteenth centuries. See Katherine Park, "Stones, Bones, and Hernias: Surgical Specialists in Fourteenth- and Fifteenth-Century Italy," in *Medicine from the Black Death to the French Disease*, pp. 110–130; Gianfranco Cruciani, *Cerusici e fisici: preciani e nursini dal XIV al XVIII secolo: storia e antologia* (Terni: Thyrus, 1999), pp. 13–18 and on Scacchi, pp. 178–187.

128 Durante Scacchi, *Sussidio di medicina* (Venice: presso Francesco Rampazzetto, 1609), fol. 36v.

129 Ibid., fol. 35v.
130 Quoted by Emilie Savage-Smith, "The Practice of Surgery in Islamic Lands: Myth and Reality," *Social History of Medicine* 13, 2 (2000): 307–321, p. 320.
131 The connection of pain representations with martyrs, anatomical models, and soldiers in the sixteenth century has been made by Moscoso, *Pain*, pp. 18–20; the cultural relationship of pain with religious, medical, and judicial truth has been stressed by Cohen, *The Modulated Scream*; on the affinities between martyrs and human dissection in medieval and Renaissance Italy, see Katharine Park, "The Life of the Corpse: Division and Dissection in Late Medieval Europe," *Journal of the History of Medicine and Allied Sciences* 50 (1995): 111–132.
132 Morris, *The Culture of Pain*, pp. 36–37.
133 E.P. Thompson, "The Moral Economy of the English Crowd in the Eighteen Century," in E.P. Thompson, ed. *Customs in Common* (New York: Norton, 1991), pp. 185–258. Significantly, historians of pre-modern pain too have made use of the notion of "economy" but in a rather unsystematic fashion: see Cohen, *The Modulated Scream*, p. 108; Moscoso, *Pain*, pp. 56–67. Lorraine Daston has used this concept to describe the epistemological relations between scientists and their objects of knowledge. Daston acknowledged that her use of the notion has very little in common with Thompson's, but nonetheless the two uses share one crucial feature: moral economies are always "legitimizing tools" that balance different elements within a system of values and beliefs. See Lorraine Daston, "The Moral Economy of Science," *Osiris* 10 (1995): 2–24, p. 3. For a different use of the phrase, see Steven Shapin, *A Social History of Truth: Civility and Science in Seventeenth-Century England* (Chicago: The University of Chicago Press, 1994), p. 27.
134 Pomata, *Contracting a Cure*, p. 93.
135 Ibid., p. 117.
136 Jean-Claude Chesnais, *Histoire de la violence de 1800 à nos jours* (Paris: Laffonte, 1980); Jonathan Davies, "Introduction," in Jonathan Davies, ed. *Aspects of Violence in Renaissance Europe* (Farnham: Ashgate, 2013), pp. 1–15.
137 Carroll, *Blood and Violence*, pp. 330–333.
138 See Chapter 1. On the tightening up and verticalization of social hierarchies in health care and poor relief institutions during the seventeenth century, see Gianna Pomata, "Medicine for the Poor in 18th and 19th Century Bologna," in Ole Peter Grell, Andrew Cunningham, and Bernd Roeck, eds. *Health Care and Poor Relief in 18th and 19th Century Southern Europe* (Aldershot: Ashgate, 2005), pp. 229–249.
139 On this point, see Mariacarla Gadebusch-Bondio, "On the Function, Utility, and Fragility of the Nose: Early Modern Patients and their Surgeons," *Nuncius* 32 (2017): 25–51, p. 51.
140 See Barbara H. Rosenwein, *Generations of Feeling: A History of Emotions, 600–1700* (Cambridge: Cambridge University Press, 2016), pp. 3–10. Rosenwein defines such communities as groups of people sharing "norms concerning the emotions that they value and deplore and the modes of expressing them" (p. 3).
141 Tagliacozzi, *De curtorum*, p. 107 (1:85).
142 Ibid., pp. 101–102 (1:80–81).
143 Bourke, *The Story of Pain*, p. 8.

CONCLUSION

The place of Tagliacozzi

Historians of plastic surgery tend to agree on the fact that such a monumental and innovative work as Tagliacozzi's *De curtorum* remained virtually without any following until the late eighteenth century. Many scholars wrote that right after its publication the book had no favorable reception at all and was, in best case, forgotten and, in the worst, ridiculed or rejected. Besides the argument based on the French disease that I examined in Chapter 1, a variety of other scarcely plausible reasons have been put into play to explain this situation. As possible culprits the following phenomena have been mentioned: the paucity of copies of the book; the premature death of Tagliacozzi; and the opposition to aesthetic practices by the Counter-Reformation Church. The problem is that Tagliacozzi and the other major Italian proponents of facial surgery and learned cosmetics were all well-established figures with no problem whatsoever with the Catholic Church.[1] As for the argument that there were too few copies of the book, a quick research on World Cat proves it wrong. I will only recall that in 1597 a pirate edition of *De curtorum* was published in Florence and another one in Frankfurt in 1598.[2]

At a closer look, it appears that Tagliacozzi's book was not at all neglected by his contemporaries and immediate followers but rather that it became the subject of a complex and fragmented reception. First, I will underline the deep resonances of reconstructive surgery and Tagliacozzi's method in two important branches of seventeenth-century medical and natural philosophical culture: teratology and the debate around mechanism and empiricism. Reconstructive surgery struck some important chords concerning the epistemology and the ontology of the "age of the new." Then I will show that in the seventeenth century this surgical method was present in two distinct kinds of medical writings or "epistemic genres." The first is that of collections of *observationes*, especially in the German-speaking lands; the second is the alchemical literature on sympathies and magnetism, especially in England. In this way, I am going to sketch a map of the geographic spread of the technique of reconstructive surgery between the fifteenth and the seventeenth centuries.

Liceti and monsters

While early modern European physicians and naturalists were notoriously highly fascinated by monsters, such creatures elicited curiosity and wonder only when they were confined to their own specific spaces in books, paintings, museum collections, or freak shows. Everyday monstrously disfigured faces would certainly cause horror.[3] Horror and repugnance formed a mixed reaction in the beholder who happened to come across disfigured people. The disfigured person was similar to a monster, but not quite like it, because its status was the product of injury or illness and not of congenital defects or its belonging to a strange, exotic race (Figure 7.1).[4]

Fortunio Liceti (1577–1657) – polymath, antiquarian, physician, natural historian, and natural philosopher – was one of the key figures of early modern

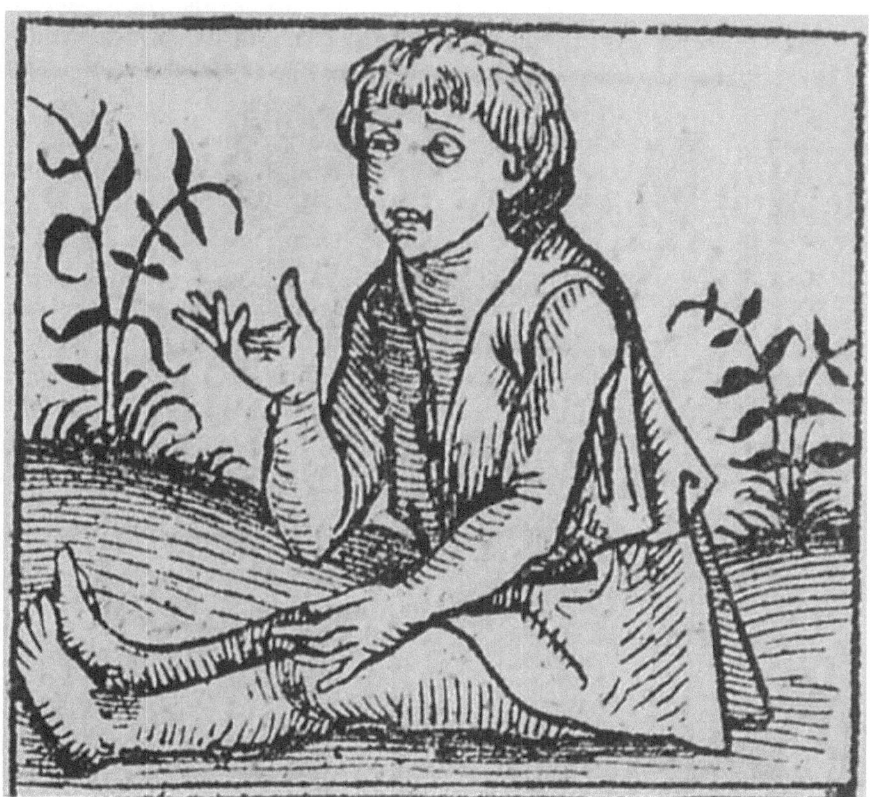

FIGURE 7.1 Hartmann Schedel, *Nuremberg Chronicles* (1493): the noseless people.

teratology. Liceti had studied arts and medicine in Bologna, where he had met Tagliacozzi as a teacher; he then moved to Padua, where he became professor of theoretical medicine.[5] His book on monsters was first published, without illustrations, in 1616; a second, beautifully illustrated edition came out in Venice in 1634. While Liceti is often credited as being one of the first thinkers who naturalized monsters, his legacy is more nuanced, because he never refrained from considering certain kinds of monsters as omens and signs of divine wrath and never fully abandoned references to the intervention of demonic forces in the course of natural life. However, it is true that Liceti made a systematic effort to classify monsters and that he attempted to follow a rather naturalistic definition. According to Liceti, a monster was

> a being under heaven which provokes in the observer horror and astonishment by the incorrect form of its members, and is produced rarely, begotten, by virtue of a secondary plan of nature, as a result of some hitch in the causes of its origin . . . [monsters are] faults of nature when she does not proceed in the right way.[6]

And he added: "It is in this [monstrous births] that I see the convergence of both nature and art, because one or the other not being able to make what they want, at least they make what they can."[7] Here one can notice the presence of ideas of nature as an artist and of monsters as products made with imperfect material. These ideas were present in Tagliacozzi's book as well, where he wrote that monsters occurred when "there is too much or too little material; it resists the artificial manipulation or is adversely affected by unaccustomed and strange humors, which hinder its inherent perfection."[8] Yet another example of the ontological proximity of art and nature.

Liceti's book made reference to grafting and monstrosities in plants and humans. He made use of Tagliacozzi's surgical procedure as a tool to clarify the status of monsters caused by an excess of matter. While discussing the tenth cause of *monstri excedenti*, which is some kind of "violent concussion of the body of the mother," Liceti described the case of a pair of twins, "already formed," who suffered from a blow to the pregnant woman's body. The parts of the bodies of the twins could be excoriated and coalesce through the union of blood – acting as glue – in unnatural shapes (Figure 7.2). To illustrate this process of excoriation, blood loss, and creation of monstrous forms, Liceti referred directly to Tagliacozzi's procedure.[9] Facial reconstructive surgery was not relevant for Liceti as a technical procedure in itself but rather as an epistemological analogy that strengthened his explanation of the cause of monsters, and it included the theme of grafting trees through analogies between blood and skin and between juices and bark.

> While we were students in Bologna, we have seen several times our master Tagliacozzi re-making human noses by excoriating the scars on the nose,

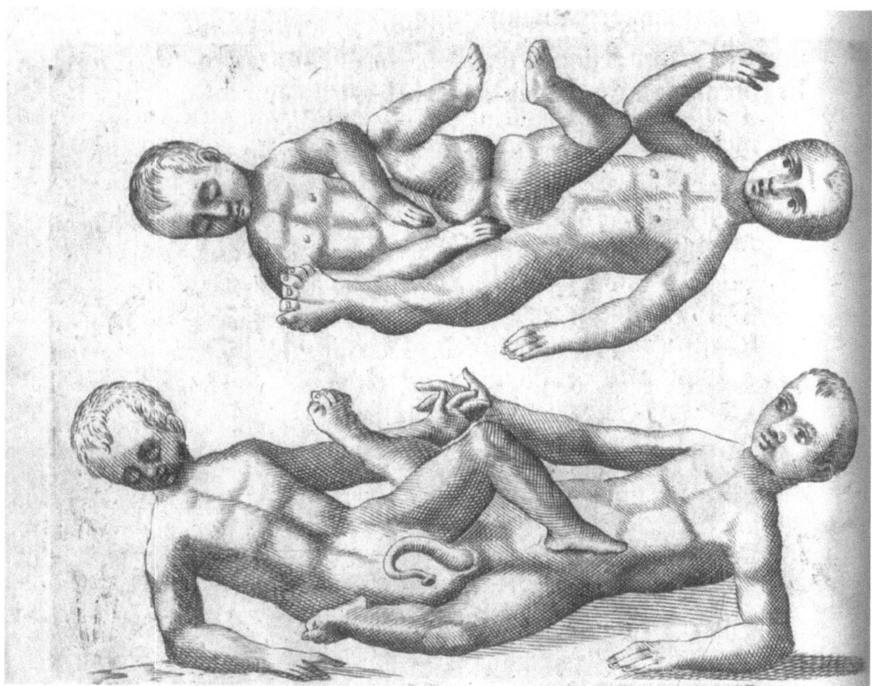

FIGURE 7.2 Fortunio Liceti, *De caussis* (1634): monstrous twins.

> and then attaching the skin of the arm to the face in the space of a few days. This can be seen even in trees when, once the bark has been removed from different parts and tied together, they are glued together through the action of the nourishing juices which flows through both parts.[10]

Liceti used his former teacher's surgical procedure as an epistemological analogy to explain the ontological status of human monsters as preternatural entities. Monsters emerged through a blind assemblage of natural causes giving way to unprecedented and singular outcomes. The artificial gave way to the preternatural, expanding the realm of the natural and, paradoxically for an Aristotelian, strengthening the dangerous analogy between natural, or divine, and human artistry.

There is more. In his discussion of "monsters with a double nature" Liceti mentioned, again with reference to Tagliacozzi, the disturbing example of man-made monsters. These were made either unintentionally by poorly skilled empirics and barber-surgeons or intentionally by the art of people seeking to make money with freak shows. The seventh cause of such *monstri ancipiti* consisted in "an imitation of nature's faults by art, not without the help of nature (*in arte peccata naturae imitante, ac non sine auxilio naturae operante*)."[11] This is a shadowing of one of the dark possibilities of the short-circuit of art and nature. Liceti could not fail to notice that "art can produce monsters." Indeed, all the works of nature were carried on by nature either alone or with some kind of cooperation. There were cases

> when art, if it is able to fashion some kind of monster, cannot help the workings of nature to this end: in fact, the origin of a monster properly depends upon nature. Indeed, the active action of the art can only apply itself to the natural things which are passive: so monsters made with the cooperation of art are to be considered as natural products. Awe can observe another benefice of the art, or in some respect a misdeed, in plants: here, living monsters can be produced; even if farmers disagree on that, they can produce one single species starting from different trees through grafting and ligations, and in this way they obtain living beings which have a monstrous nature.

Once again, the reference to plant grafting brought to Liceti's mind the memory of Tagliacozzi:

> And then our most solicitous teacher Tagliacozzi suddenly comes to mind, who used to remake ears, lips, and noses who had been cut off by joining the excoriated parts of the arm to these parts; no matter the scar that had been brought about in those parts, he could not leave the connection in a monstrous shape, as it appears in his most eloquent book.[12]

Liceti used Tagliacozzi's principle of grafting to illustrate the monstrous potential of the combination of human shapes, also alluding to artificially created monsters made through the human art of grafting. For example, Liceti reported a 1466 case of two boys in France who were struck by lightning and found attached together in one single body through their burning parts. Patients with burnings who were not treated properly could assume monstrous shapes too. And there were people who showed off monstrous humans for money.[13]

The fact that Tagliacozzi was mentioned in this context tells us something more about his difficulties and uncertainties in conceptualizing his own surgical procedure, because dangerous associations could be established between grafting, monsters, and the dishonest arts of creating artificial deformities for showing them off in freak shows. Liceti always mentioned Tagliacozzi with the greatest respect, and he used his procedure as part of his epistemology of the preternatural. But it is also clear that Tagliacozzi was operating on the dangerously porous borders between art and nature, where human artists had to intervene if they did not want to leave nature alone producing monstrous faces, as well as strong feelings of horror in the beholder.

Mechanism versus empiricism

One of Tagliacozzi's main concerns in writing a monograph on reconstructive surgery was to demonstrate that he was able to give the whole procedure a rational and normative scientific explanation. Tagliacozzi had to get rid of the association of the procedure with the empirics and the culture of secrets that surrounded it. This dichotomy between rational method and empirical practice resurfaced in the late seventeenth century, undergoing a deep conceptual shift. Grafting and reconstructive surgery were debated in a famous polemic between one of the champions of mechanical philosophy and the new microscopic anatomy, Marcello Malpighi (1628–1694), and the defender not only of the Hippocratic-Galenic tradition but also of a clinical, observation-based, pragmatic approach to medicine, Giovanni Girolamo Sbaraglia (1641–1710). One of the points of disagreement between the two Bolognese professors was precisely their interpretation of Tagliacozzi's work.

The Sbaraglia-Malpighi dispute, despite its origins in local academic and personal issues, gained European-wide visibility and at the same time both reflected and contributed to the most up-to-date debates on the new anatomy.[14] Malpighi's long reply to Sbaraglia's criticism was a reflective work, and it summarized the results of very intense decades of new anatomical research based on the principle of matter and motion, of filtration of the liquids, and on the microscopic observation of all beings, including animals and plants. Ever present throughout the whole work was the theme of nature's uniformity and of its action in terms of mechanical devices or *artifici*.[15]

In his *Anatome plantarum* (1675), Malpighi had been keen on comparing the circulation of blood and the circulation of sap in plants. In the reply to Sbaraglia, Malpighi mentioned Tagliacozzi's method as one of the examples of the usefulness of studying plant anatomy – strongly denied by Sbaraglia – because in this case the example of grafting led to find a method for reconstructing human facial parts through surgery. He explained:

> If the author requires some kind of advantage in terms of therapeutics from the examination of plant economy, he only has to look at grafting, and he will learn a method to heal wounds with no bandage and the mechanics of remaking the mutilated parts, which our own Tagliacozzi has explained so well making use of the analogy with grafting plants.[16]

Tagliacozzi's procedure was not explained in mechanical terms, but it was listed in the same paragraph and it was included under the examples of animal-plants mechanistic analogy. In the following pages Malpighi explained the similarities of blood circulation and the passing of nourishment through the veins according to hydraulic principles, valves, and so forth and referred specifically to the formations of swellings and inflated limbs.[17]

Sbaraglia replied that such a procedure came not from observation of the anatomy of plants and scientific reasoning but from mere experience and therefore could not be accounted for as a mechanical philosopher would have. Malpighi's opponent added three points against the idea that *curtorum chirurgia* actually derived from careful observation of plants and argued there was a great difference between grafting plants and treating animal wounds: the material is different; the method of fixing the parts is different; and the essence of grafting is not comparable. At best, only an a posteriori justification could be given.[18] The point is that Sbaraglia wanted to prove that such a procedure, as others, came not from observation of the anatomy of plants and scientific reasoning but from blind chance and experience and therefore could not be accounted for as Malpighi and the mechanical philosophers would have. In a way, Sbaraglia did not put into question the feasibility of facial reconstruction, but he denied it was based on rational mechanistic principles.

Reconstructive surgery could legitimately appear in one of the most advanced scientific debates of the late seventeenth century. Despite being on the "wrong" side of history, in underlining the contingency of the origins of the reconstructive method Sbaraglia proved the better epistemologist. On the other hand, the long-term role played by learned, anatomically informed surgery in the demise of Galenic physiology and the rise of mechanism and the new philosophies of the seventeenth century must be further investigated.[19] Domenico Bertoloni Meli has shown that by the beginning of the eighteenth century surgeons could identify "different cognitive horizons" than those of the physicians in that they focused on the conformation of body parts rather than on humoralism or iatrochemistry.[20] Well before that, learned surgeons like Tagliacozzi, while struggling to place their work within a Galenic-Aristotelian physiological framework centered on humors and "vital heat," contributed to shift the focus on solid organs and the circulation of fluids through such solid organs. Moreover, learned surgery contributed to the collapse of the natural and artificial distinction that was thematized by mechanical philosophers and physicians. In this respect, it is no surprise that a mechanist like Malpighi would consider Tagliacozzi's procedure with great interest.[21]

Observationes and sympathetic noses: epistemic genres

In Gianna Pomata's formulation, an "epistemic genre" is a structured and recognizable social and cultural convention for the transmission of cognitive content that can be used to trace historical changes in medical culture.[22]

Now, among the most fortunate genres of the early modern period we do not find the erudite, voluminous, humanistic monograph on one single surgical technique. Sixteenth- and early seventeenth-century European surgical works tended to be of four kinds or sub-genres. They could be comprehensive textbooks; short treatises on one single case or procedure (often occasioned by a polemic among surgeons); brief technical manuals on particularly difficult procedures (like extracting stones and treating skull fractures), new injuries (like firearms wounds), or important techniques (such as bloodletting); and edited collections of observations and/or works.[23] Tagliacozzi's book was eccentric in that it was a hybrid: part erudite commentary, part humanistic natural-history-style treatise, part technical surgical book. Moreover, this hybrid was applied to one single surgical practice and not a general medical topic. As we have seen,

Tagliacozzi's subject emerged as a unified topic, worthy of a book-length effort, from a series of dispersed cases circulating in the Renaissance. I argue that the unity he gave his topic broke down immediately thereafter and the reconstructive procedure started circulating again in the form of cases, but within new epistemic genres.

By looking at the rising epistemic genres of *curationes, observationes, consultationes*, and *consilia*, one finds that reconstructive surgery of facial mutilations was often present in these works, which followed a peculiar distribution centered on northern Europe rather than on the more conservative Italian medical circles. Consequently, Tagliacozzi's procedure was described in short paragraphs, rarely accompanied by new cases, and detached from the complex culture of the face that informed the Bolognese's book. Early seventeenth-century examples include *Consilia Medicinalia, cum Mixtim Praestantissimorum Italiae Medicorum*, published in Frankfurt in 1605, collected and edited by Joseph Lautenbach, with *consilia* by Antonio Maria Venosti and Giulio Cesare Claudini from Bologna;[24] Johannes Schenck von Grafenberg's *Observationum medicarum rariorum*, published different parts in Frankfurt between 1594 and 1599 and reprinted many times, a well-received anthology of cases by a very famous and influential physician;[25] the *Observationum et curationum chirurgicarum* by Fabricius Hildanus, published posthumously in Frankfurt in 1646 but collected between the late sixteenth and the early seventeenth century;[26] Vincenzo Gosio's *Observationes*, published in Turin in 1606 and later included by Albrecht Haller in his *Bibliotheca Chirurgica*; and Philippus Salmuth's *Observationum medicarum*, published in Brunschvig in 1648, reporting a new case of a man who received a blow while fencing.[27]

The second channel of the reception of reconstructive surgery is less easily identifiable as an epistemic genre but nonetheless possessed a remarkable coherence. In the literature on alchemical, sympathetic, or magnetic medicine a story circulated of an "allo-graft," a skin grafting procedure involving the nose from a donor, generally a nobleman "borrowing" the skin or the flesh from one of his slaves or servants. The story always ended with the death of the donor, which corresponded to the fall of the nobleman's nose. Probably, the origin of this late sixteenth-century story is a 1558 letter sent by Elisio Calenzio to his friend Orpianus after he had his nose restored by the Brancas in Tropea, reported in 1580 by Etienne Gourmelain in his *Chirurgicae artis*. The letter included the following passage: "Branca, a man of genius and skill, has learnt to graft on noses (*nares inserere*) by either taking part of the arm or by borrowing one from a slave."[28] However, the most complete and entertaining story was written by the Flemish iatrochemist and moderate Paracelsian Jean-Baptiste Van Helmont in 1621.

> This one experiment [i.e., the slave donor graft] of all others, cannot but be free from all suspect of imposture, and illusion of the Devil. A certain inhabitant of Bruxels, in a combat had his nose mowed off, addressed himself to Tagliacozzius a famous Chirurgeon, living at Bononia, that he might procure a new one; and when he feared the incision of his own arm,

> he hired a Porter [servant] to admit it, out of whose arm, having first given the reward agreed upon, at length he dig'd a new nose. About thirteenth months after his return to his own Contrey, on a sudden the ingrafted nose grew cold, putrified, and within a few days, dropt off. To those of his friends, that were curious in the exploration of the cause of this unexpected misfortune, it was discovered, that the Porter expired, neer about the same punctilio of time, wherein the nose grew frigid and cadaverous. There are at Bruxels, yet surviving, some of good repute, that were eyewitnesses of these occurrences. Is not this Magnetism of manifest affinity with mumy, whereby the nose, enjoying, by title and right of inoculation, a community of life, on a sudden mortified on the other side of the Alpes? I pray what is there in this Superstition? What of attent and exalted Imagination?[29]

Van Helmont referred here to the concept of *mumia*, an alchemical idea that "guaranteed the connection, unity, and solidarity of the organic parts thanks to which the procedure is destined to succeed" by granting the mutual action of invisible forces and material particles at a distance.[30] These ideas had developed from the debate on the "weapon salve," "an ointment that supposedly cured wounds through magical sympathies after being applied not to the wound itself but to the weapon that had caused it."[31] Thomas Browne (1605–1682) used the concept of "magnetism" to explain this allo-graft of a nose in his *Pseudodoxia epidemica*, published in London in 1646. In general, unseen forces were also classified under the rubric of "sympathy," as argued by Kenelm Digby (1603–1665), a botanist and an early member of the Royal Society, in his 1658 *Late Discourse*, whose 1661 Frankfurt edition was accompanied by an illustration of the sympathetic nose.[32]

It is this story that gave later English writers outside of the medical profession, from Samuel Butler (1613–1680) to Joseph Addison (1672–1719), the occasion to heavily satirize Tagliacozzi and reconstructive surgery in general.[33] Significantly enough, natural philosophers engaged in experiments on animal grafting performed with dogs and cocks at the Royal Society in the years 1663 and 1664 did not mention Tagliacozzi at all.[34]

The most important reason for the dissemination of this story in the regions in which iatrochemistry was most popular is its connection with an alchemical and specifically Paracelsian imagery of cultivating artificial life and the myth of the *homunculus*. This imagery became popular especially in the first part of the seventeenth century, before being played down as dangerous and potentially associated with demonic forces by alchemists themselves in the second half of the century.[35] It was indeed by the middle of the seventeenth century that satires on Tagliacozzi began to be written. Given that Tagliacozzi's book was present in all major European libraries, I believe it was within this context that stories began to circulate with reference to the falling of the nose when the donor died. Probably, Tagliacozzi's work came to be considered an example of a tradition focused on rebirth and artificial life – dangerous or ridiculous fantasy of replicating or even improving upon nature's creativity.

The story of the sympathetic nose traveled south of the Alps too. Tommaso Campanella (1568–1639) mentioned it as "the Magic of the Tropeans" in his 1620 *De sensu rerum et magia*, where he interpreted it on the basis of the theory of universal sympathies and antipathies he had found in Della Porta.[36] The Rome-based Jesuit and polymath Athanasius Kircher (1602–1680), while repeating it with an abundance of details and the playful pleasure that he often displayed in his works, considered it a fake, good only for the *vulgus*, and believed that no communication at a distance was possible in surgery.[37]

In this literature on nose allo-grafts Tagliacozzi's procedure was not always reported correctly, and especially his insistence on grafting skin instead of flesh was ignored. Reconstructive surgery was practiced in Italy and beyond, from Padua to Naples to Madrid[38] to Tropea (in Calabria), by empirical, workshop-trained surgeons, and not all of them respected the technical norms described by Tagliacozzi. It is also a fact that the language of marvels and wonders has constantly been associated with the procedure. For example, the German traveler Johannes Heinrich Pflaumern (1585–1671) wrote about Bologna in a 1625 travel guide to Italy:

> You will see a monument in honor of Tagliacozzi placed there when he was still alive. He excelled in a new method of healing: he replaced lacking lips, ears and noses so skillfully that his work was almost miraculous.[39]

Now, this undecided ontology of nature puts reconstructive surgery in close touch with Renaissance "natural magic," which among other things was associated too with agricultural techniques and the idea of perfecting nature. Campanella's "magia tropiensis" might have been more than a casual remark. After all, the language of marvels and wonders has constantly been associated with the procedure. For example, the German traveler Johannes Heinrich Pflaumern (1585–1671) wrote about Bologna in a 1625 travel guide to Italy: "You will see a monument in honor of Tagliacozzi placed there when he was still alive. He excelled in a new method of healing: he replaced lacking lips, ears and noses so skillfully that his work was almost miraculous,"[40] a word often used in connection with natural magic.

Finally, there is the story of the posthumous trial of Tagliacozzi. The story, narrated by two chronicles and one sheet of paper found within a Bolognese copy of *De curtorum*, goes like this: early in 1600, just a couple of months after his burial in the church of San Giovanni Battista in Bologna, a group of nuns would have heard a voice speaking in the church telling them about Tagliacozzi's damnation. The Inquisition took interest in the thing, unearthed the body from its tomb, but the trial was quickly dismissed and the body soon placed in its rightful place in San Giovanni Battista (the church has been subsequently destroyed).[41] No documentation exists of this trial, and all evidence of Tagliacozzi's relationship with church authorities highlights that he never had any problem with them. But two respected chroniclers reported this story, which, therefore, I am not inclined to consider as the fruit of invention. Instead, I think the Inquisition very quickly found out this was a completely bogus accusation and dismissed all the charges. Still, the story tells us something about the fact that reconstructive surgery had the ring of magic, at least for some.

From Marsilio Ficino (1433–1499) and Pico della Mirandola (1463–1494) to Giovanbattista Della Porta – an author very well known by learned physicians gathering in the house and museum of natural historian Ulisse Aldrovandi in the late sixteenth century – natural magic had been carefully distinguished from black or demonic magic. The latter aimed at producing physical effects with the active help of demons, while the former was described as the operative part of natural philosophy or the way of acting upon nature and producing wondrous effects with the help of natural forces alone.[42] As we have seen in Chapter 5, for Della Porta natural magic was an observation of the operations of nature and an imitation of them, a definition that resonated with what many writers on medicine and agriculture had said.

The same tension between surpassing nature and worshipping nature's creativity, combined with the tension between knowing the regularity of nature and producing wondrous and singular effects, is shared by Tagliacozzi's surgery and natural magic. These suggestions are strengthened by the fact that both made a reference to agriculture; that both had to do with cosmetics and the production or restoration of beauty without identifying themselves with them; and that both could not fully explain their practical way of doing things.[43] Just as traditional Galenism and Galenic surgery could not fully account for a technique Tagliacozzi "rationalized" from the empirics, in the same way the secrets and recipes Della Porta took from artisans could not be fully explained by a new theoretical physics, even if they were entirely "rational" and "natural."

Both Tagliacozzi's surgery and Della Porta's natural magic – besides their differences – offer the historian a precise perspective on the "birth of modern science," one that follows the bodily engagement with procedures and practices of manipulating human and natural matter, rather than theoretical speculation or mathematization. In both the cases of learned surgery and natural magic one can observe a historical process of appropriation and reproduction of artisanal ways of doing and knowing under the label of "medicine," "natural philosophy" – or, to employ an anachronistic term, "science."

In the seventeenth century, Tagliacozzi's procedure lost its coherence and became an element in different genres and other writers' bricolage. The historical conditions under which facial reconstructive surgery emerged and attracted attention had changed.

I have explained the publication of a book like *De cutorum* in late sixteenth-century Bologna by taking into account several factors: the political and ideological definitions of nobility; the social mobility of surgeons and physicians; the peculiar cultural dynamics of the history of the gendered face; the appeal of marvelous horticultural practices; and the Italian tradition of learned surgery.

I have argued that the publication of this book was something quite exceptional. The first book on reconstructive surgery of the face was inspired by the dissemination of information concerning one specific technique that spread from fifteenth-century Southern Italy to sixteenth-century Imperial Spain and, from there, to Bologna and Padua. At that point the technique solidified into a book. In turn, from the centers of learning and of the elaboration of nobility's culture and ideology of northern Italy, the description of the technique traveled north, to Switzerland and Germany, secondhand via the diffusion of genres of compilations of particulars and observations. The technique was also discussed/mentioned in Italian learned circles of physicians and natural philosophers' writings on teratology, empiricism, and mechanism. Through the development of alchemy applied to the human body, it traveled to England, where it became an object of ridicule and, finally, of political disdain. In fact, from an early eighteenth-century perspective *curtorum chirurgia* was satirized as involving the exploitation of a "poor man" by a nobleman. The Enlightenment philosopher Voltaire (1694–1778) wrote in 1752:

> Ainsi Talicotius,
> grand Esculapc d'Etrurie,
> répara tous les nez perdus
> par une nouvelle industrie:
> il vous prenoit adroitement
> un morceau du cul d'un pauvre homme,
> l'appliquait au nez proprement;
> enfin il arrivait qu'en somme,
> tout juste è la mort du préteur,
> tombait le nez de l'emprunteur,
> et souvent dans la meme bière,
> par justice et par bon accord,
> on remettait au gré du mort
> le nez auprès de son derrière.[44]

Throughout the early modern period, the technique was effectively applied very few times, but its scholarly power and its male gendering were passed on through time and space. Reconstructive surgery of the face remained mostly a male affair until well into the twentieth century, when it became an elective practice and got entangled with different contexts of selfhood, gender, and power. Contemporary science and technology keep working on the human face. Only to mention a few examples: facial recognition procedures promise to make digital data repositories safer (even if they generate new fears about identity theft);[45] since 2010 surgeons are able to make face transplants;[46] neuroscientists intensely study neural paths associated to facial recognition in animals and humans.[47] So much has changed from the sixteenth century, but the sciences of the face are still linked to issues of identity, gender, power, and knowledge.

Notes

1 Right after his death and burial in the church of San Giovanni Battista, the body of Tagliacozzi was taken away from its tomb under suspicion of heresy and magic; the documents of the Inquisition were lost, but the surgeon's body was placed again in its place by 1600, and therefore the investigation must have led nowhere. See Teach-Gnudi and Webster, *The Life and Times*, pp. 236–247.

2 Tomba et al., "Gaspare Tagliacozzi, Pioneer," pp. 446–447. Before the nineteenth century, the English surgeon Alexander Read published a partial vernacular translation in 1678, and another Latin edition was published in Geneva in 1721. See Alexander Read, *Chirurgorum Comes: Or the Whole Practice of Chirurgery* (London: Printed by Edw. Jones, for Christopher Wilkinson, 1678); Jean Manget, *Bibliotheca Chirugica* (Geneva: sumptibus Gabriel de Tournes, 1721).

3 On monsters, see Daston and Park, *Wonders*; Arnold I. Davidson, "The Horror of Monsters," in Arnold I. Davidson, ed. *The Emergence of Sexuality* (Cambridge: Harvard University Press, 2001); A.W. Bates, *Emblematic Monsters: Unnatural Conceptions and Deformed Births in Early Modern Europe* (New York: Rodopi, 2005), pp. 11–41; Peter Burke, "Frontiers of the Monstrous," in Laura Lunger Knoppers and Joan B. Landes, eds. *Monstrous Bodies/Political Monstrosities in Early Modern Europe* (Ithaca: Cornell University Press, 2004), pp. 25–39. On the cultural and aesthetic links between normal and monstrous faces in early modern Italy, see Sandra Cheng, "The Cult of the Monstrous: Caricature, Physiognomy, and Monsters in Early Modern Italy," *Preternature: Critical and Historical Studies on the Preternatural* 1, 2 (2012): 197–231.

4 On monstrous races and the myths of the wild man, see Campbell, *Wonder & Science*, pp. 221–317; Roger Bartra, *Wild Men in the Looking Glass: The Mythic Origins of European Otherness*, tr. Carl T. Berrisford (Ann Arbor: The University of Michigan Press, 1994), pp. 149–169; Surekha Davies, *Renaissance Ethnography and the Invention of the Human: New Worlds, Maps and Monsters* (Cambridge: Cambridge University Press, 2016).

5 On Liceti and teratology, see A.W. Bates, "The *De Monstrorum* of Fortunio Liceti: A Landmark of Descriptive Teratology," *Journal of Medical Biography* 9, 1 (2001): 49–54; Enrico Fulcheri, "Fortunio Liceti: un punto di svolta negli studi sui 'mostri' e l'inizio della moderna teratologia," *Pathologica* 94 (2002): 263–268.

6 Liceti, *De monstrorum caussis* (Padua: apud P. Frambottus, 1634), pp. 4–5. For example, Aldrovandi's, *Monstrorum Historia* – published and edited by Bartolomeo Ambrosini in 1642 – still remained attached to the traditional etymology of monstrare (to show), thus considering monsters as both showing something and as beings to be shown; see Ezio Antonelli, "Ulisse Aldrovandi e la metamorfosi del mostruoso," *Studi e memorie per la storia dell'Università di Bologna* 3 (1983): 196–242.

7 Liceti, *De monstrorum*, p. 43.

8 Tagliacozzi, *De curtorum*, p. 119 (2:3).

9 Liceti, *De monstrorum*, p. 108.

10 Ibid., pp. 108–109: "Vidimus enim saepe, dum Bononiae studiis operam navaremus, eximium praeceptorem Taliacotium nares hominum praecisas refecturum prius excoriare cicatrices nasi, deinde brachii partem decorticatam naso ad unionem coaptare, ac fuere ad plusculos dies. Quin & arborum variarum partes decorticatae, ac invicem ligatae coeunt in unum corpus glutine succi alimentaris ad eas partes ab utraque arbore defluentis."

11 Ibid., p. 125.

12 Ibid., pp. 125–126: "quando ars, si aliqua est monstra effingere valens, hoc ipsum fine opera naturae praestare nequeat: immo vero quum origo monstrorum a natura praecipue pendeat. artis autem operatio sit solum applicare activa passivis naturalibus: iam physici muneris est monstra in viventium genere artis ministerio facta considerare. Porro artis beneficio, seu verius maleficio, viventia monstra effingi posse primum observamus in stirpibus; siquidem agricolae variarum arborum insitione, colligationeve, quo magis unitae stirpes specie invicem dissideant, eo ex iis coniunctis vivens monstrosam magis

naturam obtinebit . . . Deinde vero in mentem subit solertissimum praeceptorem Taliacotium per insitionem consuevisse curtas aures, & nares, curtaque labia curare, brachio primum partibus illis excoriatis coniuncto; quod poterat nullo negocio inducta cicatrice iis partibus, coniunctum relinquere in monstrosam effigiem: ut apparet ex eius disertissimo libello."

13 Ibid., pp. 126–127. By the fifteenth century, in Italy parents of monstrous children regularly showed them for money. By 1531, such displays began to be officially licensed, and over the course of the sixteenth century references to licenses were to be found in France, England, and Germany as well. Early modern viewers of monsters could react with either pleasure or horror, depending on the circumstances. One can suppose that such shows were frequent enough. Bolognese chronicler Francesco Ghiselli reported that in May 1594 "a 12-year old monster was brought to Bologna, short (at the level of a not to tall man's knee), with a beautiful face, with one hand similar to a duck's leg and the other flattened with only two fingers, the arms were like a tree's branch, and he walked on his knees bringing his legs similar to a goat's legs, and he used to carry more than 50 libbre of weight in his mouth walking around a room, and those who wanted to see him had to pay 4 coins (*Fu condotto in Bologna mostro di circa dodici anni piccolo alla ginocchia d'huomo, non grande, bello di faccia, mani l'una somigliante a piedi d'oca e l'altra per il mezzo appiattita con solamente due dita per ciascuna parte, e le braccia come tronchi d'arbori, giva con le ginocchia tirandosi dietro le gambe fatte a guisa di quelle di capra, che altrimenti non poteva, portava caminando per le stanze più di 50 libre di peso in bocca, e chi lo voleva vedere pagava sei quattrini*)." See BUB 770, Ghiselli, *Memorie*, vol. 19 (1591–1595), fol. 668; Daston and Park, *Wonders*, pp. 190–191.

14 The first blow was Girolamo Sbaraglia, *De recentiorum medicorum studio dissertatio epistolaris ad amicum* (Parma: per Galeazzo Rosati, 1690). This pamphlet was intended to make an intervention within an already existing controversy involving a supposed opposition to a reform of the studio promoted by Malpighi at Bologna. Among other things that were going on between them, we should be aware that in 1659 Malpighi's brother Bartolomeo had killed Sbaraglia's brother Tommaso in a dispute over real estate between the two families. So it is clear enough that any reading of this polemic must be informed by the context of a longer dispute between the traditionalists and the neoterics in Bologna, which put at stake not only intellectual prestige but real power in the city and in the university. For example, Malpighi was admitted to the College of Physicians only in 1691, after he had been appointed Papal archiater of Innocent XII (ruled 1691–1700), 38 years after graduation. Moreover, Malpighi was never appointed official anatomist for the public dissection, but he always taught "practical medicine" in Bologna. Historian Marta Cavazza has rightly argued that Malpighi has been too easily depicted as a hero of *libertas philosophandi* against the dark forces of scholastic obscurantism. On this controversy, see Marta Cavazza, "The Uselessness of Anatomy: Mini and Sbaraglia versus Malpighi," in Domenico Bertoloni Meli, ed. *Malpighi Anatomist and Physician* (Florence: Olschki, 1997), pp. 129–145; and Domenico Bertoloni Meli, *Mechanism, Experiment, Disease: Marcello Malpighi and Seventeenth-Century Anatomy* (Baltimore: Johns Hopkins University Press, 2011), pp. 307–330. On the history of the metaphor of the body as machine, see the survey by Jessica Riskin, "Medical Knowledge: The Adventures of Mr. Machine with Morals," in Carole Reeves, ed. *A Cultural History of the Human Body in the Age of Enlightenment* (London: Bloomsbury, 2014), pp. 73–91; and Domenico Bertoloni Meli, "Machines of the Body in the Seventeenth Century," in *Early Modern Medicine*, pp. 91–116.

15 Bertoloni Meli, *Mechanism, Experiment, Disease*, pp. 199–226.

16 Marcello Malpighi, *Opera posthuma* (Londini: impressis A. & J. Churchill, 1697), p. 170: "Se l'autore essige di vantaggio dalla considerazione dell'economia delle piante, in ordine a remedii, ch'è quello, che li preme, osservi l'inserire, che cavarà un metodo per sanare le ferite senza tasta, la mecanica di rifare le parti multilate, tanto illustrata dal nostro Tagliacozzio coll'analogia dell'inserire le piante."

17 Ibid., pp. 172–173.

18 Giovanni Girolamo Sbaraglia, *Oculorum et mentis vigiliae ad distinguendum studium anatomicum et adpraxin medicam diridendam* (Bologna: typis P. M. Monti, 1704), pp. 196–201.

19 Oswei Temkin's classic account of the influence of surgery in the "rise of modern medicine" focused exclusively on the late eighteenth century and the early nineteenth century: see Oswei Temkin, "The Role of Surgery in the Rise of Modern Medical Thought," *Bullettin of the History of Medicine* 25, 3 (1951): 248–259. Accounts of the seventeenth-century transformation of the Galenic body into the mechanical body generally refer to the theory of circulation and the use of microscopes, but surgery is rarely ever mentioned; see, for example, Rafael Mandressi, *Le regard de l'anatomiste: Dissections et invention du corps en Occident* (Paris: Seuil, 2003), pp. 147–154. Even studies that focus on the manual character of pre-modern anatomy and its impact on physiology fail to take into account the role of surgery and surgeons. See, for example, Andrew Cunningham, "The Pen and the Sword: Recovering the Disciplinary Identity of Physiology and Anatomy before 1800: II: Old Anatomy: The Sword," *Studies in History and Philosophy of Biological & Biomedical Sciences* 34, 1 (2003): 51–76. Giovanna Ferrari has underlined the social and intellectual prestige of Italian learned surgeons in the sixteenth century but claimed that they had no impact on the changes of seventeenth-century medicine: Giovanna Ferrari, "Tra medicina e chirurgia: la rinascita dell'anatomia e la dissezione come spettacolo," in *Il Rinascimento italiano e l'Europa*, 341–366, especially pp. 365–366.

20 Domenico Bertoloni Meli, *Visualizing Disease: The Art and History of Pathological Illustrations* (Chicago: The University of Chicago Press, 2018), p. 41.

21 In recent times, historians have begun to stress the importance of medicine to understand the reality and changes of early modern times: see Cook, "The History of Medicine and the Scientific Revolution"; Nancy Siraisi, "Medicine, 1450–1620, and the History of Science," *Isis* 103, 3 (2012): 491–514.

22 Gianna Pomata, "Sharing Cases: The *Observationes* in Early Modern Medicine," *Early Science and Medicine* 15, 3 (2010): 193–236; Gianna Pomata, "The Medical Case Narrative: Distant Reading of an Epistemic Genre," *Literature and Medicine* 32, 1 (2014): 1–23; see also Carlo Ginzburg, "Our Words, and Theirs: A Reflection on the Historian's Craft, Today," *Cromohs* 18 (2014): 97–114, especially pp. 104–109.

23 See Adalberto Pazzini, *Bio-Bibliografia di Storia della Chirurgia* (Rome: Cosmopolita, 1948); Salvatore De Renzi, *Storia della medicina*, vol. 3, pp. 626–687; Vivian Nutton, "The Humanist Surgeon," in Andrew Wear, Roger K. French, and Iain M. Lonie, eds. *The Medical Renaissance of the Sixteenth Century* (Cambridge: Cambridge University Press, 1985), pp. 75–100; Cosmacini, *La vita nelle mani*, pp. 93–133; Bertoloni Meli, *Visualizing Disease*, pp. 24–36.

24 Lautenbach, *Consilia medicinalia*, "Consilium 136. On remaking noses (*De Naribus reficiendis*)."

25 Schenck von Grafenberg, *Observationum*, "Observationes VIII–X."

26 Von Hilden, *Observationum*, "Observatio XXXI: A cut off nose which has been restored (*Nasus abscissus quomodo restitutus*)."

27 Philip Salmuth, *Observationum medicarum* (Brunschvig: sumptibus Göttfried Müller, 1648), Centuria II, p. 69.

28 Quoted by Corradi, "Dell'antica autoplastica," p. 266. See also Delaporte, *Figures of Medicine*, p. 46.

29 Jean Baptiste Van Helmont, *A Ternary of Paradoxes: The Magnetick Cure of Wounds, Nativity of Tartar in Wine, Image of God in Man* [1621], tr. Walter Charleton (London: printed by James Flescher, 1650), pp. 13–14; quoted by David A. Hamilton, *A History of Organ Transplantation: Ancient Legends to Modern Practice* (Pittsburgh: University of Pittsburgh Press, 2012), p. 22.

30 Delaporte, *Figures of Medicine*, p. 47.

31 Bruce Moran, *Distilling Knowledge: Alchemy, Chemistry, and the Scientific Revolution* (Cambridge: Harvard University Press, 2005), p. 90. On Van Helmont's chemical medicine and cosmology, see Walter Pagel, *Joan Baptista Van Helmont: Reformer of Science and Medicine* (Cambridge: Cambridge University Press, 1982), pp. 9–13.

32 See Hamilton, *A History of Organ Transplantation*, pp. 22–23.
33 On this satirical literature, see Ibid., pp. 26–30; Teach-Gnudi and Webster, *The Life and Times*, pp. 297–302.
34 Hamilton, *A History of Organ Transplantation*, pp. 24–29. On animal experimentation in the seventeenth century, see Domenico Bertoloni Meli, "Early Modern Experimentation on Live Animals," *Journal of the History of Biology* 46, 2 (2013): 199–226.
35 See Newman, *Promethean Ambitions*, pp. 221–227.
36 Tommaso Campanella, *Del senso delle cose e della magia* [1603], ed. Germana Ernst (Rome: Laterza, 2007), pp. 259–260.
37 Athanasius Kircher, *Magnes, sive de arte magnetica* (Cologne: apud I. Kalcoven, 1643), pp. 333–334.
38 Dionisio Daza Chacon, *Pràctica y téorica de cirugia* (Madrid: Martin, 1626), p. 278; "Pedro de Heredia," in *Biografìas y vidas*, www.biografiasyvidas.com/biografia/h/heredia_pedro.htm
39 Johann Heinrich von Pflaumern, *Mercurius Italicus* (Augsburg: typis Andreaa Aperger, 1625), p. 84.
40 Ibid.
41 This story has been documented and described in detail by Teach Gnudi and Webster, *The Life and Times*, pp. 236–247.
42 See Paola Zambelli, *White Magic, Black Magic in the European Renaissance: Ficino, Pico, Della Porta to Trithemius, Agrippa, and Bruno* (Leiden: Brill, 2007), pp. 24–26.
43 See Luisa Muraro, *Giambattista Della Porta mago e scienziato* (Milan: Feltrinelli, 1978), pp. 21–58.
44 Voltaire's lines from *Micromegàs* are actually an almost verbatim French translation of Samuel Butler, *Hudibras* (London: Meriot, 1663), p. 11.
45 Luke Dormehl, "Facial Recognition: Is the Technology Taking Away Your Identity?," *The Guardian*, Sunday 4 May 2014.
46 Alan Yuhas and Martin Pangelly, "Firefighter Receives Full Face Transplant in Surgery Called 'Historic'," *The Guardian*, Monday 16 November 2015.
47 Le Chang and Doris Y. Tsao, "The Code for Facial Identity in the Primate Brain," *Cell* 169, 6 (2017): 1013–1028.

BIBLIOGRAPHY

Adani, Giuseppe and Gastone Tamagnini, eds., *Cultura popolare nell'Emilia Romagna. Medicina, erbe, magia* (Milan: Silvana Editoriale, 1981).

Affò, Ireneo, *Memorie degli scrittori e letterati parmigiani* (Parma: dalla Stamperia reale, 1789–1797).

Agrimi, Jole, *Ingeniosa scientia nature. Studi sulla fisiognomica medievale* (Florence: Sismel/ Edizioni del Galluzzo, 2002).

Albergati, Fabio, *Trattato del modo di ridurre a pace l'inimicitie private* (Rome: per Francesco Zannetti, 1583).

Albini, Giulinana, "La gestione dell'Ospedale Maggiore di Milano nel Quattrocento: un esempio di concentrazione ospedaliera," in Grieco and Sandri, eds. *Ospedali e città*.

Aldrovandi, Ulisse, *Monstrorum Historia* (Bologna: Bernia, 1642).

Aldrovandi, Ulisse, *Dendrologiae naturalis scilicet arborum historiae libri duo* (Bologna: ex typographia Ferroniana, 1667).

Ambrosoli, Mauro, *The Wild and the Sown: Botany and Agriculture in Western Europe, 1350–1850* (Cambridge: Cambridge University Press, 1997).

Ambrosoli, Mauro, "Cultivation and Diffusion of Species Diversity in Northern Italy: Peasant Gardeners of the Renaissance and After," in Cronan and Kress, eds. *Botanical Progress*, 177–198.

Angelozzi, Giancarlo, "Cultura dell'onore, codici di comportamento nobiliare e Stato nella Bologna pontificia: un'ipotesi di lavoro," *Annali dell'Istituto Storico Italo-Germanico in Trento* 8 (1982): 305–324.

Angelozzi, Giancarlo, "Nobili, mercanti, dottori, cavalieri, artigiani: stratificazione sociale e ideologia a Bologna nei secoli XVI e XVIII," in Tega, ed. *Storia Illustrata di Bologna*, 41–60.

Angelozzi, Giancarlo, "La proibizione del duello: Chiesa e ideologia nobiliare," in Prodi and Reinhard, eds. *Il concilio di Trento e il moderno*, 271–308.

Angelozzi, Giancarlo and Cesarina Casanova, *La nobiltà disciplinata: violenza nobiliare, procedure di giustizia e scienza cavalleresca a Bologna nel XVII secolo* (Bologna: CLUEB, 2003).

Angelozzi, Giancarlo and Cesarina Casanova, *La giustizia criminale in una città di antico regime: Il tribunale del Torrone di Bologna, secc. XVI–XVII* (Bologna: CLUEB, 2008).

Angelozzi, Giancarlo and Cesarina Casanova, *Donne criminali: Il genere nella storia della giustizia* (Bologna: Patron, 2015).

Antonelli, Ezio, "Ulisse Aldrovandi e la metamorfosi del mostruoso," *Studi e memorie per la storia dell'Università di Bologna* 3 (1983): 196–242.

Aquinas, Thomas, *Summa theologiae* (Bologna: Edizioni Studio Domenicano 1984).

Aranzi, Giulio Cesare, *Anatomicarum observationum liber, ac de tumoribus secundum locos affectos liber* (Venice: apud Iacobum Brechtanum, 1587).

Arcangeli, Alessandro and Vivian Nutton, eds., *Girolamo Mercuriale: medicina e cultura nell'Europa del Cinquecento* (Florence: Olschki, 2008).

Aristotle, *Minor Works*, tr. W.S. Hett (Cambridge: Harvard University Press, 1936).

Aristotle, *Parts of Animals*, tr. A.L. Peck (Cambridge: Harvard University Press, 1937).

Arrizabalaga, Jon, John Henderson, and Roger French, *The Great Pox: The French Disease in Renaissance Europe* (New Haven: Yale University Press, 1997).

Ars Chirurgica (Venice: apud Iuntas, 1546).

Avelini, Luisa, Roberto Finzi, and Leonardo Quaquarelli, eds., *Testi agronomici d'area emiliana e Rinascimento europeo* (Bologna: CLUEB, 2007).

Avicenna, *Canon medicinae* (Venice: industria ac sumptibus Juntarum, 1608).

Aziz, E., B. Nathan, and J. McKeever, "Anesthetic and Analgesic Practices in Avicenna's Canon of Medicine," *The American Journal of Chinese Medicine* 28, 1 (2000): 147–151.

Azzolini, Monica, "Leonardo da Vinci's Anatomical Studies in Milan: A Re-Examination of Sites and Sources," in Givens, Reeds, and Towaide, eds. *Visualizing Medieval Medicine*, 147–176.

Azzolini, Monica, *The Duke and the Stars: Astrology and Politics in Renaissance Milan* (Cambridge: Harvard University Press, 2013).

Bacon, Francis, *Descriptio globi intellectualis* in *The Works of Francis Bacon*, ed. James Spedding, Robert Leslie Ellis, and Doglas Henon Heath, 15 vols. (Boston: Houghton, Mifflin, and Company, 1857).

Bacon, Francis, "The New Atlantis," in *The Works of Francis Bacon*, ed. James Spedding, Robert Leslie Ellis, and Doglas Henon Heath, 15 vols. (Boston: Houghton, Mifflin, and Company, 1857).

Baker, Naomi, *Plain Ugly: The Unattractive Body in Early Modern Culture* (Oxford: Oxford University Press, 2010).

Bakhtin, Mikhail, *Rabelais and His World*, tr. Hélène Iswosky (Bloomington: Indiana University Press, 1984).

Baldini, Enrico, "Prodigi, simulacri e mostri nell'eredità botanica di Ulisse Aldrovandi," in Olmi, Tongiorgi Tomasi, and Zanca, eds. *Natura-cultura*, 215–243.

Bartolini, Donatella, "On the Borders: Surgeons and Their Activities in the Venetian State (1540–1640)," *Medical History* 59, 1 (2015): 83–100.

Bartra, Roger, *Wild Men in the Looking Glass: The Mythic Origins of European Otherness*, tr. Carl T. Berrisford (Ann Arbor: The University of Michigan Press, 1994).

Basile, Bruno, "'Riflessi dell'anima.' La fisiognomica prima e dopo Della Porta," in Santoro, ed. *La "mirabile" natura*, 57–70.

Bates, A.W., "The *De Monstrorum* of Fortunio Liceti: A Landmark of Descriptive Teratology," *Journal of Medical Biography* 9, 1 (2001): 49–54.

Bates, A.W., *Emblematic Monsters: Unnatural Conceptions and Deformed Births in Early Modern Europe* (New York: Rodopi, 2005), 11–41.

Battisti, Eugenio, *L'antirinascimento* (Milan: Feltrinelli, 1962).

Battisti, Eugenio, "*Natura artificiosa* to *Natura artificialis*," in Coffin, ed. *The Italian Garden*, 63–80.

Baxandall, Michael, *Painting and Experience in Fifteenth Century Italy: A Primer in the Social History of Pictorial Style*, 2nd ed. (Oxford: Clarendon Press, 1988).

Becchi, Egle and Monica Ferrari, eds., *Formare alle professioni. Sacerdoti, principi, educatori* (Turin: Codice, 2009).

Beck, Thomas, "Gardens as a 'Third Nature': The Ancient Roots of a Renaissance Idea," *Studies in the History of Gardens & Designed Landscapes* 22, 4 (2002): 327–334.

Beja de Pestrelo, Luiz, *Responsionum casuum conscientiae* (Venice: apud Io. Baptistam, Io. Bernardum Sessam, 1597).

Belfanti, Carlo Marco and Fabio Giusberti, eds., *Storia d'Italia. Annali vol. 19: La moda* (Turin: Einaudi, 2003).

Belloni, Gabriella, "Conoscenza magica e ricerca scientifica in Giambattista Della Porta," in Giambattista Della Porta, ed. *Criptologia* (Rome: Centro Internazionale di Studi Umanistici, 1982), 45–101.

Bellorini, Cristina, *The World of Plants in Renaissance Tuscany: Medicine and Botany* (Farnham: Ashgate, 2016).

Belting, Hans, *Facce. Una storia del volto*, tr. Cristina Baldacci and Pietro Conte (Rome: Carocci, 2014).

Benedetti, Alessandro, *Historia Corporis Humani sive Anatomice*, ed. and tr. Giovanna Ferrari (Florence: Giunti, 1998).

Berco, Cristian, *From Body to Community: Venereal Disease and Society in Baroque Spain* (Toronto: University of Toronto Press, 2016).

Berenson, Bernard, "The Effigy and the Portrait," in Bernard Berenson, ed. *Aesthetics and History in the Visual Arts* (Pantheon: New York, 1948).

Beretta, Marco, *La rivoluzione culturale di Lucrezio. Filosofia e scienza nell'antica Roma* (Rome: Carocci, 2015).

Bertoloni Meli, Domenico, ed., *Malpighi Anatomist and Physician* (Florence: Olschki, 1997).

Bertoloni Meli, Domenico, *Mechanism, Experiment, Disease: Marcello Malpighi and Seventeenth-Century Anatomy* (Baltimore: Johns Hopkins University Press, 2011).

Bertoloni Meli, Domenico, "Early Modern Experimentation on Live Animals," *Journal of the History of Biology* 46, 2 (2013): 199–226.

Bertoloni Meli, Domenico, "Machines of the Body in the Seventeenth Century," in Distelzweig, Goldberg, and Ragland, eds. *Early Modern Medicine*, 91–116.

Bertoloni Meli, Domenico, *Visualizing Disease: The Art and History of Pathological Illustrations* (Chicago: The University of Chicago Press, 2018).

Betri, Maria Luisa and Edoardo Bressan, eds., *Gli ospedali in area padana fra Settecento e Novecento: atti del III Congresso italiano di storia ospedaliera Montecchio Emilia, 14–16 marzo 1990* (Milano: FrancoAngeli, 1992).

Bettella, Patrizia, "The Marked Body as Otherness in Renaissance Italian Culture," in Kalof and Bynum, eds. *A Cultural History of the Human Body in the Renaissance*, 149–181.

Billacois, François, *The Duel: Its Rise and Fall in Early Modern France*, tr. Trista Selous (New Haven: Yale University Press, 1990).

Biow, Douglas, *The Culture of Cleanliness in Renaissance Italy* (Ithaca: Cornell University Press, 2006).

Biow, Douglas, "The Beard in Sixteenth-Century Italy," in Hairston and Stephens, eds. *The Body in Early Modern Italy*, 176–195.

Biringuccio, Vannoccio, *De la pirotechnia* (Milan: Polifilo, 1977).

Bonhomme, Guy, "Le cheval comme instrument du movement humain à la Renaissance," in Céard, Fontaine, and Margolin, eds. *Le corps à la Renaissance*.

Bono, Salvatore, *Schiavi musulmani nell'Italia moderna* (Naples: Edizioni Scientifiche Italiane, 1999).

Bourke, Joanna, *The Story of Pain: From Prayer to Painkillers* (Oxford: Oxford University Press, 2014).

Brady, Sean and John H. Arnold, eds., *What Is Masculinity? Historical Dynamics from Antiquity to the Contemporary World* (New York: Palgrave Macmillan, 2011).

Brizzi, Gian Paolo, "Lo Studio di Bologna tra *orbis academicus* e mondo cittadino," in Prosperi, ed. *Storia di Bologna*, vol. 3.2.

Brizzi, Gian Paolo, ed., *Imago Universitatis: celebrazioni e autorappresentazioni di maestri e studenti nella decorazione parietale dell'Archiginnasio*, 2 vols. (Bologna: Bononia University Press, 2014).

Brown, Alison, *The Return of Lucretius to Renaissance Florence* (Cambridge: Harvard University Press, 2010).

Brown, Judith C. and Robert Charles Davis, eds., *Gender and Society in Renaissance Italy* (London: Longman, 1998).

Brunelli, Giampiero, *Soldati del papa: politica militare e nobiltà nello Stato della Chiesa (1560–1644)* (Rome: Carocci, 2003).

Bruno da Longobucco, *Ars Chirurgica, in Maestro Bruno da Longobucco, chirurgo*, ed. Alfredo Focà (Reggio Calabria: Laruffa, 2004).

Burke, Peter, "The Presentation of Self in the Renaissance Portrait," in Peter Burke, ed. *The Historical Anthropology of Early Modern Italy: Essays on Perception and Communication* (Cambridge: Cambridge University Press, 1987), 150–167.

Burke, Peter, "Frontiers of the Monstrous," in Lunger Knoppers and Landes, eds. *Monstrous Bodies/Political Monstrosities*, 25–39.

Bussato, Marco, *Giardino di agricoltura . . . nel quale con bellissimo ordine si tratta tutto quello, che s'appartiene a sapere a un perfetto Giardiniero* (Venice: appresso Giovanni Fiorina, 1592).

Butler, Samuel, *Hudibras* (London: Meriot, 1663).

Bylebyl, Jerome, "The School of Padua: Humanistic Medicine in the Sixteenth Century," in Webster, ed. *Health, Medicine, and Mortality.*

Cabré, Monsterrat, "Beautiful Bodies," in Linda Kalof, ed. *A Cultural History of the Human Body in the Middle Ages* (Oxford: Berg, 2010), 127–148.

Cadden, Joan, *The Meanings of Sex Difference in the Middle Ages: Medicine, Science, and Culture* (Cambridge: Cambridge University Press, 1993).

Camerata da Randazzo, Girolamo, *Trattato dell'honor vero et del vero dishonore* (Bologna: per Alessandro Benacci, 1567).

Campanella, Tommaso, *The City of the Sun: A Poetical Dialogue*, tr. and ed. Daniel J. Donno (Berkeley: University of California Press, 1981).

Campanella, Tommaso, *Del senso delle cose e della magia*, ed. Germana Ernst (Rome: Laterza, 2007).

Campbell, Mary Baine, *Wonder & Science: Imagining Worlds in Early Modern Europe* (Ithaca: Cornell University Press, 2004).

Camporesi, Piero, *Camminare il mondo. Vita e avventure di Leonardo Fioravanti, medico del cinquecento* (Milan: Garzanti, 1997).

Camporesi, Piero, *Le officine dei sensi* (Milan: Garzanti, 2009).

Theodore Alois Buckley, ed., *The Canons and Decrees of the Council of Trent* (London: George Routlege & co., 1852).

Cardano, Girolamo, "De subtilitate," in Girolamo Cardano, ed. *Opera Omnia* (Lyon: Jean Antoine Huguetan et Marc Antione Ravaud, 1663).

Cardini, Roberto and Mariangela Regoliosi, eds., *Umanesimo e medicina: il problema dell'individuale* (Rome: Bulzoni, 1996).

Carlino, Andrea, *Books of the Body: Anatomical Ritual and Renaissance Learning*, tr. John Tedeschi and Ann C. Tedeschi (Chicago: The University of Chicago Press, 1994).

Carpue, Joseph Constantine, *An Account of Two Successful Operations for Restoring a Lost Nose* . . . (London: Longman, Hurst, Reese, Horme, and Brown, 1816).

Carrithers, Michael, Steven Collins, and Steven Lukes, eds., *The Category of the Person: Anthropology, Philosophy, History* (Cambridge: Cambridge University Press, 1985).

Carroll, Stuart, *Blood and Violence in Early Modern France* (Oxford: Oxford University Press, 2006).

Casali, Elide, "Catechesi di villa tra *oeconomica* e *res rustica*," in Avelini, Finzi, and Quaquarelli, eds. *Testi agronomici d'area emiliana*, 7–34.

Castelli, Patrizia, *L'estetica del Rinascimento* (Bologna: Il mulino, 2005).

Castelnuovo, Enrico, *Ritratto e società in Italia* (Turin: Einaudi, 2015).

Castiglione, Baldassar, *The Book of the Courtier*, tr. Leonard E. Opdyke (New York: Scribner's, 1903).

Cavallo, Sandra, *Charity and Power in Early Modern Italy: Benefactors and Their Motives in Turin, 1541–1789* (Cambridge: Cambridge University Press, 1995).

Cavallo, Sandra, *Artisans of the Body in Early Modern Italy: Identities, Families and Masculinities* (Manchester: Manchester University Press, 2010).

Cavallo, Sandra and Tessa Storey, *Healthy Living in Late Renaissance Italy* (Oxford: Oxford University Press, 2013).

Cavazza, Marta, "The Uselessness of Anatomy: Mini and Sbaraglia versus Malpighi," in Bertoloni Meli, ed. *Malpighi Anatomist and Physician*, 129–145.

Cavina, Marco, *Il sangue dell'onore: storia del duello* (Rome: Laterza, 2005).

Cavina, Marco, "I luoghi della giustizia," in Prosperi, ed. *Storia di Bologna*, vol. 3.1, 367–411.

Céard, Jean, Marie Madeleine Fontaine, and Jean-Claude Margolin, eds., *Le corps à la Renaissance* (Paris: Aux amateurs des livres, 1990).

Celsus, *De medicina*, 3 vols., tr. W.G. Spencer (Cambridge: Harvard University Press, 1935–38).

Cesalpino, Andrea, *De plantis libri XVI* (Florence: apud Georgium Marescottum, 1583).

Chamberland, Celeste Catherine, "Honor, Brotherhood, and the Corporate Ethos of London's Barber-Surgeons' Company, 1570–1640," *Journal of the History of Medicine and Allied Sciences* 64, 3 (2009): 300–332.

Chang, Le, and Doris Y. Tsao, "The Code for Facial Identity in the Primate Brain," *Cell* 169, 6 (2017): 1013–1028.

Chauliac, Guy de, *Inventarium, sive Chirurgia magna*, 2 vols., ed. Michael McVaugh (Leiden: E.J. Brill, 1997).

Cheng, Sandra, "The Cult of the Monstrous: Caricature, Physiognomy, and Monsters in Early Modern Italy," *Preternature: Critical and Historical Studies on the Preternatural* 1, 2 (2012): 197–231.

Chesnais, Jean-Claude, *Histoire de la violence de 1800 à nos jours* (Paris: Laffonte, 1980).

Chojnacki, Stanley, *Women and Men in Renaissance Venice* (Baltimore: Johns Hopkins University Press, 2000).

Cicero, *De finibus bonorum at malorum*, tr. H. Rackham (Cambridge: Harvard University Press, 1931).

Cicero, *On the Nature of Gods*, tr. H. Rackham (Cambridge: Harvard University Press, 1933).

Clericuzio, Antonio and Germana Ernst, eds., *Il Rinascimento italiano e l'Europa. Volume 5: Le scienze* (Treviso: Angelo Colla Editore, 2008).

Close, A.J., "Commonplace Theories of Art and Nature in Classical Antiquity and in the Renaissance," *Journal of the History of Ideas* 30, 4 (1969): 467–486.

Cock, Emily, "Lead[ing] 'Em by the Nose into Publick Shame and Derision': Gaspare Tagliacozzi, Alexander Read and the Lost History of Plastic Surgery, 1600–1800," *Social History of Medicine* 28, 1 (2015): 1–21.

Coffin, David C., ed., *The Italian Garden* (Washington, DC: Dumbarton Oaks, 1972).

Cohen, Elizabeth S., "Honor and Gender in the Streets of Early Modern Rome," *Journal of Interdisciplinary History* (1992): 597–625.

Cohen, Esther, *The Modulated Scream: Pain in Late Medieval Culture* (Chicago: The University of Chicago Press, 2009).

Cohen, Thomas V., "The Lay Liturgy of Affront in Sixteenth-Century Italy," *Journal of Social History* 25, 4 (1992): 857–877.

Coiter, Volcher, *Externarum et internarum principalium humani corporis partium tabulae* (Norimbergae: in officina Theodorici Gerlazeni, 1573).

Columella, *On agriculture*, 3 vols., tr. Harrison Boyd Ashe (Cambridge: Harvard University Press, 1941–1955).

Conforti, Maria, "Chirurghi, mammane, ciarlatani. Pratica medica e controllo delle professioni," in Clericuzio and Ernst, eds. *Il Rinascimento italiano e l'Europa*, 323–340.

Conforti, Maria, "Medicine, History and Religion in Naples in the Seventeenth and Eighteenth Centuries," in Grell and Cunningham, eds. *Medicine and Religion*, 63–78.

Cook, Harold J., *Matters of Exchange: Commerce, Medicine, and Science in the Dutch Golden Age* (New Haven: Yale University Press, 2008).

Cook, Harold J., "The History of Medicine and the Scientific Revolution," *Isis* 102, 1 (2011): 102–108.

Corradi, Alfonso M.E., "Dell'antica autoplastica Italiana," *Memorie del Regio Istituto Lombardo di Scienze e Lettere, classe di Scienze matematiche e naturali* 13 (1877): 225–273.

Cortesi, Giovanni Battista, *Epistola qua in simplici sede teli calvariae, os ipsius non abradendum nec perfornadum esse demonstratur, ad Ill.rem ac Excell.mum Virum D. Ioannem Cechium nostrae tempestatis Medicum celeberrimum* (Bologna: apud Faustum Bonardum, 1590).

Cortesi, Giovanni Battista, *Miscellaneorum medicinalium decades denae* (Messina: ex typographia Petri Breae, 1625).

Cortesi, Giovanni Battista, *Pharmacopeia, seu Antidotarium Messanense* (Messina: ex typis Petri Breae, 1629).

Cortesi, Giovanni Battista, *In Universam Chirurgiam absolutam Institutio* (Messina: apud haeredes Petri Breae, 1633).

Cosmacini, Giorgio, *La vita nelle mani. Storia della chirurgia* (Rome-Bari: Laterza, 2003).

Courtine, Jean-Jacques and Claudine Haroche, *Histoire du visage: exprimer et taire ses emotions (xvi-début xix siècle)* (Paris: Payot & Rivages, 1988).

Cox, Jennifer Anne, "Disability as Enacted Parable," *Journal of Religion, Disability & Health* 15, 3 (2011): 241–253.

Crasso, Girolamo, *Diario empirico. Nel quale si dimostra il modo di curare ogni sorte di ferita nel corpo humano* (Venice: appresso gli heredi di Francesco Rampazzetto, 1577).

Crisciani, Chiara, "L'individuale nella medicina tra Medioevo e Umanesimo: i 'Consilia'," in Cardini and Regoliosi, eds. *Umanesimo e medicina*, 1–32.

Crisciani, Chiara and Agostino Paravicini Bagliani, eds., *Alchimia e medicina nel Medioevo* (Florence: SISMEL/Edizioni del Galluzzo, 2003).

Croce, Giulio Cesare, *Lettera mandata da Narciso alli più belli, vaghi, et profumati giovani di questa città* (Bologna: per Vittorio Benassi, 1590).

Croce, Giulio Cesare, *Le sottilissime astuzie di Bertoldo. Le piacevoli e ridicolose simplicità di Bertoldino col Dialogus Salomonis et Marcolphi e il suo primo volgarizzamento a stampa*, ed. Piero Camporesi (Turin: Einaudi, 1978).

Cronan, Michael and W. John Kress, eds., *Botanical Progress, Horticultural Innovation and Cultural Change* (Washington, DC: Dumbarton Oaks Research Library and Collection, 2007).

Cruciani, Gianfranco, *Cerusici e fisici: preciani e nursini dal XIV al XVIII secolo: storia e antologia* (Terni: Thyrus, 1999).

Cunningham, Andrew, "The Culture of Gardens," in Jardine, Spary, and Secord, eds. *Cultures of Natural History*, 38–56.

Cunningham, Andrew, "The Pen and the Sword: Recovering the Disciplinary Identity of Physiology and Anatomy before 1800: II: Old Anatomy: The Sword," *Studies in History and Philosophy of Biological & Biomedical Sciences* 34, 1 (2003): 51–76.

Daenens, Francine, "Superiore perché inferiore: il paradosso della superiorità della donna in alcuni trattati italiani del Cinquecento," in Gentili, ed. *Trasgressione tragica*, 7–50.

Dalla Croce, Giovanni Andrea, *Cirugia universale e perfetta* (Venice: Giordano Ziletti, 1583).

Dall'Osso, Eugenio, "Un contributo al pensiero scientifico di Giulio Cesare Aranzio: La sua opera chirurgica," *Annali di medicina navale e tropicale* 61, 5 (1956): 617–627.

D'Amato, Cinzio, *Prattica nuova et utilissima. Di tutto quello, ch'al diligente Barbiero s'appartiene: cioè di cavar sangue, medicar ferrite, & balsamar corpi humani* (Venice: appresso Gio. Battista Brigna, 1669).

Daston, Lorraine, "The Moral Economy of Science," *Osiris* 10 (1995): 2–24.

Daston, Lorraine, "The Nature of Nature in Early Modern Europe," *Configurations* 6, 2 (1998): 149–172.

Daston, Lorraine and Katharine Park, *Wonders and the Order of Nature, 1150–1750* (New York: Zone Books, 1997).

Daston, Lorraine and Katharine Park, "Introduction: The Age of the New," in Daston and Park, eds. *The Cambridge History of Science*, 1–17.

Daston, Lorraine and Katharine Park, eds., *The Cambridge History of Science, Volume 3: Early Modern Science* (Cambridge: Cambridge University Press, 2006).

Daston, Lorraine and Fernando Vidal, eds., *The Moral Authority of Nature* (Chicago: The University of Chicago Press, 2003).

Davidson, Arnold I., "The Horror of Monsters," in Arnold I. Davidson, ed. *The Emergence of Sexuality* (Cambridge: Harvard University Press, 2001).

Davies, Jonathan, "Introduction," in Davies, ed. *Aspects of Violence in Renaissance Europe*, 1–15.

Davies, Jonathan, ed., *Aspects of Violence in Renaissance Europe* (Farnham: Ashgate, 2013).

Davies, Surekha, *Renaissance Ethnography and the Invention of the Human: New Worlds, Maps and Monsters* (Cambridge: Cambridge University Press, 2016).

Daza Chacon, Dionisio, *Pràctica y téorica de cirugia* (Madrid: Martin, 1626).

De Benedictis, Angela, "Il governo misto," in Prosperi, ed. *Storia di Bologna*, vol. 3.1, 201–270.

De Chaney, Edward P., "Giudizi inglesi su ospedali italiani, 1545–1789," in *Timore e carità: i poveri nell'Italia moderna. Atti del Convegno "Pauperismo e assistenza negli antichi stati italiani" (Cremona, 28–30 marzo 1980)* (Cremona: Biblioteca statale e libreria civica di Cremona, 1982), 77–101.

De Ferrari, Augusto, "Giovanni Battista Cortesi," in *Dizionario Biografico degli Italiani*, vol. 29 (Rome: Treccani, 1983).

Degli Esposti, Stefania, "Giovanni Battista Cortesi (1553–1636): da garzone-barbiere a illustre chirurgo e anatomico," *Strenna storica Bolognese* 42 (1992): 173–187.

Delaporte, François, *Figures of Medicine: Blood, Face Transplants, Parasites*, tr. Nils F. Schott (New York: Fordham University Press, 2013).

Della Casa, Giovanni, *Galateo, or the Rules of Polite Behavior*, ed. M.F. Rusnak (Chicago: The University of Chicago Press, 2013).

Della Porta, Giovanni Battista, *De i miracoli et miracolisi effetti dalla natura prodotti* (Venice: appresso Ludovico Avanzi, 1560).

Della Porta, Giovanni Battista, *Phytognomonica* (Naples: apud Horatium Salvianum, 1588).

Della Porta, Giovanni Battista, *Magiae naturalis libri XX* (Naples: Orazio Salviani, 1589).

Della Porta, Giovanni Battista, *Della fisionomia dell'uomo libri sei*, 2 vols. (Naples-Rome: Edizioni Scientifiche Italiane, 2013).

Demaitre, Luke, "Skin and the City: Cosmetic Medicine as a Urban Concern," in Nance and Florence, eds. *Between Text and Patient*, 97–120.

De Moulin, Daniel, "A Historical-Phenomenological Study of Bodily Pain in Western Man," *Bulletin of the History of Medicine* 48, 4 (1974): 540–570.

De Moulin, Daniel, *A History of Surgery: With Emphasis on the Netherlands* (Dordrecht: Maryinus Nijhoff Publishers, 1988).

De Renzi, Salvatore, *Storia della medicina in Italia* (Naples: Tip. del Filiatre-Sebezio, 1845–48).

Descartes, Renée, *L'homme* (Paris: chez Charles Angot, 1664).

Descartes, Renée, "Discours de la méthode," in Charles Adam and Paul Tannery, eds. *Oeuvres de Descartes* (Paris: Cerf, 1897–1913), vol. 5.

Descimon, Robert, "The Birth of the Nobility of the Robe: Dignity versus Privilege in the Parlement of Paris, 1500–1700," in Wolfe, ed. *Changing Identities*.

De Serres, Olivier, *Le Théatre d'Agriculture et de mesnages des champs* [1600] (Arles: Thesaurus Actes-Sud, 2001).

De Vivo, Filippo, *Information and Communication in Venice: Rethinking Early Modern Politics* (Oxford: Oxford University Press, 2007).

De Vries, Jan, "The Limits of Globalization in the Early Modern World," *Economic History Review* 63, 3 (2010): 710–733.

De Vries, Joyce, *Caterina Sforza and the Arts of Appearance* (Aldershot: Ashgate, 2010).

DeVries, Kelly, "Military Surgical Practice and the Advent of Gunpowder Weaponry," *Canadian Bulletin of Medical History* 7, 2 (1990): 131–146.

Dewald, Jonathan, *The European Nobility, 1400–1800* (Cambridge: Cambridge University Press, 1996).

Di Matteo, Berardo, Vittorio Tarabella, Giuseppe Filardo, Anna Viganò, Patrizia Tomba, and Maurilio Marcacci, "The Renaissance and the Universal Surgeon: Giovanni Andrea Della Croce, a Master of Traumatology," *International Orthopaedics* 37, 12 (2013): 2523–2528.

Dingwall, Helen M., *Physicians, Surgeons and Apothecaries: Medicine in Seventeenth-Century Edinburgh* (East Linton: Tuckwell Press, 1995).

Distelzweig, Peter, Peter Benjamin Goldberg, and Evan R. Ragland, eds., *Early Modern Medicine and Natural Philosophy* (Dordrecht: Springer, 2016).

Dolfi, Pompeo Scipione, *Cronologia della famiglie nobili di Bologna* (Bologna: G.B. Ferroni, 1670).

Dollo, Corrado, "Fra tradizione e innovazione. L'insegnamento messinese della medicina e delle scienze nei secoli XVI e XVII," *Annali di storia delle università italiane* 2 (1998): 107–122.

Donati, Claudio, *L'idea di nobiltà in Italia. Secoli XIV-XVIII* (Rome: Laterza, 1988).

Donati, Claudio, "A Project of Expurgation by the Congregation of the Index: Treatises on Dueling," in Fragnito, ed. *Church, Censorship and Culture*, 134–161.

Dormehl, Luke, "Facial Recognition: Is the Technology Taking Away Your Identity?," *The Guardian*, Sunday 4 May 2014.

Duindam, Jeroen Frans Jozef, *Myths of Power: Norbert Elias and the Early Modern European Court* (Amsterdam: Amsterdam University Press, 1994).

Dumézil, Bruno, "Faire honte dans les sources normatives du haut Moyen Age (V-VIIe siècle)," in Sère and Wettlaufer, eds. *Shame Between Punishment and Penance*, 49–64.

Eamon, William, *Science and the Secrets of Nature: Books of Secrets in Medieval and Early Modern Culture* (Princeton: Princeton University Press, 1994).

Eamon, William, *The Professor of Secrets: Mystery, Medicine, and Alchemy in Renaissance Italy* (Washington, DC: National Geographics, 2010).

Eckstein, Nicholas A. and Nicholas Terpstra, eds., *Sociability and Its Discontents: Civil Society, Social Capital, and Their Alternatives in Late Medieval and Early Modern Europe* (Turnhout: Brepols, 2009).

Eco, Umberto, *Storia della bellezza* (Milan: Bompiani, 2004).

Elias, Norbert, *The History of Manners*, tr. Edmund Jephcott (New York: Urizen Books, 1979).

Erspamer, Francesco, *La biblioteca di don Ferrante: Duello e onore nella cultura del Cinquecento* (Rome: Bulzoni, 1982).

Esposito, Anna, "Stufe e bagni pubblici a Roma nel Rinascimento," in Esposito, ed. *Taverne, locande e stufe*, 77–91.

Esposito, Anna, ed., *Taverne, locande e stufe a Roma nel Rinascimento* (Rome: Roma nel Rinascimento, 1999).

Fabiani Giannetto, Raffaella, "Types of Gardens," in Hyde, ed. *A Cultural History of Gardens in the Renaissance*, 43–72.

Fabrizi d'Acquapendente, Girolamo, *L'opere chirurgiche* (Padua: appresso Giacomo Cadorino, 1671).

Fairchild Ruggles, Douglas, *Gardens, Landscapes, & Vision in the Palaces of Islamic Spain* (University Park: The Pennsylvania State University Press, 2006).

Falloppio, Gabriele, "De decoratione," in Gabriele Falloppio, ed. *Opuscula* (Padua: apud Lucam Bertellum, 1566).

Fantappié, Carlo, "La professionalizzazione del sacerdozio cattolico nell'età moderna," in Becchi and Ferrari, eds. *Formare alle professioni*, 39–69.

Fanti, Mario, "Le classi sociali e il governo di Bologna all'inizio del secolo XVII in un'opera inedita di Camillo Baldi," *Strenna Storica Bolognese* 11 (1961): 133–179.

Fantuzzi, Giovanni, *Notizie degli scrittori bolognesi*, 9 vols. (Bologna: Stamperia di S. Tommaso d'Aquino, 1781–94).

Federici Vescovini, Graziella, "L'individuale nella medicina tra Medioevo e Umanesimo: la fisiognomica di Michele Savonarola," in Cardini and Regoliosi, eds. *Umanesimo e medicina*, 63–87.

Feher, Michael, ed., *Fragments for a History of the Human Body*, 3 vols. (New York: Zone Books, 1989).

Ferrara, Gabriele, *Nova selva di cirugia* (Venice: per Bartolomeo carampello, 1596).

Ferrari, Giovanna, "Public Anatomy Lessons and the Carnival: The Anatomy Theatre of Bologna," *Past and Present* 117 (1987): 50–106.

Ferrari, Giovanna, "Tra medicina e chirurgia: la rinascita dell'anatomia e la dissezione come spettacolo," in Clericuzio and Ernst, eds. *Il Rinascimento italiano e l'Europa*, 341–366.

Findlen, Paula, "Jokes of Nature and Jokes of Knowledge: The Playfulness of Scientific Discourse in Early Modern Europe," *Renaissance Quarterly* 43, 2 (1990): 292–331.

Findlen, Paula, *Possessing Nature: Museums, Collecting, and Scientific Culture in Early Modern Italy* (Berkeley: University of California Press, 1996).

Finucci, Valeria and Kevin Brownlee, eds., *Generation and Degeneration: Tropes of Reproduction in Early Modern Europe* (Durham: Duke University Press, 2001).

Finucci, Valeria, *The Prince's Body: Vincenzo Gonzaga and Renaissance Medicine* (Cambridge: Harvard University Press, 2015).

Fioravanti, Leonardo, *Il Tesoro della vita humana* (Venice: appresso gli heredi di Melchior Sessa, 1570).

Fioravanti, Leonardo, *La Cirugia* (Venice: appresso gli heredi di Melchior Sessa, 1570).

Fioravanti, Leonardo, *Del compendio dei secreti rationali* [first edition 1564] (Turin: appressi gli heredi del bevilacqua, 1580).

Forni, Giuseppe G., *L'insegnamento della chirurgia nello studio di Bologna: dalle origini a tutto il secolo XIX* (Bologna: Cappelli, 1948).

Fosi, Irene, *La società violenta: il banditismo nello Stato pontificio nella seconda metà del Cinquecento* (Rome: Edizioni dell'Ateneo, 1985).

Fragnito, Gigliola, ed., *Church, Censorship and Culture in Early Modern Italy* (Cambridge: Cambridge University Press, 2001).

Franco, Pierre, *Chirurgie*, ed. Edouard Nicaise (Paris: Félix Alcan, 1895).

French, Roger Kenneth, ed., *Medicine from the Black Death to the French Disease* (London: Ashgate, 1998).

Fulcheri, Enrico, "Fortunio Liceti: un punto di svolta negli studi sui 'mostri' e l'inizio della moderna teratologia," *Pathologica* 94 (2002): 263–268.

Gabriele da Barletta, *Sermonum celeberrimi* (Venice: ex officina Ioan. Bapt. Somaschi, 1571).

Gadebusch-Bondio, Mariacarla, *Medizinische Ästhetik: Kosmetik und plastische Chirurgie zwischen Antike und früher Neuzeit* (München: WFink, 2005).

Gadebusch-Bondio, Mariacarla, "I pericoli della bellezza 'mangonica'. Aspetti del dibattito su protesi, trucchi e chirurgia estetica tra 500 e 600," in Paravicini Bagliani, ed. *Le corps et sa parure*, 425–449.

Gadebusch-Bondio, Mariacarla, "On the Function, Utility, and Fragility of the Nose: Early Modern Patients and Their Surgeons," *Nuncius* 32 (2017): 25–51.

Gagné, John, "Counting the Dead: Traditions of Enumeration and the Italian Wars," *Renaissance Quarterly* 67, 3 (2014): 791–840.

Galen, "De compositione medicamentorum secundum locos," in Karl Gottlob Kühn, ed. *Opera omnia* (Leipzig: Cnobloch, 1821–1833).

Galen, *On the Natural Faculties*, tr. Arthur John Brock (London: Heinemann, 1947).

Galen, *On the Usefulness of the Parts of the Body*, 2 vols., tr. Margaret Tallmadge May (Ithaca: Cornell University Press, 1968).

Galen, "Letter to Thrasiboulos," in Peter Singer, tr. *Selected Writings* (Oxford: Oxford University Press, 1997).

Gallo, Agostino, *Le vinti giornate dell'agricoltura* (Venice: Appresso Camillo Borgominerio, 1578).

García Ballester, Luis, ed., *Practical Medicine from Salerno to the Black Death* (Cambridge: Cambridge University Press, 1994).

Gardi, Andrea, *Lo Stato in Provincia: L'amministrazione Della Legazione Di Bologna Durante Il Regno Di Sisto V (1585–1590)* (Bologna: Istituto per la storia di Bologna, 1994).

Garzoni, Tommaso, *La piazza universale di tutte le professioni del mondo*, 2 vols., ed. Paolo Cherchi and Beatrice Collina (Turin: Einaudi, 1996).

Gaurico, Pomponio, *De sculptura*, ed. Paolo Cutolo (Naples: Edizioni Scientifiche Italiane, 1999).

Gautherie, Aurélien, "Physical Pain in Celsus' *On Medicine*," *Studies in Ancient Medicine* 42 (2014): 137–154.

Gautier, Léon, *La médecine à Genève jusqu'à la fin du dix-huitième siècle* (Genève: Jullien, 1906).

Gehl, Paul F., "Military Courtesy in Sixteenth-Century Lithuania: Il Cavaliere of Domenico Mora," *Archivum Lithuanicum* 3 (2001): 55–76.

Gelfand, Toby, *Professionalizing Modern Medicine: Paris Surgeons and Medical Science and Institutions in the 18th Century* (Westport: Greenwood Press, 1980).

Gentilcore, David, "'All That Pertains to Medicine': Protomedici and Protomedicati in Early Modern Italy," *Medical History* 38, 2 (1994): 121–142.

Gentilcore, David, *Medical Charlatanism in Early Modern Italy* (Oxford: Oxford University Press, 2006).

Gentili, Giulio, *La vita e l'opera di Bartolomeo Maggi (1516–1552)* (Bologna: Università di Bologna, 1967).

Gentili, Vanna, ed., *Trasgressione tragica e norma domestica: esemplari di tipologie femminili dalla letteratura europea* (Rome: Edizioni di Storia e Letteratura, 1983).

Ghilini, Girolamo, *Theatro d'huomini letterati* (Venice: per il Guerigli, 1647).

Ghirardi, Angela, *Bartolomeo Passerotti, pittore, 1529–1592: Catalogo generale* (Rimini: Luisè, 1990).

Ghirardi, Angela, "Bartolomeo Passerotti, il culto di Michelangelo e l'anatomia nell'età di Ulisse Aldrovandi," in Olmi, ed. *Rappresentare il corpo*, 151–164.

Gilman, Sander L., *Making the Body Beautiful: A Cultural History of Aesthetic Surgery* (Princeton: Princeton University Press, 1999).

Gil-Sotres, Pedro, "Derivation and Revulsion: The Theory and Practice of Medieval Phlebotomy," in García Ballester, ed. *Practical Medicine*, 110–155.

Ginzburg, Carlo, "Microhistory: Two of Three Things That I Know about It," *Critical Inquiry* 20, 1 (1993): 10–35.

Ginzburg, Carlo, "Our Words, and Theirs: A Reflection on the Historian's Craft, Today," *Cromohs* 18 (2014): 97–114.

Givens, Jean A., Karen M. Reeds, and Alain Towaide, eds., *Visualizing Medieval Medicine and Natural History, 1250–1550* (Aldershot: Ashgate, 2006).

Goelicke, Andreas Ottomar, *Historia chirurgiae* (Magdeburg: in Officina Rengeriana, 1713).

Gordon, Bonnie, "It's Not about the Cut: The Castrato's Instrumentalized Song," *New Literary History* 46, 4 (2015): 647–667.

Grafton, Anthony and Nancy Siraisi, eds., *Natural Particulars: Nature and the Disciplines in Renaissance Europe* (Cambridge, MA: MIT Press 1999).

Greco, Manfredi et al., "The Primacy of the Vianeo Family in the Invention of Nasal Reconstruction Technique," *Annals of Plastic Surgery* 64 (2010): 702–705.

Green, Monica, ed., *The Trotula: A Medieval Compendium of Women's Medicine* (Philadelphia: University of Pennsylvania Press, 2001).

Green, Monica, *Making Women's Medicine Masculine: The Rise of Male Authority in Pre-Modern Gynaecology* (Oxford: Oxford University Press, 2008).

Greig, Aina, Andreas Gohritz, Max Geishauser, and Wolfgang Mühlbauer, "Heinrich von Pfalzpaint, Pioneer of Arm Flap Nasal Reconstruction in 1460, More Than a Century Before Tagliacozzi," *Journal of Craniofacial Surgery* 26, 4 (2015): 1165–1168.

Grell, Ole Peter and Andrew Cunningham, eds., *Medicine and Religion in Enlightenment Europe* (Aldershot: Ashgate, 2007).

Grell, Ole Peter, Andrew Cunningham, and Bernd Roeck, eds., *Health Care and Poor Relief in 18th and 19th Century Southern Europe* (Aldershot: Ashgate, 2005).

Grendler, Paul, *The Universities of the Italian Renaissance* (Baltimore: Johns Hopkins University Press, 2002).

Grieco, Allen J., "The Social Politics of Pre-Linnaean Botanical Classification," *I Tatti Studies* 4 (1991): 131–149.

Grieco, Allen J., Michael Rocke, and Fiorella Superbi Gioffredi, eds., *The Italian Renaissance in the Twentieth Century* (Florence: Leo S. Olschki, 2002).

Grieco, Allen J. and Lucia Sandri, eds., *Ospedali e città: l'Italia del Centro-Nord, XIII–XVI secolo* (Florence: Le Lettere, 1997).

Groebner, Valentin, *Defaced: The Visual Culture of Violence in the Late Middle Ages* (New York: Zone Books, 2004).

Groebner, Valentin, *Who Are You? Identification, Deception, and Surveillance in Early Modern Europe* (New York: Zone Books, 2007).

Gurunluoglu, Raffi and Aslin Gurunluoglu, "Giulio Cesare Arantius (1530–1589): A Surgeon and Anatomist: His Role in Nasal Reconstruction and Influence on Gaspare Tagliacozzi," *Annals of Plastic Surgery* 60, 6 (2008): 717–722.

Gurunluoglu, Raffi, Maziar Shafighi, Aslin Gurunluoglu, and Safiye Cavdar, "Giulio Cesare Aranzio (Arantius) (1530–89) in the Pageant of Anatomy and Surgery," *Journal of Medical Biography* 19, 2 (2011): 63–69.

Haeger, Knut, *The Illustrated History of Surgery* (New York: Bell, 1988).

Hairston, Julia J. and Walter Stephens, eds., *The Body in Early Modern Italy* (Baltimore: Johns Hopkins University Press, 2010).

Hamilton, David A., *A History of Organ Transplantation: Ancient Legends to Modern Practice* (Pittsburgh: University of Pittsburgh Press, 2012).

Hanlon, Gregory, "In Praise of Refeudalization: Princes and Feudataries in North-Central Italy from the Sixteenth to the Eighteenth Century," in Eckstein and Terpstra, eds. *Sociability and Its Discontents*, 213–225.

Harvey, Karen, "The History of Masculinity, circa 1650–1800," *Journal of British Studies* 44 (2005): 296–311.

Heller, Thomas, Morton Sosna, and David Wellbery, eds., *Reconstructing Individualism: Autonomy, Individuality, and the Self in Western Thought* (Stanford: Stanford University Press, 1986).

Henderson, John, *The Renaissance Hospital: Healing the Body and Healing the Soul* (New Haven: Yale University Press, 2006).

Henri de Mondeville, *Chirurgie*, ed. Edouard Nicaise (Paris: Félix Alcan, 1893).

Hilden (Hildanus), Fabry von, *Observationum et curationum cheirurgicarum centuria tertia* (Basel: Typis Hieronymi Galleri, 1614).

Hilden (Hildanus), Fabry von, *Observationum et curationum cheirurgicarum centuria tertia* (Basel: Sumptibus Johannis Theodori de Bry, typis Hieron. Galleri, 1619).

Honeck, Mischa, Martin Klimke, and Anne Kuhlmann, eds., *Germany and the Black Diaspora: Points of Contact 1250–1914* (New York, Oxford, Berghahn Books, 2013).

Horden, Peregrine, "Pain in Hippocratic Medicine," in Porter, ed. *Religion Health & Suffering*, 295–315.

Horstmanshoff, Manfred, Helen King, and Claus Zittel, eds., *Blood, Sweat, and Tears: The Changing Concepts of Physiology from Antiquity into Early Modern Europe* (Leiden: Brill, 2012).

Hunt, John Dixon, *Garden and Grove: The Italian Renaissance Garden in the English Imagination, 1600–1750* (Philadelphia: University of Pennsylvania Press, 1996).

Hunter, Michael, *Science and Society in Restoration England* (Cambridge: Cambridge University Press, 1981).

Hyde, Elizabeth, ed., *A Cultural History of Gardens in the Renaissance* (London: Bloomsbury, 2013).

Ingrassia, Giovanni Filippo, *Methodus dandi relationes pro mutilates, torquendis, aut a tortura excusandis*, ed. G. Curcio (Catania: Romeo Prampolini, 1939).

Jacquart, Danielle and Claude Thomasset, *Sexuality and Medicine in the Middle Ages*, tr. Matthew Adamson (Princeton: Princeton University Press, 1988).

Janssen, Diederik, "Can the Hegemon Speak? Reading Masculinity Through Anthropology," in Brandy and Arnold, eds. *What Is Masculinity?*, 35–56.

Jardine, Nicholas, Emma Spary, and Jim A. Secord, eds., *Cultures of Natural History* (Cambridge: Cambridge University Press, 1996).

Kalof, Linda and William Bynum, eds., *A Cultural History of the Human Body in the Renaissance* (Oxford: Berg, 2010).

King, Helen, "The Early Anodynes: Pain in the Ancient World," in Mann, ed. *The History of the Management of Pain*, 51–62.

King, Helen, *The One-Sex Body on Trial: The Classical and Early Modern Evidence* (Farnham: Ashgate, 2013).

Kircher, Athanasius, *Magnes, sive de arte magnetica* (Cologne: apud I. Kalcoven, 1643).

Klestinec, Cynthia, *Theaters of Anatomy: Students, Teachers, and Traditions of Dissection in Renaissance Venice* (Baltimore: Johns Hopkins University Press, 2011).

Klestinec, Cynthia, "Renaissance Surgeons: Anatomy, Manual Skill, and the Visual Arts," in Distelzweig, Goldberg, and Ragland, eds. *Early Modern Medicine*, 43–58.

Kolsky, Stephen, *Courts and Courtiers in Renaissance Northern Italy* (Aldershot: Ashgate, 2003).

Koslofsky, Craig, "Knowing Skin in Early Modern Europe, c. 1450–1750," *History Compass* 12, 10 (2014): 794–806.

Landazuri, Hildebrando, "Plastic Surgery Pioneers," *British Journal of Plastic Surgery* 15, (1962): 117–122.

Laqueur, Thomas, *Making Sex: Body and Gender from the Greeks to Freud* (Cambridge: Harvard University Press, 1990).

Lasagni, Roberto, ed., *Dizionario Biografico dei Parmigiani* (Parma: PPS, 1999).

Laughran, Michelle, "Oltre la pelle. I cometici e il loro uso," in Belfanti and Giusberti, eds. *Storia d'Italia. Annali vol. 19: La moda*, 43–82.

Lautenbach, Joseph, *Consilia medicinalia cum mixtim praestantissimorum Italiae medicorum* (Frankfurt: Officina typographica Wolfgangi Richteri, impressis Iohannis Sartorii, 1605).

Lazzarini, Elena, "Alle origini della chirurgia plastica nei 'libri dei segreti' e nei trattati del XVI Secolo," *Genesis*, 10, 1 (2011): 39–62.

Lazzaro, Claudia, *The Italian Renaissance Garden: From the Conventions of Planting, Design, and Ornament to the Grand Gardens of Sixteenth-Century Central Italy* (New Haven: Yale University Press, 1990).

Le Gall, Jean-Marie, *Un idéal masculin. Barbes et moustaches, xv-xviii siècles* (Paris: Payot & Rivages, 2011).

Le Goff, Jacques, "Head or Heart? The Political Use of Body Metaphors in the Middle Ages," in Michael Feher, ed. *Fragments for a History of the Human Body*, vol. 3 (New York: Zone Books, 1989), 12–27.

Leonard, Amy and Karen L. Nelson, eds., *Masculinities, Childhood, Violence: Attending to Early Modern Women- and Men: Proceedings of the 2006 Symposium* (Newark: University of Delaware Press, 2011).

Leong, Elaine, *Recipes and Everyday Knowledge: Medicine, Science, and the Household in Early Modern England* (Chicago: The University of Chicago Press, 2018).

Leriche, Renée, *The Surgery of Pain*, tr. Archibald Young (London: Baillière, Tindall, & Cox, 1939).

Liceti, Fortunio, *De monstrorum caussis* (Padua: apud P. Frambottus, 1634).

Liebaut, Jean, *Trois livres appurtenant aux infirmitez et maladies des femmes*, in *Pregnancy and Childbirth in Early Modern France.*

Lincoln, Elizabeth, "Curating the Renaissance Body (Pietro Paolo Magni's Illustrated Treatise 'Discorsi Sopra Il Modo Di Sanguinare, Attaccar Le Sanguisughe, & Le Ventose, Far Le Fregagioni Vessicatorij a Corpi Humani')," *Word&Image* 17, 1–2 (2001): 42–61.

Lippi, Daniela, "Medicina e chirurgia nell'opera di Tarduccio Salvi da Macerata," in Fabiola Zurlini, ed. *Medici e medicina nelle Marche: Lo studio Firmano e la storia della medicina* (Fermo: Andrea Livi Editore, 2005), 89–94.

Lomazzo, Giovanni Paolo, *Trattato dell'arte de la pittura* (Milan: appresso paolo Gottardo Pontio, 1584).

Long, Pamela O., "Trading Zones in Early Modern Europe," *Isis* 106, 4 (2015): 840–847.

Lowe, Kate, "The Stereotyping of Black Africans in Renaissance Europe," in Lowe and Earle, eds. *Black Africans in Renaissance Europe*, pp. 17–47.

Lowe, Kate, "The Black Diaspora in Europe in the Fifteenth and Sixteenth Centuries, with Special Reference to German-Speaking Areas," in Honeck, Klimke, and Kuhlmann, eds., *Germany and the Black Diaspora*, pp. 38–56.

Lowe, Kate and T.F. Earle, eds., *Black Africans in Renaissance Europe* (Cambridge: Cambridge University Press, 2005).

Lucretius, *De rerum natura*, tr. W.H.D. Rouse (Cambridge: Harvard University Press, 1943).

Luigini, Luigi, *De morbo Gallico omnia quae extant apud omnes medicos cuiuscumque nationis* (Venice: G. Ziletti, 1566–67).

Lundquist, Kjell, "Reconstruction of the Planting in Uraniborg, Tycho Brahe's Renaissance Garden on the Island of Ven," *Garden History* 32, 2 (2004): 152–166.

Lunger Knoppers, Laura and Joan B. Landes, eds., *Monstrous Bodies/Political Monstrosities in Early Modern Europe* (Ithaca: Cornell University Press, 2004).

MacLean, Ian, *The Renaissance Notion of Woman: A Study in the Fortunes of Scholasticism and Medical Science in European Intellectual Life* (Cambridge: Cambridge University Press, 1985).

Maggi, Bartolomeo, *De vulnerum, a bombardarum, & sclopetorum globulis illatorum, & de eorum symtpomatum curatione, & medicamenta ipsis ulceribus curandis idonea*, in *De sclopettorum et tormentariorum vulnerum natura, et curatione, libri IIII* (Venice: apud Guglielmum Valgrisium, 1566).

Magli, Patrizia, "The Face and the Soul," in Feher, ed. *Fragments for a History of the Human Body*, vol. 2.

Magni, Pietro Paolo, *Discorsi intorno al sanguinar i corpi humani* (Rome: appreso Bartolomeo Bonfadino & Tito Diani, 1584).

Malagola, Carlo, *Statuti delle Università e dei Collegi dello Studio Bolognese*, 2 vols. (Bologna: Zanichelli, 1888).

Malcomson, Cristina, *Studies of Skin Color in the Early Royal Society: Boyle, Cavendish, Swift* (London: Routledge, 2016).

Malfi, Tiberio, *Nuova prattica della decoratoria manuale e della sagnia; l'una a barbieri, et l'altra a chirurgici singolarmente necessaria* (Naples: appresso Ottavio Beltrano, 1629).

Malpighi, Marcello, *Opera posthuma* (London: impressis A. & J. Churchill, 1697).

Mandressi, Rafael, *Le regard de l'anatomiste: Dissections et invention du corps en Occident* (Paris: Seuil, 2003).

Manget, Jean, *Bibliotheca Chirugica* (Geneva: sumptibus Gabriel de Tournes, 1721).

Manget, Jean, *Bibliotheca scriptorum medicorum* (Geneva: sumptibus Perachon et Cramer, 1731).

Mann, Ronald D., ed., *The History of the Management of Pain: From Early Principles to Present Practice* (Carnforth: Parthenon, 1988).

Marcocci, Giuseppe, "L'Italia nella prima età globale (ca 1300–1700)," *Storica* 60 (2014), 7–50.

Marinello, Giovanni, *Le medicine pertinenti alle infermità delle donne* (Venice: appresso Francesco de Franceschi, 1563).

Marino, Giovan Battista, *La samprognia* (Venice: presso Gio. Pietro Bigonci, 1575).

Marino, Salvatore, *Ospedali e città nel Regno di Napoli. Le Annunziate: istituzioni, archivi e fonti (secc. XIV-XIX)* (Florence: Olschki, 2014).

Marinozzi, Silvia, "The Vianeo and Gaspare Tagliacozzi," *Medicina nei secoli* 11 (1999): 603–610.

Martin, Craig, *Renaissance Meteorology: Pomponazzi to Descartes* (Baltimore: Johns Hopkins University Press, 2011).

Martin, Craig, *Subverting Aristotle: Religion, History, and Philosophy in Early Modern Science* (Baltimore: Johns Hopkins University Press, 2014).

Mason, Peter, *Before Disenchantment: Images of Exotic Animals and Plants in the Early Modern World* (London: Reaktion, 2009).

Mattioli, Pietro Andrea, *Commentarii inex libros Pedacii Dioscorides Anarzabei de materia medica* (Venice: apud Vincentium Valgrisium, 1554).

Mauss, Marcel, "A Category of the Human Mind: The Notion of Person, the Notion of Self," in Carrithers, Collins, and Lukes, eds. *The Category of the Person.*

Mazo Karras, Ruth, *From Boys to Men: Formation of Masculinity in Late Medieval Europe* (Philadelphia: University of Pennsylvania Press, 2003).

Mazoyer, Marcel and Laurence Roudart, *A History of World Agriculture: From the Neolithic to the Current Crisis* (London: Earthscan, 2006).

McVaugh, Michael, "Treatment of Hernia in the Later Middle Ages: Surgical Correction and Social Construction," in French, ed. *Medicine from the Black Death*, 131–155.

McVaugh, Michael, *The Rational Surgery of the Middle Ages* (Florence: Sismel/Edizioni del Galluzzo, 2006).

Meier Reeds, Karen, "Renaissance Humanism and Botany," *Annals of Science* 33, 6 (1976): 519–542.

Meldrum, Marcia, ed., *Opioids and Pain Relief: A Historical Perspective* (Seattle: IASP Press, 2003).

Mercuriale, Girolamo, *De morbis cutaneis et omnibus corporis humani excrementis tractatus locupletissimi* (Venice: apud Gratiosum Perchacinum, 1572).

Mercuriale, Girolamo, *De decoratione liber* (Frankfurt: apud Ioannem Wechelum, 1587).

Mercuriale, Girolamo, *De morbis cutaneis* (Venice: apud Iuntam, 1601).

Mercurio, Scipione, *La commare o raccoglitrice* (Venice: appresso Gio. Battista Cion, 1596).

Mercurio, Scipione, *De gli errori popolari d'Italia libri sette* (Padua: ad'Istanza di Francesco Bolzetta, 1645).

Metzler, Irina, *Disability in Medieval Europe: Thinking about Physical Impairment during the High Middle Ages, C. 1100–1400* (New York: Routledge, 2006).

Micali, Giovanni, "The Italian Contribution to Plastic Surgery," *Annals of Plastic Surgery* 31, 6 (1993): 566–571.

Milligan, Gerry, "The Politics of Effeminacy in *Il Cortegiano*," *Italica* 83, 3/4 (2006): 345–366.

Milligan, Gerry and Jane Tylus, eds., *The Poetics of Masculinity in Early Modern Italy and Spain* (Toronto: Centre for Reformation and Renaissance Studies, 2010).

Minadoi, Tomaso, *De humani corporis turpitudinibus cognoscendis et curandis* (Padua: apud Franciscum Bolzettam, 1600).

Mitchell, Piers D., *Medicine in the Crusades: Welfare, Wounds and the Medieval Surgeon* (Cambridge: Cambridge University Press, 2004).

Mondino de' Liuzzi, *Anotomia*, ed. Piero P. Gorgi and Gian Franco Pasini (Bologna: Istituto per la Storia dell'Università di Bologna, 1992).

Monga, Luigi, "Odeporica e medicina: I viaggiatori del Cinquecento e la rinoplastica," *Italica* 69, 3 (1992), 37893.

Montaigne, Michel de, *Journal de voyage en Italie* (Paris: Les Belles Lettres, 1946).

Montaigne, Michel de, *The Complete Essays*, tr. Donald M. Frame (Stanford: Stanford University Press, 1965).

Montalbani, Ovidio, *L'honore de Collegi dell'arti della città di Bologna. Brieve trattato Fisicopolitico e Legale Storico* (Bologna: Benacci, 1670).

Montanile, Milena, ed., *L'edizione nazionale del teatro e l'opera di G. B. Della Porta: atti del Convegno, Salerno, 23 maggio 2002* (Pisa: Istituti editoriali e poligrafici internazionali, 2004).

Moran, Bruce, *Distilling Knowledge: Alchemy, Chemistry, and the Scientific Revolution* (Cambridge: Harvard University Press).

Morel, Philippe, *Les Grotesques. Les figures de l'imaginaire dans la peinture Italienne de la fin de la Renaissance* (Paris: Flammarion, 1997).

Morgan, Luke, *The Monster in the Garden: The Grotesque and the Gigantic in Renaissance Landscape Design* (Philadelphia: University of Pennsylvania Press, 2016).

Morozzo, Achille, *Opera nova* (Venice: ad instanza de Melchior Sessa, 1550).

Morris, David B., *The Culture of Pain* (Berkeley: University of California Press, 1991).

Morton, A.G., *History of Botanical Science* (London: Academic Press, 1981).

Moscheo, Rosario, "Istruzione superiore e autonomie locali nella Sicilia moderna: Apertura e sviluppi dello 'Sudium urbis Messanae' (1590–1641)," *Archivio storico messinese* 59 (1991): 75–221.

Moscoso, Javier, *Pain: A Cultural History*, tr. Sarah Thomas and Paul House (New York: Palgrave Macmillan, 2012).

Moulinier-Brogi, Laurence, "Esthétique et soins du corps dans les traités médicaux latins à la fin du Moyen Âge," *Médiévales* 46 (2004): 55–72.

Moulton, Ian Frederick, "Castiglione: Love, Power, and Masculinity," in Milligan and Tylus, eds. *The Poetics of Masculinity*, 119–142.

Mudge, Ken, Jules Janick, Steven Scofield, and Eliezer E. Goldschmidt, "History of Grafting," *Horticultural Reviews* 35 (2009): 437–493.

Muir, Edward, *Mad Blood Stirring: Vendetta in Renaissance Italy* (Baltimore: Johns Hopkins University Press, 1998).

Münster, Ladislao, "Un precursore bolognese quattrocentesco della chirurgia plastica," in *Atti del Convegno medico dell'amicizia italo-svizzera* (Bologna: Zanichelli, 1953), 1–5.

Muraro, Luisa, *Giambattista Della Porta mago e scienziato* (Milan: Feltrinelli, 1978).

Murphy, Caroline, *Lavinia Fontana: A Painter and Her Patrons in Sixteenth-Century Bologna* (New Haven: Yale University Press, 2003).

Murphy, Hannah, *A New Order of Medicine: The Rise of Physicians in Reformation Nuremberg* (Pittsburgh: University of Pittsburgh Press, 2019).

Muurling, Sanne and Marion Pluskota, "The Gendered Geography of Violence in Bologna, 17–19th Centuries," in Simonton, ed. *Routledge History Handbook of Gender and the Urban Experience*, 153–164.

Muzio, Girolamo, *Il duello* (Venice: appresso Gabriel Giolito de Ferrari e fratelli, 1550).

Nance, Brian and Eliza Glaze Florence, eds., *Between Text and Patient: The Medical Enterprise in Medieval & Early Modern Europe* (Florence: SISMEL/ Edizioni del Galluzzo, 2011).

Nauert, Charles G., "Humanists, Scientists, and Pliny: Changing Approaches to a Classical Author," *The American Historical Review* 84 (1979): 72–85.

Newman, William R., *Promethean Ambitions: Alchemy and the Quest to Perfect Nature* (Chicago: University of Chicago Press, 2004).

Niccoli, Ottavia, *Storie di ogni giorno in una città del Seicento* (Rome: Laterza, 2000).

Novarese, Daniela, *I capitoli dello Studio della nobile città di Messina* (Messina: Università degli Studi di Messina, 1990).

Nutton, Vivian, "The Humanist Surgeon," in Wear, French, and Lonie, eds. *The Medical Renaissance of the Sixteenth Century*, 75–100.

Ochs, Kathleen H., "The Royal Society of London's History of Trades Programme: An Early Episode in Applied Science," *Notes and Records of the Royal Society of London* 39, 2 (1985): 129–158.

Ogilvie, Bernard W., *The Science of Describing: Natural History in Renaissance Europe* (Chicago: The University of Chicago Press, 2006).

Olmi, Giuseppe and Paolo Prodi, "Science and Nature in Bologna Circa 1600," in *The Age of Correggio and the Carracci: Emilian Painting of the Sixteenth and Seventeenth*

Centuries (Bologna/Washington/New York: Pinacoteca Nazionale/National Gallery of Art/The Metropolitan Museum of Art, 1986), 213–235.

Olmi, Giuseppe, *L'inventario del mondo: catalogazione della natura e luoghi del sapere nella prima età moderna* (Bologna: Il Mulino, 1992).

Olmi, Giuseppe, ed., *Rappresentare il corpo: arte e anatomia da Leonardo all'Illuminismo* (Bologna: Bononia University Press, 2004).

Olmi, Giuseppe, "L'agronomia illustrata. Osservazioni sull'iconografia dei trattati agronomici della prima età mdoerna," in *Testi agronomici*, 89–126.

Olmi, Giuseppe, Luca Tongiorgi Tomasi, and Attilio Zanca, eds., *Natura-cultura: L'interpretazione del mondo fisico nei testi e nelle immagini* (Florence: Olschki, 2000).

Olmi, Marco Antonio, *Physiologia barbae humanae* (Bologna: apud Iannem Baptistam Bellagambam, 1602).

Ongaro, Giuseppe and Elda Martellozzo Forin, "Girolamo Mercuriale e lo studio di Padova," in Arcangeli and Nutton, eds. *Girolamo Mercuriale*, 29–50.

O'Rourke Boyle, Marjorie, *Senses of Touch: Human Dignity and Deformity from Michelangelo to Calvin* (Leiden: Brill, 1998).

Padoani, Elideo, *Processus, Curationes et Consilia in curandis particularibus morbis, quæ prosperos habuerunt eventus . . . Medicinæ Candidatis in praxi cum sequentibus communicata* (Leipzig: Nicholas Nerlicht, 1607).

Pagel, Walter, *Joan Baptista Van Helmont: Reformer of Science and Medicine* (Cambridge: Cambridge University Press, 1982).

Pagel, Walter, *Paracelsus: An Introduction to Philosophical Medicine in the Era of the Renaissance*, 2nd ed. (New York: Karger, 1982).

Paleotti, Gabriele, *Discorso intorno alle immagini sacre e profane* (Bologna: per Alessandro Benacci, 1582).

Palmer, Ada, *Reading Lucretius in the Renaissance* (Cambridge: Harvard University Press, 2014).

Palmer, Richard, "Physicians and Surgeons in Sixteenth-Century Venice," *Medical History* 23, 4 (1979): 451–460.

Palmer, Richard, "Medical Botany in Northern Italy in the Renaissance," *Journal of the Royal Society of Medicine* 78 (1985): 149–157.

Pancino, Claudia, "Malati, medici, mammane e saltimbanchi. Malattia e cura nella Bologna moderna," in Prosperi, ed. *Storia di Bologna 3.2*, 683–769.

Panofsky, Erwin, "The History of the Theory of Human Proportions as a Reflection of the History of Styles," in Erwin Panofsky, ed. *Meaning in the Visual Arts: Papers in and on Art History* (Garden City: Anchor Books, 1955), 55–109.

Paolella, Alfonso, "L'autore delle illustrazioni delle *Fisiognomiche* di Della Porta e la ritrattistica. Esperienze filologiche," in Santoro, ed. *La "mirabile" natura*, 81–94.

Paracelsus, *Opera omnia medico-chemico-chirurgica, vol. III: Chirurgica opera complectens* (Geneva: Jean-Antoine and Samuel De Tournes, 1658).

Paravicini Bagliani, Agostino, ed., *Le corps et sa parure/The Body and Its Adornment* (Firenze: SISMEL/Edizioni del Galluzzo, 2007).

Paravicini Bagliani, Agostino, ed., *Le monde vegetal: Médecine, botanique, symbolique* (Florence: Sismel/Edizioni del Galluzzo, 2009).

Paré, Ambroise, *Oeuvres completes*, 3 vols., ed. Jean-François Malgaigne (Paris: Baillière, 1840).

Park, Katharine, "The Life of the Corpse: Division and Dissection in Late Medieval Europe," *Journal of the History of Medicine and Allied Sciences* 50 (1995): 111–132.

Park, Katharine, "Was There a Renaissance Body?," in Grieco, Rocke, and Superbi Gioffredi, eds. *The Italian Renaissance in the Twentieth Century* (Florence: Leo S. Olschki, 2002), 321–335.

Park, Katharine, "Natural Particulars: Medical Epistemology, Practice, and the Literature of Healing Springs," in Grafton and Siraisi, eds. *Natural Particulars*.

Park, Katharine, "Nature in Person: Medieval and Renaissance Allegories and Emblems," in Daston and Vidal, eds. *The Moral Authority of Nature*, 50–73.

Park, Katherine, "Stones, Bones, and Hernias: Surgical Specialists in Fourteenth- and Fifteenth-Century Italy," in French, ed. *Medicine from the Black Death*, 110–130.

Park, Katharine, *Secrets of Women: Gender, Generation, and the Origins of Human Dissection* (New York: Zone Books, 2006).

Park, Katharine, "Cadden, Laqueur, and the 'One-sex Body'," *Medieval Feminist Forum* 46, 1 (2010): 96–100.

Pastore, Alessandro, *Il medico in tribunale: la perizia medica nella procedura penale d'antico regime (secoli XVI-XVIII)* (Bellinzona: Casagrande, 1998).

Pastore, Alessandro, "Gli ospedali in Italia fra Cinque e Settecento: evoluzione, caratteri, problemi," in Betri and Bressan, eds. *Gli ospedali in area padana*, 71–87.

Pastore, Alessandro and Giovanni Rossi, eds., *Paolo Zacchia: Alle origini della medicina legale: 1584–1659* (Milano: Franco Angeli, 2008).

Paul of Aegina, *The Seven Books of Paulus Aegineta*, 3 vols., tr. Francis Adams (London: The Sydenham Society, 1844–1847).

Payne, Alyna, "*Mescolare, Composti* and Monsters in Italian Architectural Theory of the Renaissance," in Secchi Tarugi, ed. *Disarmonia, bruttezza*, 273–294.

Payne, Lynda, *With Words and Knives: Learning Medical Dispassion in Early Modern England* (Aldershot: Ashgate, 2007).

Pazzini, Adalberto, *Bio-Bibliografia di Storia della Chirurgia* (Rome: Cosmopolita, 1948).

Pelling, Margaret, *The Common Lot: Sickness, Occupations and the Urban Poor in Early Modern England* (London: Longman, 1998).

Perouse, Gabriel-André, "La Renaissance et la beauté masculine," in Céard et al., eds. *Le corps à la Renaissance*, 61–76.

Pertile, Antonio, *Storia del diritto italiano dalla caduta dell'Impero romano alla codificazione*, 5 vols. (Bologna: Forni, 1965).

Peruzzi, Enrico, "La concezione della bellezza nel *De decoratione*," in Arcangeli and Nutton, eds. *Girolamo Mercuriale*, 247–256.

Pesenti, Tiziana, "'Professores chirurgie', 'medici ciroici' e 'barbitonsores' a Padova nell'età di Leonardo Buffi da Bertapaglia († dopo il 1448)," *Quaderni per la Storia dell'Università di Padova* 11 (1978), 1–38.

Phillippy, Patricia Berrahou, *Painting Women: Cosmetics, Canvases, and Early Modern Culture* (Baltimore: Johns Hopkins University Press, 2006).

Pico, Ranuccio, *Appendice de' vari soggetti Parmigiani* (Parma: appresso Mario Vigna, 1642).

Plato, *Timaeus, Critias, Cleitophon, Menexenus, Epistles*, tr. G. Bury (Cambridge: Harvard University Press, 1929).

Pliny, *Natural History*, 10 vols., tr. H. Rackham (Cambridge: Harvard University Press, 1938–1963).

Polverini Fosi, Irene, *Papal Justice: Subjects and Courts in the Papal State, 1500–1750* (Washington, DC: Catholic University of America Press, 2011).

Poma, Roberto, "*Dolorifica voluptas*: Pain and Pleasure in Early Modern Medicine," presentation at the 2015 RSA meeting in Berlin, Humboldt University, March 27, 2015.

Pomata, Gianna, "Barbieri e comari," in Adani and Tamagnini, eds. *Cultura popolare nell'Emilia Romagna*, 161–183.

Pomata, Gianna, *Contracting a Cure: Patients, Healers, and the Law in Early Modern Bologna* (Baltimore: Johns Hopkins University Press, 1998).

Pomata, Gianna, "Menstruating Men: Similarity and Difference of the Sexes in Early Modern Medicine," in Finucci and Brownlee, eds. *Generation and Degeneration*, 109–152.

Pomata, Gianna, "Medicine for the Poor in 18th and 19th Century Bologna," in Grell, Cunningham, and Roeck, eds. *Health Care and Poor Relief*, 229–249.

Pomata, Gianna, "Sharing Cases: The *Observationes* in Early Modern Medicine," *Early Science and Medicine* 15, 3 (2010): 193–236.
Pomata, Gianna, "The Medical Case Narrative: Distant Reading of an Epistemic Genre," *Literature and Medicine* 32, 1 (2014), 1–23.
Pomata, Gianna and Nancy G. Siraisi, "Introduction," in Pomata and Siraisi, eds. *Historia*, 1–38.
Pomata, Gianna and Nancy G. Siraisi, eds., *Historia: Empiricism and Erudition in Early Modern Europe* (Cambridge: MIT Press, 2005).
Poni, Carlo, *La seta in Italia. Una grande industria prima della rivoluzione industriale* (Bologna: Il Mulino, 2009).
Pontano, Giovanni, *Dialogues*, tr. Julia Haig Gaisser (Cambridge: Harvard University Press, 2012), 129.
Pormann, Peter E., ed., *Islamic Medical and Scientific Tradition*, vol. 2 (London/New York: Routledge, 2010).
Porter, Martin, *Windows of the Soul: Physiognomy in European Culture 1470–1780* (Oxford: Oxford University Press, 2005).
Porter, Roy, ed., *Religion Health & Suffering* (London: Routledge, 2013).
Porzio, Simone, *De dolore* (Florence: apud Laurentium Torrentinum, 1551).
Pouchelle, Marie-Christine, *Corps et chirurgie à l'apogée du Moyen Age: savoir et imaginaire du corps chez Henri de Mondeville, chirurgien de Philippe le Bel* (Paris: Flammarion, 1983).
Prodi, Paolo, ed., *Disciplina dell'anima, disciplina del corpo e dsiciplina della società tra medioevo ed età moderna* (Bologna: Il mulino, 1994).
Prodi, Paolo and Wolfgang Reinhard, eds., *Il concilio di Trento e il moderno* (Bologna: Il mulino, 1996).
Prosperi, Adriano, *Dalla peste nera alla guerra dei trent'anni* (Turin: Einaudi, 2000).
Prosperi, Adriano, ed., *Storia di Bologna, Vol. 3.1: Bologna nell'età moderna, istituzioni, forme del potere, economia e società* (Bologna: Bononia University Press, 2008).
Quétel, Claude, *The History of Syphilis*, tr. Judith Braddock and Brian Pike (Baltimore: Johns Hopkins University Press, 1990).
Quint, David, "Duelling and Civility in Sixteenth Century Italy," *I Tatti Studies in the Italian Renaissance* 7 (1997): 231–278.
Quondam, Amedeo, *Forma del vivere. L'etica del gentiluomo e i moralisti italiani* (Bologna: Il mulino, 2010).
Ray, Meredith, *Daughters of Alchemy: Women and Scientific Culture in Early Modern Italy* (Cambridge: Harvard University Press, 2015).
Read, Alexander, *Chirurgorum comes: or the whole practice of chirurgery* (London: Printed by Edw. Jones, for Christopher Wilkinson, 1678).
Reeves, Carole, ed., *A Cultural History of the Human Body in the Age of Enlightenment* (London: Bloomsbury, 2014).
Rinieri, Giacomo, *Cronaca 1535–1549* (Bologna: Studio Costa, Fondazione del Monte di Bologna e Ravenna, 1998).
Ripa, Cesare, *Iconologia*, ed. Sonia Maffei (Turin: Einaudi, 2012).
Riskin, Jessica, "Medical Knowledge: The Adventures of Mr. Machine with Morals," in Reeves, ed. *A Cultural History of the Human Body*, 73–91.
Rocke, Michael, *Forbidden Friendships: Homosexuality and Male Culture in Renaissance Florence* (Oxford: Oxford University Press, 1996).
Rodríguez, Moreno, Rosa María, and Luis García Ballester, "El dolor en la teoría y práctica médicas de Galeno," *Dynamis* 12 (1982): 3–24.
Romano, Ruggiero, *Tra due crisi: l'Italia del Rinascimento* (Turin: Einaudi, 1971).

Rombolà, Franco, *La chirurgia plastica in Calabria nei secoli XV e XVI: I fratelli Vianeo* (Cosenza: Galassia, 1997).

Rosenwein, Barbara, *Generations of Feeling: A History of Emotions, 600–1700* (Cambridge: Cambridge University Press, 2016).

Ross, Sarah G., *The Birth of Feminism: Woman as Intellect in Renaissance Italy and England* (Cambridge: Harvard University Press, 2009).

Rossi, Paolo, *Francesco Bacone. Dalla magia alla scienza* (Rome: Laterza, 1957).

Rossi, Paolo, *I filosofi e le macchine 1400–1700* (Milan: Feltrinelli, 1962).

Rousset, François, *Traitté nouveau de l'hysterotomotokie [1581]*, tr. Valerie Worth-Stylianou, *Pregnancy and Childbirth in Early Modern France. Treatises by Caring Physicians and Surgeons (1581–1625)* (Toronto: The Other Voice in Early Modern Europe: The Toronto Series, 2013).

Sabuco de Nantes Barrera, Oliva, *The True Medicine*, ed. and tr. Gianna Pomata (Toronto: Center for Reformation and Renaissance Studies, 2010).

Salmuth, Philip, *Observationum medicarum* (Brunschvig: sumptibus Göttfried Müller, 1648).

Saltini, Antonio, *Storia delle scienze agrarie. Venticinque secoli di pensiero agronomico*, 4 vols. (Bologna: Edagricole, 1984).

Salvi da Macerata, Tarduccio, *Il chirurgo* (Rome: appresso Gio. Battista Robletti, 1643).

Salvi da Macerata, Tarduccio, *Il ministro del medico* (Rome: appresso Gio. Battista Robletti, 1650).

Samaden, Lucia, "Giovanni Tommaso Minadoi (1548–1615): da medico della 'nazione' veneziana in Sira a professore universitario a Padova," *Quaderni per la storia dell'Università di Padova* 31 (1998): 91–164.

Sammern, Romana, "Red, White and Black: Colors of Beauty, Tints of Health and Cosmetic Materials in Early Modern English Art Writing," *Early Science and Medicine* 20, 4–6 (2015): 397–427.

Samson, Alexander, "Locus Amoenus: Gardens and Horticulture in the Renaissance," *Renaissance Studies* 25, 1 (2011): 1–23.

Santoni-Rugiu, Paolo and Philip J. Sykes, *History of Plastic Surgery* (Berlin/New York: Springer, 2007).

Santoro, Marco, ed., *La "mirabile" natura. Magia e scienza in Giovan Battista Della Porta (1615–2015)* (Pisa: Serra, 2016).

Saraf, Sanjay and Ravi S. Parihar, "Sushruta: The First Plastic Surgeon in 600 B.C.," *The Internet Journal of Plastic Surgery* 4, 2 (2006).

Sarti, Raffaella, "Bolognesi schiavi dei 'Turchi' e 'Turchi' schiavi dei Bolognesi tra Cinque e Settecento: alterità etnico-religiosa e riduzione in schiavitù," *Quaderni storici* 107, 2 (2001): 437–473.

Sarton, George, *Introduction to the History of Science*; 3 vols. (Washington: The Carnegie Institute, 1927–48).

Savage-Smith, Emilie, "The Practice of Surgery in Islamic Lands: Myth and Reality," *Social History of Medicine* 13, 2 (2000): 307–321.

Savoia, Paolo, "The *Book of the Sick* of Santa Maria della Morte in Bologna and the Medical Organization of a Hospital in the Sixteenth Century," *Nuncius* 31 (2016): 163–235.

Savoia, Paolo, "Skills, Knowledge, and Status: The Career of An Early Modern Italian Surgeon," *Bulletin of the History of Medicine* 93, 1 (2019): 27–54.

Sbaraglia, Giovanni Girolamo, *Oculorum et mentis vigiliae ad distinguendum studium anatomicum et adpraxin medicam diridendam* (Bologna: typis P. M. Monti, 1704).

Sbriccoli, Mario, "Fonti giudiziarie e fonti giuridiche. Riflessioni sulla fase attuale degli studi di storia del crimine e della giustizia criminale," *Studi Storici* 29, 2 (1988): 491–501.

Scacchi, Durante, *Sussidio di medicina* (Venice: presso Francesco Rampazzetto, 1609).

Schalick III, Walton O., "To Market, to Market: The Theory and Practice of Opiates in the Middle Ages," in Meldrum, ed. *Opioids and Pain Relief*, 5–20.

Schenck von Grafenberg, Johannes, *Observationum medicarum rariorum libri VII* (Frankfurt: E. Paltheniana, 1665).

Schiefsky, Mark, "Galen's Theleology and Functional Explanation," *Oxford Studies in Ancient Philosophy* 33 (2007): 369–400.

Schmitt, Jean-Claude, "For a History of the Face: Physiognomy, Pathognomy, Theory of Expression," *Kritische Berichte* 40, 1 (2012): 7–20.

Secchi Tarugi, Luisa, ed., *Disarmonia, bruttezza e bizzarria nel Rinascimento* (Florence: Franco Cesari, 1995).

Sère, Bénédicte and Jörg Wettlaufer, eds., *Shame between Punishment and Penance/La honte entre peine et penitence* (Florence: SISMEL/Edizioni del Galluzzo, 2013).

Shapin, Steven, *A Social History of Truth: Civility and Science in Seventeenth-Century England* (Chicago: The University of Chicago Press, 1994).

Shapin, Steven, *The Scientific Revolution* (Chicago: The University of Chicago Press, 1998).

Shepard, Alexandra, "Manhood, Patriarchy, and Gender in Early Modern History," in Leonard and Nelson, eds. *Masculinities, Childhood, Violence*, 77–95.

Silverman, Lisa, *Tortured subjects: Pain, Truth, and the Body in Early Modern France* (Chicago: The University of Chicago Press, 2001).

Simili, Alessandro, *Gerolamo Mercuriale lettore e medico a Bologna. Nota II: Il soggiorno e gli insegnamenti* (Bologna: Azzoguidi, 1966).

Simili, Alessandro, *Girolamo Cardano lettore e medico a Bologna* (Bologna: Azzoguidi, 1969).

Simons, Patricia, *The Sex of Men in Premodern Europe: A Cultural History* (Cambridge: Cambridge University Press, 2011).

Simonton, Deborah, ed., *Routledge History Handbook of Gender and the Urban Experience* (Abington: Routledge, 2017).

Siraisi, Nancy, "Vesalius and Human Diversity in De humani corporis fabrica," *Journal of the Warburg and Courtauld Institutes* 57 (1994): 60–88.

Siraisi, Nancy, *Medieval and Early Renaissance Medicine* (Chicago: The University of Chicago Press, 1990).

Siraisi, Nancy, *The Clock and the Mirror: Girolamo Cardano and Renaissance Medicine* (Princeton: Princeton University Press, 1997).

Siraisi, Nancy, *History, Medicine, and the Traditions of Renaissance Learning* (Ann Arbor: University of Michigan Press, 2007).

Siraisi, Nancy, "Medicine, 1450–1620, and the History ofScience," *Isis* 103, 3 (2012): 491–514.

Skinner, Patricia, "The Gendered Nose and Its Lack: 'Medieval' Nose-Cutting and Its Modern Manifestations," *Journal of Women's History* 26, 1 (2014): 45–67.

Skinner, Patricia, *Living with Disfigurement in Early Medieval Europe* (New York: Palgrave Macmillan, 2017).

Smith, Pamela, *The Body of the Artisan: Art and Experience in the Scientific Revolution* (Chicago: The University of Chicago Press, 2004).

Soto-Miranda, Miguel Angel, Andrés Romero-Y-Huesca, Alberto Goné-Fernández, and Jaime Soto-González, "Tagliacozzi: no sólo cirujano plástico," *Gaceta médica de México* 142, 5 (2006): 423–429.

Sperati, Giorgio, "Amputation of the Nose Throughout History," *Acta otorhinolaryngologica Italica* 29, 1 (2009): 44–50.

Sprengel, Kurt, *Geschichte der Chirurgie* (Halle: Kümmel, 1819).

Starn, Randolph, "The Early Modern Muddle," *Journal of Early Modern History* 6, 3 (2002): 296–307.

Statuta civilia et criminalia civitatis Bononiae (Bologna: Pisarri, 1735–1736).

Stiker, Henri-Jacques, *A History of Disability*, tr. William Sayers (Ann Arbor: The University of Michigan Press, 1999).

Stolberg, Michael, "A Woman Down to Her Bones: The Anatomy of Sexual Difference in Early Modern Medicine," *Isis* 94 (2003): 274–299.

Stolberg, Michael, "Bedside Teaching and the Acquisition of Practical Skills in Mid-Sixteenth-Century Padua," *Journal of the History of Medicine and Allied Sciences* 69, 4 (2014): 633–661.

Subrhamanyan, Sanjay, "Connected Histories: Notes towards a Reconfiguration of Early Modern Eurasia," *Modern Asian Studies* 31 (1997): 735–762.

Taegio, Bartolomeo, *La villa* (Milan: dalla stampa di Francesco Moscheni, 1559).

Tagault, Jean, *Institutione di cirugia* (Venezia: appresso Giorgio Angelieri, 1570).

Tagliacozzi, Gaspare, *De curtorum chirurgia per insistionem libri duo* (Venice: apud G. Bindonum iuniorem, 1597).

Tagliacozzi, Gaspare, *De curtorum chirurgia per insitionem*, tr. Joan H. Thomas (New York: The Classics of Medicine Library Gryphon Editions, 1996).

Tateo, Francesco, "Arte e scienza della 'villa' in Giambattista Della Porta," in Montanile, ed. *L'edizione nazionale del teatro e l'opera di G. B. Della Porta*, 9–17.

Teach-Gnudi, Martha and Jerome Pierce Webster, *The Life and Times of Gaspare Tagliacozzi, Surgeon of Bologna 1545–1599* (New York: Herbert Reichner, 1950).

Tega, Walter, ed., *Storia Illustrata di Bologna*, vol. 2 (Bologna: Nuova Editoriale AIEP, 1989).

Temkin, Oswei, "The Role of Surgery in the Rise of Modern Medical Thought," *Bullettin of the History of Medicine* 25, 3 (1951): 248–259.

Terpstra, Nicholas, *Lay Confraternities and Civic Religion in Renaissance Bologna* (Cambridge: Cambridge University Press, 1995).

Thompson, E.P., "The Moral Economy of the English Crowd in the Eighteen Century," in E.P. Thompson, ed. *Customs in Common* (New York: Norton, 1991), 185–258.

Tilney, Nicholas L., *Invasion of the Body: Revolutions in Surgery* (Cambridge: Harvard University Press, 2011).

Tinagli, Paola, *Women in Italian Renaissance Art: Gender, Representation and Identity* (Manchester: Manchester University Press, 1997).

Toledo-Pereyra, Luis H., "Galen's Contribution to Surgery," *Journal of the History of Medicine and Allied Sciences* 28, 4 (1973): 357–375.

Tomai, Tomaso, *Idea del giardino del mondo* (Venice: appresso Domenico Imberti, 1611).

Tomba, P., A. Viganò, P. Ruggieri, and A. Gasbarrini, "Gaspare Tagliacozzi, Pioneer of Plastic Surgery and the Spread of His Technique throughout Europe in *De Curtorum Chirurgia per Insitionem*," *European Review for Medical and Pharmacological Sciences* 18, 4 (2014): 445–450.

Tosh, Peter, "The History of Masculinity: An Outdated Concept?," in Brady and Arnold, eds. *What Is Masculinity?*, 17–34.

Tosi, Renzo, *Dizionario delle sentenze latine e greche* (Milan: BUR, 2017).

Touber, Jetze, "Articulating Pain: Martyrology, Torture, and Execution in the Works of Antonio Gallonio (1556–1605)," in Van Dijkhuizen and Enenkel, eds. *The Sense of Suffering*, 59–89.

Tramelli, Barbara, *Giovanni Paolo Lomazzo's* Trattato dell'Arte della Pittura*: Color, Perspective and Anatomy* (Leiden: Brill, 2017).

Trombara, Carlo, *Memorie e documenti sulla cattedra di anatomia umana normale dell'Università di Parma* (Parma: Tipografia parmense, 1958).

Truitt, Elly R., *Medieval Robots: Mechanism, Magic, Nature, and Art* (Philadelphia: University of Pennsylvania Press, 2015).

Turchini, Angelo, "La nascita del sacerdozio come professione," in Prodi, ed. *Disciplina dell'anima*, 225–256.

Valensi, Lucette, *Ces étrangers familiers. Musulmans en Europe, xvi-xviii siècles* (Paris: Payot, 2012).

Val Valdivieso, María Isabel del, "Catilina García, la Cantorala. Una actitud decidida tras la agresión," in María Jesús Fuente and Remedios Morán, eds. *Raíces Profundas. La violencia contra las mujeres (Antigüedad y Edad Media)* (Madrid: Polifemo, 2011), 255–276.

Van Dijkhuizen, Jan Frans and Karl A.E. Enenkel, "Introduction," in Van Dijkhuizen and Enenkel, eds. *The Sense of Suffering*, 1–18.

Van Dijkhuizen, Jan Frans and Karl A.E. Enenkel, eds., *The Sense of Suffering: Constructions of Physical Pain in Early Modern Culture* (Leiden: Brill, 2009).

Van Helmont, Jean Baptiste, *A Ternary of Paradoxes: The Magnetick Cure of Wounds, Nativity of Tartar in Wine, Image of God in Man*, tr. Walter Charleton (London: printed by James Flescher, 1650).

Van't Land, Karine, "Sperm and Blood, Form and Food: Late Medieval Medical Notions of Male and Female in the Embryology of *Membra*," in Horstmanshoff, King, and Zittel, eds. *Blood, Sweat, and Tears*, 363–392.

Varchi, Benedetto, *Storie fiorentine*, 3 vols., ed. Leandro Perini and Roberto Bigazzi (Rome: Edizioni di storia e letteratura, 2003).

Varolio, Costanzo, *Anatomiae sive De resolution corporis humani* (Frankfurt: apud Iannem Wechelum & Petrum Fischerum consortes, 1591).

Veneziani, Sabrina, "Le lezioni dermatologiche di Girolamo Mercuriale," in Arcangeli and Nutton, eds. *Girolamo Mercuriale*, 203–215.

Venturi, Gianmaria, *Trattato degli innesti* (Reggio: G. Davolio, 1816).

Verardi Ventura, Sandra, "'L'ordinamento Bolognese Dei Secoli XVI-XVII.' Introduzione all'edizione del Ms. B 1114," *L'Archiginnasio* 76 (1981), 349–354.

Vesalius, Andreas, *On the Fabric of the Human Body*, 3 vols., tr. William Frank Richardson (San Francisco: Norman Publishing, 1998).

Vidal, Fernando, "Brains, Bodies, Selves, and Science: Anthropologies of Identity and the Resurrection of the Body," *Critical Inquiry* 28, 4 (2002): 930–974.

Vigarello, Georges, "The Upward Training the Body from the Age of Chivalry to Courtly Civility," in Feher, ed. *Fragments for a History of the Human Body*, vol. 2, 148–199.

Vigarello, Georges, *Histoire de la beauté: Le corps et l'art d'embellir de la Renaissance à nos jours* (Paris: Points, 2014).

Viviani, Vincenzo, *Vita di Galileo* (Rome: Salerno, 2001).

Von Pflaumern, Johann Heinrich, *Mercurius Italicus* (Augsburg: typis Andreaa Aperger, 1625).

Walker, Katherine, "Pain and Surgery in England, circa 1620-circa 1740," *Medical History* 59, 2 (2015), 255–274.

Walker Bynum, Caroline, "Material Continuity, Personal Survival, and the Resurrection of the Body: A Scholastic Discussion in Its Medieval and Modern Contexts," in Caroline Walker Bynum, ed. *Fragmentation and Redemption: Essays on Gender and the Human Body in Medieval Religion* (New York: Zone Books, 1992), 239–297.

Walker Bynum, Caroline, *The Resurrection of the Body in Western Christianity* (New York: Columbia University Press, 1995).

Walter, Claus, "The Evolution of Rhinoplasty," *The Journal of Laryngology and Otology* 102, 1988: 1079–1085.

Wangensteen, Owen H., Sarah D. Wangensteen, and John Wiita, "Lithotomy and Lithotomists: Progress in Wound Management from Franco to Lister," *Surgery* 66, 5 (1969): 929–952.

Wear, Andrew, *Knowledge and Practice in English Medicine, 1550–1680* (Cambridge: Cambridge University Press, 2000).

Wear, Andrew, Roger K. French, and Iain M. Lonie, eds. *The Medical Renaissance of the Sixteenth Century* (Cambridge: Cambridge University Press, 1985).

Webster, Charles, ed., *Health, Medicine, and Mortality in the Sixteenth Century* (Cambridge: Cambridge University Press, 1979).

Wechsler, Judith, *A Human Comedy: Physiognomy and Caricature in Nineteenth-Century Paris* (Chicago: The University of Chicago Press, 1982).

Weinstein, Donald, "Crusade, Chivalry, Millennium and Utopia: The Vision of Domenico Mora," *Acta Histriae* 10 (2002): 601–610.

Welch, Evelyn, "Art on the Edge: Hair, Hats, and Hands in Renaissance Italy," *Renaissance Studies* 23, 3 (2009): 241–268.

Whitaker, Iain S. et al., "The Birth of Plastic Surgery: The Story of Nasal Reconstruction From the *Edwyn Smith Papyrus* to the Twenty-First Century," *Plastic and Reconstructive Surgery* 120 (2007): 327–336.

Wilson, Bronwen, *The World in Venice: Print, the City, and Early Modern Identity* (Toronto: University of Toronto Press, 2005).

Wolfe, Michael, ed., *Changing Identities in Early Modern France* (Durham: Duke University Press, 1996).

Yuhas, Alan and Martin Pangelly, "Firefighter Receives Full Face Transplant in Surgery Called 'Historic'," *The Guardian*, Monday 16 November 2015.

Zacchia, Paolo, *Quaestiones medico-legales [1621–1635]* (Nuremberg: Johannes Georg Lochner, 1726).

Zambelli, Paola, *White Magic, Black Magic in the European Renaissance: Ficino, Pico, Della Porta to Trithemius, Agrippa, and Bruno* (Leiden: Brill, 2007).

Zemon Davies, Natalie, *The Return of Martin Guerre* (Cambridge: Harvard University Press, 1983).

Zemon Davis, Natalie, "Boundaries and the Sense of Self in Sixteenth-century France," in Heller, Sosna, and Wellbery, eds. *Reconstructing Individualism*, 53–63.

Ziegler, Joseph, "Philosophers and Physicians on the Scientific Validity of Latin Physiognomy, 1200–1500," *Early Science and Medicine* 12, 3 (2007): 285–312.

Zilsel, Edgar, "The Genesis of the Concept of Scientific Progress and Scientific Cooperation," in Edgar Zilsel, ed. *The Social Origins of Modern Science* (Dordrecht: Springer, 2003).

INDEX

Note: Page numbers in *italic* indicate a *figure* on the corresponding page.